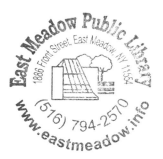

YOU ARE

WHAT YOUR

GRANDPARENTS

ATE

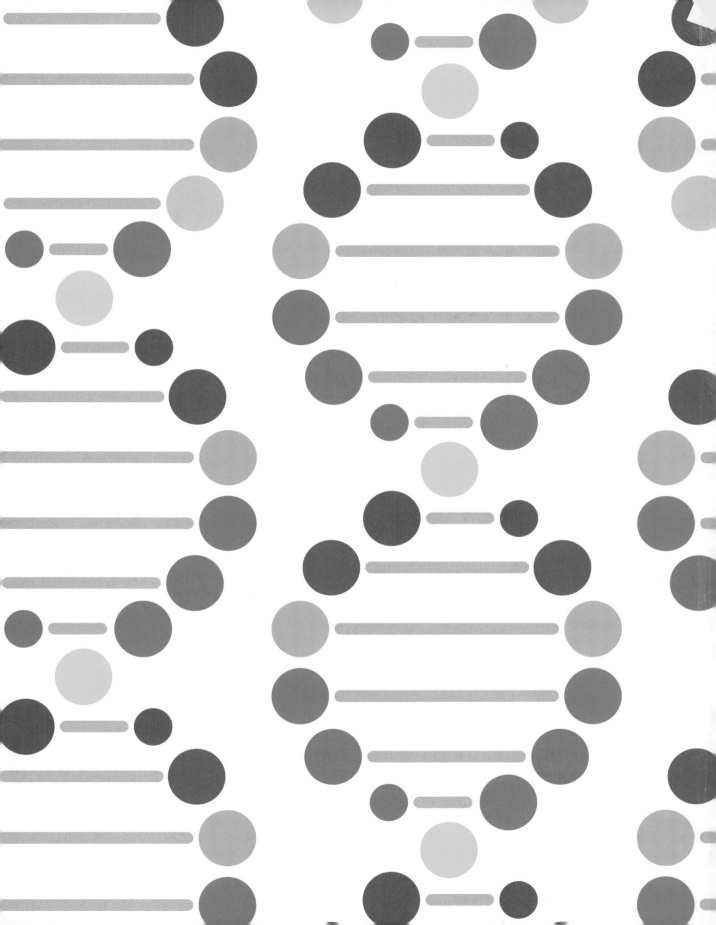

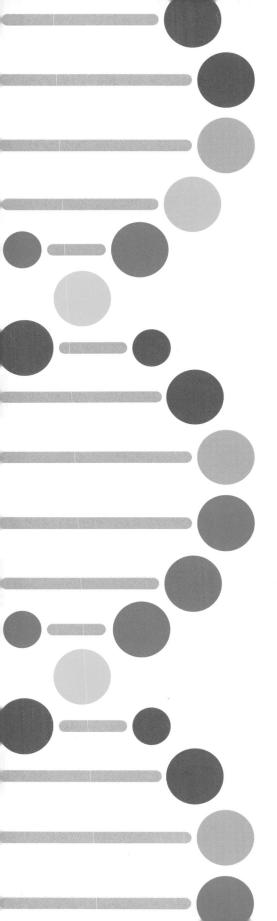

YOU ARE
WHAT YOUR
GRANDPARENTS
ATE

What You Need to Know About
Nutrition, Experience, Epigenetics
& the Origins of Chronic Disease

JUDITH FINLAYSON

Foreword by Dr. Kent Thornburg

Robert
ROSE

For complete cataloguing information, see page 320.

DISCLAIMER
This book is a general guide only and should never be a substitute for the skill,
knowledge and experience of a qualified medical professional dealing with the facts,
circumstances and symptoms of a particular case.

The nutritional, medical and health information presented in this book is based on the research, training
and professional experience of the author, and is true and complete to the best of her knowledge.
However, this book is intended only as an informative guide for those wishing to know more about health,
nutrition and medicine; it is not intended to replace or countermand the advice given by the reader's
personal physician. Because each person and situation is unique, the author and the publisher urge
the reader to check with a qualified health-care professional before using any procedure where there
is a question as to its appropriateness. A physician should be consulted before beginning any exercise
program. The author and the publisher are not responsible for any adverse effects or consequences
resulting from the use of the information in this book. It is the responsibility of the reader to consult
a physician or other qualified health-care professional regarding their personal care.

At the time of publication, all URLs linked to existing websites. Robert Rose Inc. is not responsible for
maintaining, and does not endorse the content of, any website or content not created by Robert Rose Inc.

Design: Laura Palese
Production: Kevin Cockburn/PageWave Graphics Inc.
Editor: Sue Sumeraj
Copy editor and indexer: Gillian Watts
Proofreader: Kelly Jones

DNA Icons: Marish/Shutterstock

The publisher gratefully acknowledges the financial support of our publishing program
by the Government of Canada through the Canada Book Fund.

Canadä

Published by Robert Rose Inc.
120 Eglinton Avenue East, Suite 800, Toronto, Ontario, Canada M4P 1E2
Tel: (416) 322-6552 Fax: (416) 322-6936
www.robertrose.ca

Printed and bound in Canada.

1 2 3 4 5 6 7 8 9 TCP 27 26 25 24 23 22 21 20 19

To Charlee Moore,
whose belief in the power of nutrition
was the genesis of this book.

CONTENTS

FOREWORD

I invite you to indulge in a story that has not previously been told in its entirety. It reveals how, in just three decades, our views on the origins of disease have dramatically changed.

MEDICINE, LIKE MOST FIELDS, is driven by dogma. Medical dogma provides a framework for understanding how diseases originate, their treatment and how relevant knowledge is packaged and passed on to the next generation. But it can also seduce us into becoming comfortable with the status quo. Everyone wants to believe we already understand human disease. Challenges to our belief system are threatening. Yet every research scientist knows our ignorance is greater than our knowledge. That's why this book is so exciting: it reveals new medical knowledge that challenges current views of disease origins and offers the inside scoop on how chronic diseases arise.

Thirty years ago, David J.P. Barker, a courageous physician-epidemiologist, challenged current thinking on the origins of human disease. Why, he wondered, did northern England have high death rates among newborns and high rates of adult death from heart disease, when the same was not true in southern England? Dr. Barker could have blamed the usual suspects — infectious agents, toxic chemicals or even genes. But he rejected these explanations. Instead, he speculated that many northern babies were physically compromised in the womb, a result of poor maternal nutrition and high stress wrought by blue-collar industrial life. He theorized that even babies who survived infancy were affected in ways that led to heart disease when they became adults.

Ultimately, Dr. Barker proved his theory, and the dogma that "bad" genes alone cause disease has been disproven.

The recent rapid rise in global rates of diabetes, obesity and hypertension is evidence of an environmental culprit, as is the geographic distribution of these conditions. But can the genetic code change fast enough to explain this? Do people in the Deep South of the United States, where chronic disease prevalence is highest in that country, carry most of the bad genes for the population? The answer is no to both questions. The precipitous rise in these conditions must be related to changing environmental factors. Poor nutrition and stress, we now know, can alter susceptible genes. This is the basis of epigenetics, a recently recognized mechanism underlying health and disease.

It would be a mistake to think that our genes are unrelated to our risk for chronic disease. As research marches forward, it is becoming clear that our genetic makeup determines the degree to which our early-life environment affects our disease risk as adults. It's neither nature nor nurture alone, but both working together.

Since Dr. Barker's discovery, our understanding of "environmental disease" has changed dramatically. We now know that poor nutrition can harm a developing embryo even before a future mother is officially pregnant. We know that changes in gene expression caused by stress and poor nutrition are passed on to offspring across more than one generation. These discoveries have changed our views on human reproduction.

Medical stories are difficult to tell. A plot can quickly become laborious if the scientific detail is mind-numbing or, worse, the story is told so superficially that accuracy is left behind. Judith Finlayson is highly informed on the science of early-life growth and nutrition, and the lifelong consequences, and she explains difficult medical concepts in a clear and friendly fashion, without compromising veracity. While many faddish health books try to argue a scientific foundation to sell their ideas, few have researched their subjects as thoroughly as she has.

This is not just another health promotion book. It explains why we are suffering the largest health epidemic in human history, why we need better wholesome foods to buy, why we need better food policy and why we must pay careful attention to the health and nutrition of our young women and men as they prepare to bear the next generation. Judith Finlayson offers a new and exciting view of how we have come to our present state of poor health and how we can reinvent ourselves as healthy.

Kent L. Thornburg, PhD
M. Lowell Edwards Chair, Professor of Medicine, Knight Cardiovascular Institute
Director, Bob and Charlee Moore Institute of Nutrition and Wellness
Oregon Health & Science University

PREFACE

In 1969 David Barker was a young doctor living in
Kampala, Uganda, studying Buruli ulcer disease.
At that time, the prevailing wisdom held that
the disfiguring condition was carried by mosquitos.

THE REALITY, DR. BARKER concluded after exploring the local shoreline, was that the illness was triggered by wounds instigated by razor-sharp weeds growing on the shores of the river Nile. It probably wasn't the first time he broke ranks with the medical establishment, but his relatively brief sojourn in Africa set the stage for a paradigm-shifting career devoted to deciphering the origins of chronic disease. This intellectual nonconformity established footing for a new model of chronic disease based on how babies develop and grow, first in the womb and then later as infants.

I came of age when the old model prevailed. In those days, the public health doctrine was (and to a large extent still is) that conditions such as obesity, diabetes, heart disease and even cancer are caused by an adult lifestyle: too much high-calorie, nutrient-deficient food, cigarettes and alcohol, and not enough physical activity.

While all of those certainly contribute to disease development, David Barker showed us that its roots lie elsewhere: in our first thousand days of life, beginning with conception — and, even more surprisingly, long before that. Who would ever have imagined that what your grandmother ate, whether your grandfather smoked at an early age, or whether your parents experienced trauma could increase your risk of developing a chronic illness decades after you were born? Not even David Barker when he set out on his journey and stumbled upon the developmental origins of health and disease.

David Barker was an epidemiologist who passed away in 2013, and his work provides the framework for this book. His early work identified connections between where people lived and their vulnerability to certain diseases. However, over the years, his research led him into epigenetics, which at that time was an emerging field. Today this gene-related science is flourishing because it is linked with virtually everything we do, from what we eat and how much we exercise or weigh to how well we age. Broadly speaking, epigenetics is the connection between our genes and the environment.

In simple terms, a wide variety of experiences have an impact on what is known as gene expression. Over the past few decades, scientists have learned more and more about how our genes react to external stimuli, such as the nutrition our bodies received when we were no more than an embryo in our mother's womb. While our DNA doesn't change, stresses, including poor nutrition, can spark reactions that change how our genes express themselves, increasing the risk for a wide variety of chronic diseases, from heart disease and diabetes to some types of cancer. These changes, some of which take place in utero (in the womb), have the potential to be passed on to future generations.

I BEGIN MY BOOK by telling the story of some of Dr. Barker's early epidemiological work, which linked geography with heart disease. In the decade that he documented in his *Atlas of Mortality from Selected Diseases in England and Wales, 1968 to 1978*, heart disease was thought to be a condition of affluence. So why, he wondered, were his maps showing that men in the poorer regions of England had significantly higher rates of the condition? Dr. Barker wasn't content with documenting statistical discrepancies; he wanted to identify what lay beneath them. He believed he was on to something when he discovered that the locations showing high rates of heart disease also had higher rates of infant mortality than the norm. Was heart disease linked with some vulnerability originating in childhood? If that was the case, he needed to know more about what those people had experienced as infants and young children.

Enter Ethel Margaret Burnside, Hertfordshire's first Chief Health Visitor and Lady Inspector of Midwives, and one of my favorite characters in this remarkable story. E. Margaret, as she liked to be called, began her work in 1911. She cycled around the county, managing her team of nurses and midwives, all of whom she had carefully trained to painstakingly document relevant details relating to the births of babies born in the county. It's thanks to his discovery of those records that David Barker was able to take his first big step along the road to identifying the fetal origins of chronic disease. The information contained in the documents led to the Barker hypothesis, which was published in the British medical journal *The Lancet* in 1986.

Unfortunately, his idea that heart disease was the end result of a long process launched by poor nutrition in the womb was deemed to be nonsense by most of the medical establishment. Some researchers (at least one of whom later became a trusted colleague and friend) set out to prove he was wrong. They were not successful. Meanwhile, Dr. Barker continued his work with various colleagues, publishing numerous studies that linked poor nutrition in pregnancy with long-lasting negative effects on the health of offspring.

For Dr. Barker, the tide began to turn around the turn of the millennium. In 2000 some prominent and previously skeptical American researchers published a paper in the journal *Paediatric and Perinatal Epidemiology*, stating that they were finally convinced by his ideas. A couple of years later, David Barker was invited to address the prestigious U.S. National Institutes of Health (NIH), the largest biomedical research agency in the world. This honor recognized that his research into the fetal origins of disease was no longer a hypothesis. It was treated as proven fact.

Over the years, many researchers continued to build upon Dr. Barker's work, using epidemiological tools to identify links between factors such as birth weight, the pace of childhood growth and chronic illnesses such as diabetes and heart disease. Today a substantial body of research can definitively link your experiences in the womb (as well as those of your parents and grandparents) with the likelihood that you will develop a chronic illness. The mechanisms by which this happens are varied and complex; they are initiated in utero and involve not only the genes you inherit from both your parents but also how your organs develop in response to factors such as adequate or inadequate nutrition, as well as the complex processes known as gene expression.

You Are What Your Grandparents Ate tells the story of this relatively new approach to chronic disease, now known as the developmental origins of health and disease (DOHaD), that was spawned by David Barker's work. Dr. Barker's analysis of the Hertfordshire data was just the first of many studies showing that malnutrition during pregnancy changes the metabolism in ways that increase the risk for certain diseases later in life. Today his ideas form the basis for many research collaborations around the world that are examining the connections between life in the womb and a wide range of chronic conditions. This research repeatedly confirms links between chronic illness as an adult and fetal experience in the womb — not only poor nutrition, but also other factors such as trauma and exposure to toxins.

This book is organized into three basic parts. Chapters 1 through 4 provide extensive background information, including the remarkable detective story, complete with twists and turns, that documents Dr. Barker's discovery of the data he needed to establish his basic principles. Chapter 2 explores the evolution of genetics and eventually epigenetics, one of the key developmental processes that link fetal experience with adult health. Chapter 3 focuses on heritability, including how familial experiences are passed on biologically through the generations. A focus on the 100-year effect explains how what your grandmother ate impacts the genetic material that made you. In chapter 4, those themes are continued, broadening the triggers for disease development well beyond nutrition to include trauma and exposure to toxins, as well as social and economic stress.

The second part of the book, chapters 5 through 8, looks at developmental health through the life cycle, from pregnancy and early childhood through adolescence, adulthood and old age. In general terms, the first thousand days of life, from the moment of conception to the time a child celebrates its second birthday, is the period of what experts call maximum developmental plasticity. A fetus is particularly susceptible to the impact of adverse environmental factors. How you grow and develop in utero will have an enormous impact on your health for decades to come. In childhood and adolescence, patterns of growth and the timing of developments such as puberty are among the changes that can signal fault lines, predicting the risk for future health problems.

Chapters 7 and 8 take an in-depth look at the major chronic illnesses of our time. There are strong connections among all these conditions, many of which can be traced back to developmental programming. The story here is fundamentally about the lifelong consequences that result from experiences in the womb and early childhood, as well as intergenerational inheritance and the negative impact of factors such as the obesogenic environment. The good news is that even small changes in diet and exercise patterns can kindle positive changes in gene expression that help to counter these challenges.

Chapter 9 zeroes in on the thriving universe of bacteria that live on and inside your body. These bacterial cells and their genes are known as the microbiome, an entity that plays such a critical role in health and well-being that it has been called our "second genome." David Barker passed away just as the microbiome was gaining traction as an area of serious research, but he had indicated he was aware of its potential, and I suspect he would have been keenly interested in this bacterial ecosystem. We now know that the microbiome is likely seeded in utero and that its influence is systemic. Our bacterial companions play key roles in body systems such as metabolism, the immune system and even the brain. Since Dr. Barker was an epidemiologist, I imagine he would have been fascinated to learn, for instance, that where you live partially determines the bacteria that reside in your gut. And I'm sure he'd be immersed in the research that links imbalances in bacterial composition with chronic illnesses such as obesity, nonalcoholic fatty liver disease and even allergies. He probably wouldn't be at all surprised to learn that the microbiome affects the epigenome, which he understood to shape the development of chronic disease.

UNTIL I DISCOVERED David Barker's work, I subscribed to the conventional wisdom that chronic illness is pretty much the result of the genes we inherit from our parents and the lifestyle we choose to live. Now I see the landscape of health and wellness in a different light. Yes, your genes are involved, but they're like actors in a starring role. From the perspective of your genome, your epigenome is the director: it calls the shots on how each gene's part shapes up.

Traditionally we've argued about the relative impacts of nature and nurture as if they were two warring camps. Now, thanks to the science of epigenetics, we know that lifestyle does play a significant role in chronic illness, but not quite as we thought. Nature and nurture are tightly entwined — the image of the double helix comes to mind. Like those two parallel strands of DNA, nature and nurture interact, affecting all aspects of your life. Moreover, their effects don't begin or end with you and your parents. Their influence extends through the generations.

Some of the information in this book is not good news. But thankfully, we now know that epigenetic changes can be reversed and that certain risks can be mitigated. With that in mind, I've included an abundance of practical information on, for instance, good nutrition when planning for pregnancy.

I believe everyone can benefit from the ideas in this book. Although the science is often complex, I've done my best to explain it in accessible language and to select the most relevant information from the wide body of burgeoning research. When you are reading through the book, you will come across terms that are italicized. Anticipating that you may need help in remembering what they mean, I've provided a glossary at the back of the book.

I hope I've managed to convey at least some of the excitement I experienced while researching this oh-so-fascinating subject, and that the information I've shared will be useful in helping you take positive steps toward managing your health.

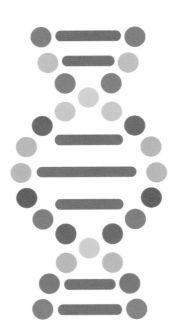

DAVID BARKER

— AND —

EPIDEMIOLOGY

Man brings all that he has or can have into the world with him.
Man is born like a garden ready planted and sown.

— WILLIAM BLAKE

THEY CALLED IT A "map of vulnerability," a vividly colored graphic that displayed at a glance how disease was distributed across England. In 1984, after spending years working on the *Atlas of Mortality from Selected Diseases in England and Wales, 1968 to 1978*, David Barker, an epidemiologist, and Clive Osmond, a statistician, could link prosperity, or lack thereof, with big differences in health. When it came to heart disease, certain areas of the country — those that were less affluent — showed large patches of red. This was a puzzling result, given that heart disease had traditionally been associated with wealth. Nevertheless, their research confirmed that over a 50-year period, people categorized as being poor because of their habitat had significantly higher rates of heart disease. They also died younger than others. Drilling down, the researchers found that 50 years earlier, those locations had also had higher rates of infant mortality than the norm.

The question is, how does being poor link with infant mortality rates and heart disease later in life? David Barker strongly suspected that the connection was some sort of vulnerability that originated in childhood. Could it be poverty? Was it possible that poor people are simply more vulnerable to the vicissitudes of life? Over time, and in some cases thanks to pure happenstance, Dr. Barker acquired the data that enabled him to connect the dots between a poor start in life, beginning with conception, and chronic disease as an adult.

How It Began

In basic terms, *epidemiology* identifies groups of people who are at risk for disease based on specific criteria — in Dr. Barker's case, the economic conditions that distinguished where they lived. Epidemiologists will tell you that one fly in the ointment of their work is migration. While the health status of migrants does not reflect the long-term conditions of an area, it has a statistical impact on the overall results. So if you expected to find high rates of neonatal death based on the information contained in the *Atlas* and found no such thing, you would likely wonder whether migration played a role. Such an anomaly is exactly what Barker and Osmond found in one of the regions they studied. In slum areas of the city of London, infant mortality rates between 1921 and 1925 were remarkably low.

Infant Mortality in Victorian London

As anyone who has read Charles Dickens knows, toward the end of the 19th century many of London's impoverished citizens lived in crowded, unsanitary conditions. Remember Oliver Twist and his heartbreaking plea for more gruel? Yet despite such dreadful circumstances, few babies died before birth.

The social reformer Charles Booth documented working-class life in London during this period, and his research hinted at an explanation for the surprisingly low infant mortality rates. He observed that most of the young people who traveled to London from the villages surrounding the city were the cream of the local crop. Like many immigrants to foreign countries, they had left home because they were looking for a better life — in Booth's words, "a known economic advantage." Robust teenage girls who had been raised on wholesome farm food were

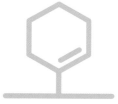

Epidemiology:

The study of disease patterns in different groups of people, with a view toward identifying the underlying causes of diseases. By studying populations rather than individuals, epidemiology lays the foundation for public health interventions directed at improving the health of large groups of people.

hired as domestic servants. Working in London's finer homes, they may have been poorly paid, but they continued to be well nourished. And when they became pregnant, they gave birth to healthy babies who weren't likely to die.

Hunches about Links

David Barker began to suspect there was a link between poor living conditions, fetal nutrition and heart disease later in life. He knew there was research that supported this belief. For instance, a 1973 study of employees of the Bell System in the United States found that those whose parents had a white-collar occupation were less likely to end up with heart disease than those whose parents were from blue-collar families. A Norwegian doctor, Anders Forsdahl, was also mining this territory. In 1977 he published a report based on statistics provided by his government that connected the dots between poverty in childhood and adult heart disease. He, too, suspected that low social and economic status in childhood created a lifelong vulnerability to poor health.

Throughout the 1970s, a wide range of social scientists were exploring the social origins of illness, both physical and mental. But despite emerging support for his hunches, Barker didn't have any concrete evidence to link nutrition in early life with adult disease. He knew his theory wouldn't stand up to scrutiny without detailed information about babies. He needed hard facts about their birth and social circumstances and how they thrived (or didn't) early in life.

An Emerging Hypothesis

At the turn of the 20th century, the government of Great Britain was very concerned about the deteriorating health of the British people. One in 10 infants did not live long enough to celebrate their first birthday, and according to press reports, as many as two-thirds of the young men who volunteered to fight in the Boer War were rejected because their health wasn't up to snuff. The medical officer of health in Hertfordshire, a county in southeast England, decided to do something about this sorry state: he appointed the country's first Chief Health Visitor and Lady Inspector of Midwives, Ethel Margaret Burnside. Little did he realize how significant that appointment would turn out to be — not only for Hertfordshire but also for people around the world almost a century later.

E. Margaret, as she liked to be called, was tall (about five foot ten) and rather imposing. She began her work in 1911 and had soon recruited an army of what we would now call midwives and public health nurses to staff her team. Their job was to deliver babies and provide advice on proper infant care after they were born. They were also required to document their work. As a manager, E. Margaret was very hands-on, traveling around the county on her bicycle and making sure her nurses recorded their activities in meaningful detail. In one year alone, the cyclometer on her bicycle recorded 2,921 miles.

Thanks to Burnside's rather formidable personality, we are told, the Hertford-shire county clerk agreed to purchase 60 spring balances for her team. Her nurses were instructed to weigh babies when they were born and when they reached the age of one. E. Margaret made sure that this information, along with pertinent details about any ill-nesses and developmental concerns, was carefully recorded on cards. When the baby had its first birthday, the card was turned in to the county office, where the information was transcribed into ledgers.

The Hertfordshire Records

The records documenting Burnside's work were maintained until 1948, when England's National Health Service was established. At that point they were archived in a public building, where they lay dormant, gathering dust. Meanwhile, in the early 1980s David Barker had begun to systemically communicate with local health officials across the country, in search of the birth records he so desperately needed. But he wasn't having much success.

Finally, a stroke of luck: a reply from the county of Hertfordshire notifying him that they had found, hidden away under the stairs, a collection of old ledgers. These registers documented the births of thousands of children between 1911 and 1945, as well as their growth patterns and what they were fed until their first birthday. True to the spirit of E. Margaret, the dusty oversized books contained detailed comments on the babies, their mothers and the social circumstances of the families involved. In fact, they contained so many personal details that officials initially declined to give Dr. Barker access to the information because of privacy concerns.

Fortunately, happenstance stepped in. The ledgers contained information on babies born in the village of Much Hadham, a place David Barker knew quite well. During the Second World War, he and his mother, like many British women and children, had been evacuated to the countryside to protect them from the London Blitz. Much Hadham was where they had ended up and where his sister was born. Since his sister's records were in the ledgers, Dr. Barker was granted access to the material.

In the spring of 2018 I made a trip to Southampton, where the ledgers are now kept. I found them fascinating, not only for the information they contain but also because they so clearly belong to a distant past. Written in pen and ink, they look like artifacts from the era of Charles Dickens, like financial accounting books with columns for recording sales and expenses. Viewing them in the flesh, so to speak, it's hard to believe they formed the basis of one of the most revolutionary health discoveries of the 20th century.

Identifying the Links

After gaining access to the ledgers, Dr. Barker needed to establish a system for making use of their information. The records were transferred to his unit at the University of Southampton, where the tedious and time-consuming work of entering the material into a computer began. Once that was finished, mortality studies based on the information were completed. At that point Dr. Caroline Fall, a physician who was working on her PhD in epidemiology, joined the team. Her task was to trace the men and women whose births the ledgers documented.

The team initiated a two-pronged approach, the first of which involved identifying those who had passed away by locating their death records. The second involved tracking down people who were still alive. "As bona fide researchers we were able to identify people whose births were recorded in the ledgers, then approach them and ask if they were interested in being part of a follow-up study," Dr. Fall commented. Once located, they were invited to attend clinics set up throughout the country. There they were interviewed in detail about their health as adults.

The first result of this research was the Barker hypothesis, which was published in *The Lancet*, a highly regarded British medical journal, in 1986. Using the Hertfordshire records, Dr. Barker and his team were able to establish a link between a less than ideal environment in the womb, low birth weight (5.5 pounds/2,500 g or less) and an increased risk for heart disease later in life.

From Hypothesis to Accepted Truth

To say that Dr. Barker's hypothesis was initially met with skepticism is an understatement. For starters, it went against then-current messages of public health that linked diet and lifestyle to heart disease. A flurry of experts set out to disprove it, but over time, more and more evidence emerged to support Dr. Barker's ideas. Eventually many doubters were won over.

The tipping point likely came in 2000, when epidemiologists Matthew W. Gillman of Harvard Medical School and Janet W. Rich-Edwards of the monumental Nurses' Health Studies, published a paper titled "The Fetal Origins of Adult Disease: From Sceptic to

Convert." Noting their previous resistance to Dr. Barker's findings, they acknowledged they had finally been convinced by the "dozens of studies" that confirmed his ideas.

The Dutch Hunger Winter

Sometime in the mid-1990s, David Barker had a conversation with a Dutch obstetrician who alerted him to the possibility that a treasure trove of birth information might be hidden away in Amsterdam: the health records of women who gave birth at the Wilhelmina Gasthuis during a unique period in the Second World War. The roots of the Gasthuis run very deep — back to the 1600s, when it was a hospital for treating victims of the plague. For decades it was the main teaching hospital in Amsterdam, and during the Second World War it also served as a maternity hospital. Given the Dutch attention to detail, when women became pregnant, significant particulars regarding their pregnancy, the birth of their babies and relevant details about the offspring were painstakingly recorded.

Tessa Roseboom, a professor of early development and health at the University of Amsterdam, has been working with this data for more than 20 years. As she told me in an interview, in Holland medical records are usually destroyed after 15 years. However, for some reason the documents from the Wilhelmina Gasthuis escaped this fate and were sent for storage in the attic of the building. In the early 1990s, when a new hospital was being built as part of the cutting-edge Academic Medical Centre, the records were found and moved to the city archive. This was the material David Barker heard about; realizing its potential, he sprang into action.

In 1996 Tessa Roseboom was still a PhD student. She was part of a team working with the Wilhelmina Gasthuis records when the senior person unexpectedly left. That thrust her into the role of head, and she began working closely with David Barker on what is now known as the Dutch Famine Birth Cohort Study. Sadly, this material owes its origins to a tragic episode during the Second World War. In the winter of 1944, the German command recognized that they were on the road to being defeated by the Allies. They decided to retaliate with a railway strike, abruptly blocking food shipments to parts of the Netherlands, including Amsterdam. The embargo, which has been described as "a conspiracy to starve a nation," lasted for seven months, until May 1945, when the country was liberated by Allied troops.

It was a particularly harsh winter, and the previously well-nourished population was quickly plunged into near starvation. Daily energy intake fell well below 1,000 calories, and at the height of the famine, provisions were so scarce that people were consuming as few as 400 calories a day. Some people were so hungry they ate tulip bulbs. The cold, the famine and constant worry set the stage for higher rates of infectious disease and increased mortality. The stress was unbearable. Women often found themselves pregnant and alone because their spouses were elsewhere, perhaps detained in concentration camps. Sometimes they had to send their existing children away because they simply couldn't feed them.

However, the Dutch Hunger Winter, as it is now called, turned out to be a fertile field for research. First, it lasted for only a few months. Second, it affected a well-defined group — everyone in the western part of the Netherlands — all of whom were malnourished during the same period. That meant researchers could investigate the effects of famine exposure on specific periods of pregnancy.

The Netherlands has long been recognized for its agricultural production, and prior to the famine the women had eaten well. Moreover, once the Allied troops arrived, they returned to their typical diet. As Tessa Roseboom commented, "People immediately realized it was a unique opportunity to study the effects of famine on pregnancy and the offspring. This was first reported in a paper published in 1947, 'The Effect of Wartime Starvation in Holland Upon Pregnancy and Its Product.'"

By the time Tessa Roseboom began working with David Barker, half a century had passed. The children whose mothers had been pregnant during the famine were now 50 years old. The proof of his theory that chronic disease originates in the womb and quietly develops over decades would be in the pudding that these subjects represented. And indeed, as a group, they were demonstrably less healthy than their counterparts. People whose mothers had been pregnant during the famine were twice as likely to have heart disease and more likely to be obese and to suffer from diabetes, high blood pressure and high cholesterol than those whose mothers had been pregnant in normal conditions.

The Helsinki Connection

As noted earlier, in the early 1990s many, if not most, people in the scientific community believed the Barker hypothesis was wrong. One was an epidemiologist named Johan Eriksson, who was based in Helsinki, Finland. "I first heard about the Barker hypothesis at a big European diabetes meeting. At that meeting people were making fun of the idea that low birth weight might be a risk factor for heart disease," he told me in an interview. "I realized I had access to hospital birth records and other data that I was sure would prove David Barker was wrong."

Sometime around 1993, before he could complete his critique of Dr. Barker's work, Dr. Eriksson ended up at a small meeting arranged by the European Union. Experts in the area of the developmental origins of disease had been invited, and David Barker was attending. "The host didn't show up, and David and I went for lunch together," Dr. Eriksson recalled. "Then we had a beer or two at the airport."

As the men got to know each other, two things started to become clear: they really liked each other personally, and Dr. Eriksson had access to massive amounts of information that could be very useful in establishing sharper links between the development of disease in adults and their earlier experiences. "David's Hertfordshire data ended by the time the baby turned one," Dr. Eriksson told me. "In Finland we could track growth throughout childhood. David became very interested and invited me to the facility at Southampton, which was the center of his research."

The next year, Dr. Eriksson invited David Barker to Finland. They met at a rooftop bar, where they wrote an application for a significant grant from the British Heart Foundation. Their proposal, based on Dr. Eriksson's treasure trove of Finnish data, was approved. That study focused not only on the importance of prenatal growth but also on the relationship between growth during childhood and coronary heart disease. The first of many publications based on data from the Helsinki Birth Cohort Study (HBCS), it was published in the *British Medical Journal* in 1997. After that, they authored more than 120 studies together. "Without David and without the British Heart Foundation, the value of the Helsinki Birth Cohort Study would never have been maximized," Dr. Eriksson commented.

The Helsinki Birth Cohort Study

For various reasons, Finland has a history of poor health, characterized in the past by high rates of infant and male mortality and high rates of type 1 diabetes, among other markers. The country also has a tradition of strong social and health services. In 1934 child welfare clinics were established in Helsinki and health-care professionals began to record the weight of newborns. Thirteen thousand children were included in that first wave of data collection. Subsequently, until they turned 11, their weight and growth patterns were recorded at regular intervals.

To people such as David Barker, those records were a cornucopia. In his book *Nutrition in the Womb*, he acknowledged their importance: for the first time researchers could explore whether people who experienced strokes or developed illnesses such as heart disease or diabetes had grown and developed differently from others. The answer was, they had.

THE VALUE OF DATA

Is it any wonder that Finland has one of the strongest health technology sectors in the world? This small northern country has become a world leader in the high-tech tracking and use of health information.

Why are Finnish people so far ahead in this burgeoning field? Perhaps it's because the country has very deep roots in public health initiatives and the collection and use of personal health data. Since 1964 every baby born in Finland has been assigned a personal identification number either at birth or during the early years. For every native-born citizen, there is a detailed record that tracks their unique health information, including data such as their illnesses, the prescription medicines they take, when they are admitted to hospital and so on. This material has provided an invaluable resource for researchers trying to sort out the links between early experiences and the development of chronic disease.

Finland also has a history of strong social programs, such as free schooling and public health interventions. For instance, in the 1920s a program of prenatal care for women living in cities was initiated; by the 1940s women from rural areas were included as well. In 1938 the "baby box" program for low-income mothers was launched, with a view to reducing the country's high infant mortality rate — about 65 out of every 1,000 babies were dying in their first year of life. The program was so well received that by 1949 it had expanded to include all mothers. Every new mother, regardless of income level, receives a box of basic infant supplies that includes clothing, blankets and toys in a sleep-worthy box, complete with mattress. The initiative is credited with helping Finland achieve one of the lowest infant mortality rates in the world: today about 2.3 babies out of every 1,000 births, according to the World Bank. By contrast, World Bank statistics peg the 2016 infant mortality rate in the United States at 6.5 per 1,000.

In the summer of 2018 I interviewed Professor Mika Gissler, an epidemiologist associated with Finland's National Institute for Health and Welfare in Helsinki. He credited a number of factors for Finland's success story, including the introduction of national health insurance in the 1960s, as well as technical innovations such as the personal identification number, which makes it easy to track people over their lifetime. These innovations provide policymakers with an abundance of detailed health information on the nation's citizens at various stages in their lives, enabling the government to identify pathways to illness or health in large segments of the population and to take large-scale corrective steps.

The North Karelia Project, which has long been recognized as one of the most successful public health interventions in the world, is a case in point. In the early 1970s the northern part of the province of Karelia had one of the highest incidences of heart disease in the world, attributable to high rates of cigarette smoking and poor dietary habits. "In the 1940s, that part of the country was quite poor. It was agriculturally based, and after the war there were food shortages for some years," Professor Gissler told me. "But once the economy improved, the people began to eat less healthy food — more fats and sugar. By the 1960s the rates of heart disease and mortality were beginning to skyrocket."

In 1972 a pilot program directed at preventing heart disease was initiated. It was a comprehensive, community-based intervention aimed at lifestyle factors, including such initiatives as reducing smoking and making dietary improvements. The results have been well documented. Between 1970 and 1995, the mortality rates from heart disease among males between the ages of 30 and 64 in North Karelia declined by 73 percent.

As noted, the country has also had a long-standing commitment to high-quality prenatal care, which includes a nutritional component. The Finnish word for their prenatal clinics is *neuvola*, places where pregnant women and children can obtain advice, always free of charge. Healthy eating is highlighted not only during the prenatal stage but also in well-baby clinics after the baby is born.

Eriksson and Barker's 1997 paper found that babies whose growth was restricted in utero because of poor maternal nutrition had an increased risk of heart disease as adults. Subsequent papers examined growth and excess weight in childhood, concluding that the highest rates of heart disease occurred in males who were thin at birth but gained weight rapidly as children. As their work progressed, Eriksson and Barker continued using the HBCS data to detect patterns of early development that identified people at greater risk for other diseases, such as diabetes and stroke.

Dr. Barker observed that none of these children would have stood out as 11-year-olds in a classroom, yet all were at risk of developing a chronic disease later in life. There is only one way such a risk can be identified early enough to allow preventive steps to be taken: if researchers collect detailed data on variables such as birth and placental weight, as well as patterns of growth and development throughout children's formative years. Based on current information, we now have insights into the links between too much, too little or the wrong kind of nutrition and the likelihood of developing chronic conditions later in life. We are also learning more about other factors that have an impact on growth, such as genes, hormones and social and psychological stress.

The Oregon Connection

In 1988 a colleague invited Kent Thornburg to speak at a conference he was organizing in Italy. At the time, Dr. Thornburg was a developmental physiologist with a special interest in heart disease, affiliated with the Oregon Health & Science University (OHSU), in Portland. His colleague urged him to make the trip because, he said, he was bringing someone Dr. Thornburg would find interesting. That someone was David Barker, and it was Dr. Thornburg's first exposure to his work.

"I was very skeptical," Dr. Thornburg told me in an interview. "I was studying biological processes and the role of the placenta in the development of disease later in life. I simply didn't know of any mechanisms that could possibly explain his theories. David suggested that we work together to find out if it was true. Now I recognize that he was placating me. He knew it was true, but he wanted to involve me in his research because he understood I had expertise that could move it forward."

That was the beginning of an abiding friendship, as well as an intense and productive working relationship that developed over the years. "We decided that the placenta had to be important," Dr. Thornburg told me. "David wanted to understand its link with heart disease and birth weight. At that point I was looking at these sorts of things in the lab but I wasn't doing human studies." The two remained in close touch, and when Dr. Thornburg became editor of the journal *Placenta* in the early 1990s, he made a practice of inviting Dr. Barker to Portland to discuss their mutual areas of interest.

"David would visit regularly, and he'd arrive with raw, unpublished data fresh off Clive's tables. Clive Osmond is the statistical brain behind David's work. David wanted to know why the relationships were occurring. We spent almost all of our time together trying to understand the relationship between Clive's data and biology. We knew, for instance, that there was a statistical connection between low birth weight and cardiovascular disease. What we didn't know was why that connection would exist."

Basically, the two men were trying to understand the regulators of human development in the womb. Dr. Thornburg understood the biology and Dr. Barker had his finger on

THE CHINESE FAMINE

In the mid-20th century, as part of a strategy to thrust China into the modern age, Chairman Mao announced a new five-year plan: the Great Leap Forward. Suddenly, with no advance warning, millions of people were uprooted and dispatched to agricultural communes, where they were expected to become farmers. One result was a prolonged period of famine.

Unlike the Dutch Hunger Winter, which lasted for only six months and affected just half the population of a tiny country, the Chinese famine continued for three years, and its impact was felt by more than half a billion people. Researchers from Brown University in the United States and Harbin Medical University in China decided to investigate whether this prolonged period of malnutrition affected glucose tolerance and, as a result, the incidence of type 2 diabetes. The resulting study was published in the *American Journal of Clinical Nutrition* in 2017.

The data are based on people whose mothers had been pregnant during the famine or who had been conceived shortly after it ended; in some cases, both parents had experienced the famine. The researchers took blood samples from more than 3,000 residents of a rural area in China. Overall, they found increased rates of hyperglycemia (high blood sugar) and type 2 diabetes in people who had been in utero during the famine. Surprisingly, they also found an increased risk of hyperglycemia in the offspring of the people who were malnourished in utero. In addition, they found that those who had been conceived shortly after it ended were at greater risk of both conditions.

The study concluded that maternal malnutrition wasn't the only factor likely to affect the metabolism of offspring. Fathers also had an impact. There were 332 people in the sample whose parents had not been exposed to the famine. The incidence of hyperglycemia in that group was 5.7 percent. The rate rose to 11.3 percent when both parents had famine exposure. But most interesting, perhaps, is the fact that when the mother alone experienced famine, the frequency was 10.6 percent — not much higher than the incidence of 10 percent for people who had only famine-exposed fathers.

While consistent with other famine studies, a key differentiator of these findings is that the study showed that the adverse effects of famine can be transmitted to the second generation. As the authors said, "To our knowledge, [this study provides] the first direct evidence in support of the notion that prenatal exposure to an adverse nutritional milieu plays an important role in affecting glucose metabolism and diabetes risk across multiple generations."

the pulse of epidemiology. Over the years, this sharing of expertise cemented their relationship. "Sometime around 2003 David was invited to speak at the National Institutes of Health. Once he received their endorsement, people pretty well stopped challenging his work," Dr. Thornburg told me. "He was loved in the US and we have a tremendous research infrastructure at OHSU. When I invited him to move to Oregon, he came."

Around that time, the two men also began to collaborate on studies. "David was really working in high gear, and many of his insights aren't reflected in publications," Dr. Thornburg commented. "In addition to the hard science work, we are working hard on the ground to improve nutrition for women and girls. One of our goals is encouraging people to change their diet with a view toward reversing the effects of poor prenatal nutrition."

For 10 years David Barker lived a binational life, spending half the year in Portland and the remainder in England. Then, in 2013, he unexpectedly passed away.

Meanwhile

When David Barker was in the early stages of discovering the fetal origins of adult disease, he wasn't entirely alone. Other researchers were also intrigued by the possibility that life before birth shapes our future health. Lars Olov Bygren, a preventive health specialist at the Karolinska Institute in Stockholm, Sweden, became interested in the topic in the early 1980s. Dr. Bygren was born in the town of Överkalix in northern Sweden. Generations of his family had lived in the town and he was very familiar with the local history, which intrigued him. In good years, thanks to long hours of sunlight, the land produced an agricultural bounty, much of which was preserved to last through the winter. But not all years were plentiful. If the harvest was poor, people didn't have enough to eat and stayed hungry throughout the frigid weather.

Dr. Bygren began to wonder if this feast-and-famine cycle was affecting the residents' health. Fortunately, the town kept detailed agricultural records in addition to census-type data. He identified 99 citizens and traced their history back for two generations. Comparing the life spans of people born in 1890, 1905 and 1920 revealed intriguing connections between feast, famine and long-term health. Males whose grandfathers had experienced a boom year just before puberty (when boys' sperm cells are being formed) died six years sooner than those whose grandfathers experienced famine during the same developmental period.

Like David Barker's, Dr. Bygren's work was initially not well received. Even though his statistics were sound, reputable journals would not publish his study. Then he teamed up with a British geneticist, Marcus Pembrey. Dr. Pembrey's own work was raising questions about the possibility that life experiences were being passed along genetically across generations. When he saw the Överkalix data, Dr. Pembrey realized it supported his speculations. Using an expanded version of Bygren's information, the scientists confirmed the original findings.

The Epigenetic Connection

As David Barker was developing his hypothesis, researchers investigating a new concept rooted in cell biology and embryology were exploring the relationship between fetal development and a process known as gene expression. Studies (at that point conducted in laboratories) were beginning to link malnutrition in the womb with systemic changes in offspring. The now-famous agouti mouse study determined that these changes involved *DNA methylation*, a mechanism that cells use to influence gene expression. As the years passed, researchers gradually began documenting similar patterns in humans. For example, certain environmental impacts, such as malnutrition, can alter gene expression, resetting body processes. Some of those changes, as Marcus Pembrey found, can be passed on through the generations. These discoveries underpin the science of epigenetics. (See chapter 2 for more on the agouti mice, methylation and epigenetics in general.)

Many recent studies are using epigenetics to show how fetal experience influences long-term health. For instance, one study of individuals conceived during the Dutch Hunger Winter, published in *Nature Communications* in 2014, looked at individuals whose mothers were exposed to famine in the early stages of pregnancy. These individuals had higher birth weights than those born before or after the famine and, later in life, were more likely to have "an unfavourable metabolic profile" — a higher *body mass index* (BMI) and blood sugar, as well as elevated LDL ("bad") cholesterol and total cholesterol levels. They were also found to have reduced DNA methylation. Interestingly, DNA methylation in individuals whose mothers were in the later stages of gestation when the famine struck was not similarly affected, possibly because the fetus is more sensitive to environmental impacts at the earlier stages in its development.

THE DEVELOPMENTAL ORIGINS OF HEALTH AND DISEASE

The idea that adverse conditions in utero could have a lifelong effect that spans generations began to take hold across the scientific community around 2000. Just before that (in 1999), Dr. Kent Thornburg convened an international conference, "The Fetal Origins of Adult Disease," in San Diego. That meeting spawned interest in establishing a global organization, and in 2003 the International Society for the Developmental Origins of Health and Disease was formed.

Today, under Dr. Thornburg's direction, the Bob and Charlee Moore Institute for Nutrition & Wellness at OHSU is one of the world centers for research into the *developmental origins of health and disease* (DOHaD). The Moore Institute is linked with research collaborations around the world that are examining the connections between life in the womb and a wide range of chronic conditions. This research repeatedly confirms associations between factors in utero — such as over- or undernutrition and exposure to toxins and various other stresses — and chronic illnesses as an adult. Given the many advancements in genetic research in the past two or three decades, scientists now have many more tools available to them than David Barker did when it all began.

2

THE
EMERGENCE
OF
EPIGENETICS

> There is no single gene; there are many and what they do depends on what is happening elsewhere in the body. Genes do one thing in one person and another thing in another. They are part of a democracy.
>
> — DAVID BARKER, *NUTRITION IN THE WOMB*

YOU PROBABLY THINK THAT, because you are human, your genome is the best! Well, think again. In terms of your gene count (about 26,000 and declining, as the science of genetics improves), you are a poor cousin to many other species. A lowly grain of rice has almost twice as many genes as you do (46,000), and collectively, the invisible bacteria that live in your gut house trillions more than that. When it comes to quantity, you're in an uphill fight to stay on the same plane as an earthworm. But here's the thing, as geneticist and author Siddhartha Mukherjee pointed out in his book *The Gene: An Intimate History*, only the human can paint a masterpiece. Thus, he noted, "It is not what you have ... but what you *do* with it."

In other words, your genes alone do not determine who you become. While the genetic inheritance you received from your parents is permanent, we now know that your genes are constantly engaging in dynamic interactions with their environment. Many different factors, such as nutrition and stress, influence how your genes are expressed. Gene expression is important because it plays a significant role in your health and well-being — in the person that is you. Its influence can be traced back to when you were in the womb: changes in gene expression are one of the ways a fetus adapts to environmental cues.

Becoming You

In very basic genetic terms, here's your story: Both of your parents contribute equally to your genome when you are conceived. Your father's sperm and your mother's egg combine to create a cell, or zygote, with 46 *chromosomes*, 23 from each parent. Those chromosomes contain your genes. Each of your genes contains two versions, known as *alleles*, one from your father and one from your mother.

As you develop in your mother's womb, the zygote begins a process of dividing itself to create an organism composed of multiple cells — the embryo. Although virtually all those cells contain the same 23 pairs of chromosomes, at various points in your development they begin to differentiate themselves, creating diverse types of cells that have specialized functions: brain cells, liver cells, *stem cells*, mast cells and so on. That's why you have hundreds of different cell types, each with its own specific set of tasks.

How does the embryo create the different kinds of cells it needs to function as a human being? Again to oversimplify, all of its cells contain DNA, a chemical that carries genetic information, which has been described as a biological version of a computer language. DNA provides the instructions that guide the process of making each cell type, and it does this by switching specific genes on or off.

The Epigenetic Landscape

Conrad Waddington, a British scientist, is credited with coining the term *epigenetics* in 1942. Fifteen years later, he applied himself to developing a metaphorical image that captured the complexities of cell differentiation. At that point many scientists seriously entertained the idea that an embryo was a kind of mini adult — that all of its adult characteristics were present from the moment of

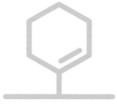

Epigenetic:

Relating to, being or involving changes in gene function that do not involve changes in DNA sequence.

Epigenetics:

A biological process resulting in heritable changes (those passed on to cells of the same type as they divide) that are transmitted to future generations of cells or offspring.

conception. Others believed that a baby was the result of a developmental process involving a long series of interactions among various constituents. Waddington belonged to the latter camp, and in 1957 he published a conceptual framework illustrating his theories.

Known as Waddington's epigenetic landscape, his compelling image suggests various developmental paths a cell might take toward differentiation, each leading to a different result. Waddington pictured the zygote as a ball positioned at the top of a hill that is intersected by a series of valleys running horizontally across the terrain. Each valley represents an intersection. As the ball rolls downward (or the cell develops), it passes different locations, and each experience is recorded on the ball (or the cell's DNA), causing it to change (become increasingly differentiated) over time. Eventually, it reaches the bottom, where it is the sum of all it has encountered.

By the time it reaches the bottom of the hill, the single cell has divided and differentiated often enough to create all the different cells (heart, brain, liver and so on) it needs to become a human being. The differentiated cells have settled into their various troughs (the valleys). The cell has maintained its original genetic material, but how those genes are expressed has changed.

Waddington developed his model before epigenetic mechanisms were understood, but scientists seem to agree that it is a useful metaphor for capturing the process of cell differentiation. It is an epigenetic phenomenon resulting from changes in the epigenetic landscape, not from genetic inheritance. Rolling the ball back up the hill would mean returning it to its stem cell state, an extremely challenging procedure. In fact, that process would take us into the territory of cloning.

The First Geneticists

The sum of all your genes comprises your *genome*. Your genes themselves are regions of your DNA, the chemical compound that carries fundamental information throughout your genome. DNA was discovered in 1953, but that's no reason to assume that genetics is a very modern science. In fact, over the centuries many different types of researchers — mathematicians, chemists and biologists, to name just three — have applied themselves to studying the science of how we become ourselves. At first glance, you'd be unlikely to include the Greek philosopher Aristotle in this group. However, his idea that children inherit characteristics from both parents was earth-shattering at a time when male semen was believed to be the fundamental life force and the sole source of hereditary information. Females, it was thought, weren't much more than nutrient-dispensing receptacles.

Although he got many of the details wrong, Aristotle's view of heredity as the transmission of information was a paradigm shift in scientific knowledge; some scientists have suggested that he should be acknowledged for identifying the principle of parental inheritance, later explained by DNA. When it comes to inherited traits, however, Gregor Mendel's studies of peas represent a further paradigm shift. In fact, this process of genetic inheritance is now called *Mendelian inheritance* (see "The Patient Gardener: Mendel's Peas," page 39).

Classic Mendelian inheritance is based on the principle that traits are passed on by the parents in a relatively straightforward fashion, via genes. The final outcome of your genome, combined with gene expression, is called your *phenotype*. Phenotype is a complicated concept, but in simplistic terms it is *you* — your physical form, personality traits, moods and, to some extent, your behavior. While genes determine your phenotype, they are regulated by epigenetic mechanisms that are modified by environmental influences. So how traits are inherited is not quite as simple as Mendel thought. As Kent Thornburg told me, "Mendel was lucky he found the color of pea flowers as an indicator of gene expression, because most phenotypic traits are more complicated in their expression."

It's More Than Genes

Remember the Swedish epidemiologist Lars Bygren and the British geneticist Marcus Pembrey from chapter 1? Their work confirmed that certain of your grandparents' life experiences could be passed on genetically to you. Using historical data from the Swedish town of Överkalix, Dr. Bygren was able to link the experiences of one generation with the health outcomes of another. The problem is, even though his data seemed sound, no one would publish his work. While the scientists who reviewed (and rejected) the paper for publication did not quibble with the statistics, they dismissed its conclusions as impossible.

As the rejections piled up from journals, Bygren started scanning scientific literature for anyone who might have had similar findings. In 2000 he came across Marcus Pembrey, a clinical geneticist at the Institute of Child Health in London. Dr. Pembrey was studying diseases in children that were linked to a missing part of the *DNA sequence* from chromosome 15. At that point Dr. Pembrey was pushing the envelope of Mendelian genetics, and the Överkalix data interested him because he was finding his own results baffling. He was studying two separate diseases, differentiated only by whether the DNA was missing from the chromosome 15 that came from the father or from the chromosome 15 that came from the mother. If the DNA deletion was inherited from the father, the child had Prader-Willi syndrome, which causes insatiable hunger and leads to extreme obesity. But if an identical DNA deletion was inherited from the mother, the offspring ended up with Angelman syndrome, a severe mental impairment that leaves children with jerky movement patterns and unable to speak.

Dr. Pembrey recognized that the DNA deletion on chromosome 15 must somehow record whether it came from the mother or father. But how could that be? There was no difference at all between the DNA sequences, so something else — some memory of where the chromosome had been — was getting passed down. The Överkalix data provided evidence of a similar *transgenerational inheritance*. It appeared to both scientists that something in addition to the DNA code itself was being transmitted between generations.

Doctors Bygren and Pembrey decided to collaborate on a two-pronged study to examine more deeply whether life experiences could be transferred across generations. In one prong, the team used England's Avon Longitudinal Study of Parents and Children (ALSPAC), which tracked the health and development of thousands of children from the time they were in utero. Included in the ALSPAC were data on 5,451 fathers who had been smokers. Of those, 166 had smoked just prior to puberty, when their sperm — the vessels that would transmit their genetic material — were forming. The sons of those men turned out to be heavier than average, and even compared to the sons of men who habitually smoked but didn't start smoking until after they had passed the sensitive phase when the testes are beginning to generate sperm. Again it seemed that a certain experience — in this case, exposure to certain toxins — at a specific time could leave some sort of record in genetic material that was passed down.

In the second prong, the researchers expanded the Överkalix data to include both men and women from multiple birth years, and what they saw was equally remarkable. As Bygren had noted before, the grandsons of men who experienced a season of feast just before puberty had a significantly increased risk of earlier death. But they also found that the granddaughters of women who had lived through a famine period when they were pregnant had a significantly increased risk of early death. In other words, grandfathers who were overnourished when their bodies were beginning to produce sperm put their grandsons at risk of early death, and grandmothers who were undernourished when pregnant — the point at which their daughter's eggs were forming — put their granddaughters at risk. The question was, how could those nongenetic messages be getting passed down?

EPIGENETIC INHERITANCE

Marcus Pembrey's discovery that a DNA deletion on chromosome 15 inexplicably recorded whether it came from the male sperm or the female egg played a significant role in the revolutionary concept of transgenerational epigenetic inheritance. While Dr. Pembrey's initial work identified the process of imprinting, whereby one copy of a gene is epigenetically silenced in offspring, it paved the way toward the possibility that a broader spectrum of epigenetic inheritance might exist.

Although Professor Pembrey's work is highly regarded and subsequent research indicates that some *epigenetic tags* may be inherited by offspring, the idea that certain experiences might leave chemical marks on genes that can be passed on to future generations is still being challenged by geneticists, in part because it clashes with the assumption that traits are transmitted by "hardwired" DNA. This research is changing almost by the minute. The current wisdom is that most methylation marks disappear at the zygote stage, but that *epigenetic modifications* resulting from other processes are inheritable.

Some of the current research is focused on identifying mechanisms by which male health at the time of conception affects the health of offspring. It turns out that factors such as a father's age, his diet and even his weight may affect his baby's well-being. As Marcus Pembrey's study of cigarette smoking in young males showed, exposure to toxins can leave a biological memory that can be passed on to future generations. Now we're beginning to get a handle on how this may work.

Charles Darwin's Legacy

Traditional wisdom holds that your genome — the complete package of DNA you were born with — is permanent throughout your lifetime. The question is, does traditional wisdom still hold? The answer is yes and no. Remember Charles Darwin? He predated the science of genetics, but he was on to something relevant almost 200 years ago. His intellectual legacy was seeing nature not as something static but rather as phenomena engaged in a continuous process of slow, steady change. Although he didn't know it, his theory of evolution is loosely based on DNA and how it changes over time.

You may recall that Charles Darwin returned from his voyages bearing a treasure trove of specimens, including what he thought were numerous species of birds. Upon closer examination he discovered they were different types of finches, but with such distinctive characteristics that it was difficult to see their underlying commonality. Their features varied according to their habitat, but since all were finches, Darwin concluded they had descended from a common ancestor. Eventually he decided that their adaptations had evolved to ensure that they could exist in the different environments they found themselves inhabiting. Over generations, the birds had passed on their most beneficial traits to their progeny, and those adaptations ensured long-term survival of their species.

Darwin wasn't alone in theorizing about evolution. Jean-Baptiste Lamarck was a French scientist who published his *Theory of Inheritance of Acquired Characteristics* in 1801. He believed that when animals adapt to their environment, those changes are passed on to future generations. He theorized, for instance, that giraffes were originally short-necked animals. As their food supply moved ever higher into the treetops, the animals had to constantly stretch to reach the leaves. Over time their necks became elongated, a physical characteristic that was passed on to offspring. His ideas were dismissed by the scientific community until fairly recently, when it became clear that their fundamental premise could be explained by epigenetics. In Lamarckian terms, just as giraffes passed on their newly elongated necks to future generations, human offspring inherit epigenetic changes resulting from environmental impacts such as malnutrition.

Darwin, like the other scientists of his time, was no stranger to selective breeding. Farmers had been doing it for centuries to achieve objectives such as increased milk production in cows, and pet lovers such as dog and guinea pig fanciers were deliberately mating their animals to produce features such as desirable coat color and long hair. Most people understood that parents pass on traits, both emotional and physical, to their children. However, during Darwin's time, their understanding of how this actually happens was spotty, to say the least.

The Patient Gardener: Mendel's Peas

Twenty years after Charles Darwin returned from his voyages at sea, Gregor Mendel, an Austrian monk, planted his first crop of "purebred" peas. Whereas Darwin sailed far and wide to collect his precious specimens, Mendel was a disappointed man who had returned to the comfort of his garden after failing the examination to qualify as a teacher in Vienna. Unlike Darwin, he was not a man of great intellect and grand vision. Probably his most radical behavior involved his early work on the mating habits of mice, which was deemed far too racy by the bishop in charge of his monastery, who shut down his research. At that point Mendel shifted his interest to peas and began breeding various types of hybrids.

It was slow, painstaking physical labor that over a period of eight years produced some 30,000 pea plants. Planting and tending the peas was just the beginning, however. Once they reached maturity, the real work began. It was characterized by endless minutiae — rigorous documentation and repeated reviews of his findings — that eventually revealed the underlying patterns of heredity.

Much of the work was tedious, but by using the tools of patient observation and meticulous record-keeping, Mendel achieved major breakthroughs in our understanding of heredity. Common sense would suggest that parental traits will be blended in offspring. However, by cross-pollinating purebred plants that had either yellow or green pods and very different characteristics (for example, tall varieties and short ones), Mendel discovered something quite different: when individual traits are passed on through the generations, certain traits will dominate.

If the traits of each purebred plant had blended as you might expect, for instance, the pods would be a chartreuse color. Instead, all the first-generation offspring of Mendel's hybrid peas had yellow pods. Green pods didn't appear until the second generation, and then in a ratio of 3:1 yellow to green; this ratio continued in later generations. Interestingly, in hybrid plants that usually produced yellow beans, a tendency to green pods could remain hidden for generations. Today we call this a recessive gene.

Mendel's results established the basis for what we now call the science of genetics. It relates to the part of your genome that is fixed, which has been described as "genetic hardwiring." By hybridizing plants he learned that traits are passed on through the generations in a regular manner, through some substance that is inherited equally from each parent. Today we call that substance genes.

The Curious Case of Identical Twins

Since Mendel's day we've learned a lot about genes and how they behave, not only in the laboratory but also by studying creatures in their natural habitats, such as honeybees, large groups of people, and individuals. Some of the most valuable things we've learned have come from studying identical twins.

You don't get much more similar than identical, or monozygotic, twins. Because they develop from the same egg, they have virtually the same DNA at birth. They shared the same prenatal environment, and the chemical tags that switch their genes on or off are alike, as are most of their early-life experiences. This makes them ideal candidates for studying the relationship between nature and nurture, which is the foundation of epigenetics.

When comparing identical twins, it's reasonable to assume they would be vulnerable to the same illnesses. It turns out that this isn't necessarily the case. Their 23 pairs of matched chromosomes account for only a percentage of disease risk for any condition. Consider schizophrenia, for instance. It is generally believed to have a strong genetic component, yet research shows that if one twin has the illness, the chances of the other being afflicted are less than half. Statistics for other conditions are even more dramatic: if one has heart disease, there is only a 30 percent likelihood the other twin will have it too, and the figure for rheumatoid arthritis, an autoimmune disease, hovers around 15 percent. In fact, research from King's College London, in England, shows that identical twins rarely die of the same disease.

This raises the age-old question, how much of our health and well-being do we owe to nature (our genes) and what role does nurture (the environment) play? We now know that a wide range of environmental influences — lifestyle factors such as diet and exercise, exposure to toxins and stress — can affect whether identical twins will be susceptible to a condition, as well as how severely it might affect them if contracted. As twins grow older and spend less time together, their lives change. They have different experiences, eat different foods and enjoy different activities. Over time they may even begin to look less and less alike. When twins reach their late seventies, they shouldn't assume that if one develops Alzheimer's disease, the other will too. That happens only about 40 percent of the time. With a view toward quantifying the effects of this differentiation, a group of Australian researchers took a look at the inventory of twin studies published over the past 50 years. Their conclusions, published in the journal *Nature Genetics* in 2015, were that genes account for 49 percent of the studied traits and 51 percent are due to environmental factors.

Comparable Inputs, Different Results

So how do we explain the puzzling phenomenon of monozygotic twins, genetically identical individuals with similar upbringings yet very dissimilar lives? Research shows that at some point their epigenetic tags began to change, which means the behavior of their genes had altered in response to their different life experiences. Those changes involve various chemical processes. The three major ones are DNA methylation, *histone modification* and *RNA signaling*. These mechanisms, which cells use to influence gene expression, are affected by a wide variety of influences such as diet, illness, medications, toxins and stress, to name just a few.

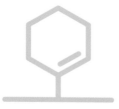

DNA methylation:

A methyl group is a structural unit found in the cells of living organisms. Methylation, a chemical reaction that takes place in cells, occurs when a methyl group attaches to DNA, usually hindering expression of the gene to which is it attached.

Histone modification:

Histones are proteins that are closely associated with DNA. They can be modified by several different molecules, as well as by methyl groups. These modifications are more dynamic than those associated with methylation. There are different types of histone modifications (including acetylation, methylation and phosphorylation) and they have diverse biological effects, from both activating and silencing genes to repairing DNA.

In the case of DNA methylation, a *methyl group* — a carbon atom plus three hydrogen atoms — attaches itself to DNA, turning the "volume" of a gene up or down. A Spanish study that looked at identical twins discovered that they were pretty similar in their levels of DNA, in terms of both methylation and *histone acetylation*, when they were infants. However, as they aged, their differences became more profound. The variances were most noticeable when the twins had lived separately for a long period of time.

Research on identical twins conducted by Dr. Tim Spector at the Department of Twin Research at King's College London shows links between specific diseases, such as breast cancer and diabetes, and methylation of the DNA that encodes certain genes. Scientists are hoping to be able to predict, for instance, which twin is likely to get a disease simply by identifying whether a group of specific genes is turned on or off. It is well known that smoking affects DNA methylation, and studies show a link between smoking and the development of a specific type of skin cancer in female twins who are smokers. Lifestyle differences such as choosing to smoke or not exercising are known to accelerate epigenetic changes in twins. The good news is that studies have also shown that when people quit smoking, their methylation status improves. However, in the end this may not mean much, because total methylation is not a very good indicator of disease risk. What matters is which genes are methylated and how much they are methylated.

With a view to getting a handle on how quickly genetic behavior can be modified, Finnish researchers studied 10 sets of identical twins who had very similar life experiences until they reached adulthood. When they were in their early twenties, their exercise habits changed. Within three years, the twins who had become sedentary began to show worrisome symptoms: less stamina, a higher percentage of body fat and indications of *insulin resistance*. Even more surprisingly, their lack of activity affected how their brains developed. The brains of the more active twins functioned better, particularly in the areas linked with motor skills and coordination.

While we may not understand how this actually works, other researchers have been linking epigenetic changes resulting from physical exercise with improved mental and physical health. Moreover, a 2017 study in *Acta Physiologica*, a Scandinavian journal, reported on mouse studies demonstrating that the positive benefits of a healthy diet and adequate exercise, adopted by either male or female parents, would be inherited by their offspring. Shades of Jean-Baptiste Lamarck!

Pet Fanciers

In Darwin's day, guinea pigs and mice were extremely popular pets. Both were bred to develop people-pleasing traits such as vibrant orange coats and long, curly hair. Using Mendel's genetic framework, these characteristics were "hardwired" into patterns that passed through generations in fairly predictable ways.

Victorian rodent fanciers preferred their mice to have a band of orange-yellow hair that was as broad and as vibrant as possible. Although they didn't understand their work in genetic terms, in order to produce the desired result, they were selecting for a mutant gene that was gradually overtaking their animals. When scientists became involved in studying these creatures, they soon focused their attention on the agouti gene, which among other functions determines the colors and patterns of mammals' coats (yes, people also have an agouti gene). It turns out that the "prettiest" pets — those with the

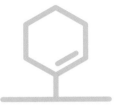

RNA signaling:

RNA stands for ribonucleic acid, a molecule that plays important roles in gene regulation and expression. It includes different subclasses, including mRNA (messenger RNA), miRNA (microRNA) and lncRNA (long noncoding RNA), which perform various functions, from carrying information from DNA to other parts of the cell to regulating gene expression.

Folate: The Tip of an Epigenetic Iceberg

Have you ever tasted Marmite? This yeast-based spread usually evokes a strong response: most British people love it, but many others aren't so sure. Even its manufacturers identify it as a "love it or hate it" product. Whatever your feelings, you may be surprised to learn that Marmite occupies a unique place in the history of nutritional science. Almost by happenstance, it can be directly linked with successful efforts to reduce the incidence of potentially deadly birth defects. Thanks to Lucy Wills, a young hematologist working in India in the early 1930s, Marmite made a significant contribution to one of the largest-scale nutritional interventions in the world.

A pioneering medical researcher, Dr. Wills was investigating pernicious anemia in pregnant women, a condition characterized by too few red blood cells that was particularly prevalent in India and often fatal in those who were impoverished. She soon became interested in the women's diet, which was rice-based and nutritionally deficient. In the process of investigating nutritional solutions, and after many false leads, she fed one of her anemic research monkeys (perhaps accidentally) some Marmite. Its recovery was immediate and complete. At that point Dr. Wills began feeding Marmite to her pregnant patients, whose recovery was equally remarkable.

Folate and Pregnancy

Although it's not clear that the nutritional factor in Marmite was folate — it's an ongoing subject of research, and some experts believe it was actually vitamin B_{12} — for various reasons this was the first step toward identifying that nutrient. After returning to England, Dr. Wills continued to successfully treat her anemic patients with yeast extract. Eventually, scientists were able to isolate folate from yeast, developing a synthetic version known as folic acid in 1941.

And here's why folate is particularly important for pregnant women: When cells are rapidly dividing, which is a characteristic of fetal growth, they use folate at a rapid rate. If a pregnant woman lacks an adequate supply of this nutrient, pernicious anemia is a likely result. Increased risks for specific types of birth defects are another outcome of folate deficiency.

Since the 1990s, a large-scale experiment has been going on throughout the world. At that point many countries began fortifying certain grain products with folic acid. Their objective was to reduce the incidence of spinal cord birth defects in infants, and in this regard folic acid supplementation appears to have been successful. Clearly, it also reduces the incidence of pernicious anemia in pregnant women. The problem is, we don't know whether folic acid supplements will benefit everyone. People with inadequate levels of B_{12} who take folic acid supplements will suffer from abnormally high levels of the amino acid homocysteine, which increases the risk of stroke and heart disease. Also, evidence now suggests that consuming too much folic acid in the form of supplements may mask the symptoms of a vitamin B_{12} deficiency.

Folate and Methylation

One thing we do know is that folate is a *methyl donor.* Research done on the agouti mice tells us that methyl donors such as folate support the functioning of specific genes. Once again, though, we don't understand how they affect the all-inclusive metabolic background in which your genes operate. That interaction is very complex. Some genes, such as the agouti, need to be methylated to promote health, while others will be inappropriately inhibited if they are overmethylated. Regardless, the body needs a constant supply of methyl groups, and experts tell us not to be concerned that genes will become "accidentally" overmethylated.

The good news is that a broad spectrum of methyl donors, including folate, is found in a wide variety of foods, such as green vegetables, onions, garlic, beets and whole grains, especially wheat, barley and rye. Rather than taking supplements, it is preferable to support your body's DNA methylation process by consuming a varied diet of *nutrient-dense* whole foods.

Today methylation is probably the most studied process with regard to nutrient–gene interactions. However, methylation is just the tip of the iceberg. Researchers are actively looking into other gene-related processes, gene–nutrient interactions and individual responses to particular foods. And a relatively new science, *nutrigenomics*, which studies the relationship between nutrients, genes and health, is a burgeoning field.

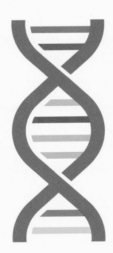

widest, most vibrant bands of color — carried a variation of the agouti gene known as "lethal yellow." These mice were very sickly and tended to die young. Less beautiful but still "pretty" mice carried a different variation known as "viable yellow." These mice lived longer but were prone to diseases such as obesity, diabetes and some types of cancer.

Why was this happening? Well, for starters, the agouti gene determines coat color by influencing how the pigment melanin acts in the body. The problem is, melanin operates in cells that reside throughout the body, not only in those affecting hair color. When agouti genes lose methyl groups (known as hypomethylation), that deficiency affects organs such as the liver and kidneys. So mice with the lethal yellow mutation died and those with the viable yellow mutation were likely to suffer from certain diseases.

Scientists soon realized that the coats of mice carrying the viable yellow mutation varied greatly in color, from a bright orange-yellow to a variegated brown. They named the brownish coloring pseudoagouti. Just as with the lethal yellow variation, the coloring of the mice signaled their health. Those on the yellow end of the spectrum were very unhealthy, whereas those with pseudoagouti coloring were in fine physical shape.

By studying the coat colors of agouti mice, scientists achieved a major breakthrough in our understanding of how nutrition can produce positive changes in gene expression and how those changes can be passed on through the generations. Researchers Rob Waterland and Randy Jirtle at Duke University, who published the results of their work in 2003, fed a group of female yellow agouti mice a diet containing vitamin B_{12}, folic acid, choline and betaine — nutrients known to carry methyl groups and thus improve methylation. Those mice gave birth to healthy brown mice. Remarkably, the benefits were achieved without altering the chemical code of DNA. Although the offspring still carried the variant of the gene associated with yellow coats, their nutrient-rich diets had switched off its expression through gene methylation. Perhaps even more surprising, when the offspring became mothers themselves, their babies were also healthy, even without further supplementation. The yellow variant was still there, but it had been silenced, and that muted effect was inherited.

Elastic Genes: The Honeybee Saga

Although Mendel's great contribution to genetics was based on identifying the hereditary patterns of how peas reproduce, he began his career by studying honeybees. The problem was, even though he designed a special mating cage for his "dearest little animal," he couldn't get his bees to mate on command. Clearly this put a damper on any research into reproduction. If he couldn't control their mating, he couldn't study how bees passed on their hereditary characteristics.

Taking the long view, this probably worked out for the best. Honeybees are much more complicated than peas, from a genetic perspective, and likely wouldn't have lent themselves to the tedious, detailed cataloging that was Mendel's stock-in-trade. They are, however, much more interesting than pea plants, and studying life in the hive certainly would have added a spark to Mendel's rather dull, dutiful life.

Even though beehives function cooperatively, like well-oiled machines, whenever I think about them, soap operas come to mind. Take the queen bee, for instance. She lives what might be described as a long, luxurious life (about 20 times longer than a plebeian bee), fed and groomed by worker bees who devote themselves to ensuring her well-being. Once she has mated, which takes place early in her life, she never leaves the hive again. And then her real work begins: laying as many eggs as possible, around 2,000 a day. When her productivity declines below a certain level, she is ousted from her throne, to be replaced by a new queen. High drama, for sure.

Meanwhile, the supporting players keep the hive humming. The worker bees (and their subset, the nurses) do the very visible work of the colony. It's these bees that build the hive, forage for food and take care of all the baby bees produced by the queen.

Given such dramatic differences in their roles, it would be reasonable to assume that queen bees are very different genetically from the other members of the hive. But that would be incorrect. Despite disparities in physical appearance — queen bees are larger, with longer legs and extended abdomens, for instance — all the bees in a hive have identical gene sequences (though males have only 16 chromosomes, while females have 32). So what determines their diverse appearance, behavior and roles?

Diet is a significant factor. Except for their first few days as larvae, worker bees consume honey, which they make from nectar gathered from flowers. Honey is very nutritious, and they thrive on it. However, because of her unique role, the queen is fed nutritionally enhanced food. From birth and throughout her lifetime, she consumes royal jelly, a secretion produced by female worker bees that is even more nutritious than honey (which is why worker bee larvae are also fed a boost of royal jelly to get them off to a good start). As a result, queen bees grow quickly, have some unique physical features, live particularly long lives and are very fertile.

The relationship between worker bees and nurses is equally interesting. By studying bees of the same age, researchers found that they divide up the work, assigning the forager role to some and the nurse role to others, based on an awareness of the hive's needs. At the point when the roles are initially assigned, the scientists identified specific patterns of DNA methylation in sample bees that were linked to their roles. They found 155 regions where the DNA tags differed between the nurse and forager bees. However, when the needs of the bee community change — for instance, if more nurses are required — some forager bees step up to the plate and switch jobs. The scientists wanted to know if their DNA tags would change when their roles did, and the answer was yes. When the forager bees began to behave like nurses, the DNA tags for 107 regions changed.

If bees can change their DNA methylation tagging by changing their behavior, it seems reasonable to believe that humans can too. We know that the activity of genes is regulated by the process of DNA tagging, which means that making changes to your lifestyle can effect change at the molecular level. In other words, you can change how your genes behave.

FOREVER YOUNG

Why does the queen bee live so much longer than the other bees? The theory is that her diet of royal jelly extends her life. It is thought to contain some magical ingredient or combination of ingredients that promotes longevity. Used in Asia for centuries, royal jelly is rich in substances (such as medium-chain fatty acids) that have been linked with various health benefits. More recently it has become a popular addition to skin-care products, where it is touted as having anti-inflammatory and skin-healing properties. Naturally, we're told it works to prevent wrinkles as well.

It would be easy to dismiss this as beauty industry hype, except that serious scientists are now studying royal jelly. And guess what? It may actually work. (A caveat: some people may develop hypersensitivity.) I won't go into the technical details, but basically royal jelly has the ability to reactivate genes associated with longevity that have been epigenetically silenced. It may boost collagen production, which some say helps to keep your skin looking young. It also appears to reduce DNA methylation and support good gut health by encouraging the development of beneficial bifidobacteria. There's more, but you get the idea. Royal jelly, which has a long and successful track record of sustaining queen bees, may well have the power to support your genes as they go about their constant and very busy work.

It's Not Hardwiring

Mendel made a great contribution to our understanding of heredity. He was able, for the first time, to predict the odds of a particular color in offspring based on traits inherited from the parents. His work forms the basis for predicting genetic inheritance based on parental genotype even today. But in keeping with his times, he took a "hardwiring" approach to biological inheritance. In today's hyper-connected world, it's much easier to recognize that many different mechanisms affect our genes and that they operate like something approaching a hectic free-trade zone. Social network theorist Nicholas Christakis has gone so far as to suggest that, rather than operating independently of each other, genetics and culture are actively engaged in a continuous dialectic.

Consider this: Historian Edmund Russell points out that, as a species, early humans were inherently lactose intolerant. He suggests that our ability to consume dairy products is an adaptive genetic variation, one that evolved in groups of people with a history of herding. He sees lactose tolerance as a developmental advantage that benefited human herders by increasing the quantity and range of nutrients available to them. It also proved particularly advantageous in times of poor agricultural yield. Although a high proportion of people of African descent are lactose intolerant, the descendants of those who herded cattle also developed the ability to digest lactose.

As the 20th century shifted into gear and physical networks such as highways, railroads and telegraph and telephone lines were constructed around the world, Mendel's descendants began to take a more dynamic approach to heredity. In the early 1900s Thomas Hunt Morgan, a cell biologist at Columbia University who studied fruit flies, helped to transition Mendel's concept of heredity to a more contemporary understanding of the way genes actually work. How to explain a fruit fly with white eyes, which he produced in his lab? Basically Morgan was able to identify the concept of mutant alleles, specific defects in genes that we now know can be linked with a wide variety of chronic illnesses. He eventually concluded that genes were not immutable. He realized that, as a gene developed, it could adapt itself to support the demands of the developing organism, an understanding that paved the way for the science of epigenetics.

Around the same time, Sewall Wright, a graduate student at Harvard University, was studying guinea pigs, specifically the agouti locus linked with the uniquely colored coat that breeders found desirable and that they bred their animals to achieve (see "Pet Fanciers," page 43). Because his background was in physiology, he was particularly interested in how genes behave as part of the entire organism. His work identified additional

Nutritional Epigenetics: An Emerging Science

Do you need a cup of coffee to get your day off to the right start? Or does a jolt of caffeine keep you awake all night? You may not realize it, but your response to your morning joe depends on your genome. People break down coffee at very different rates, and there is more than disrupted sleep at stake. Numerous genes participate in how your body metabolizes coffee, which helps explain why studies on the possible benefits of drinking coffee produce conflicting results. It's not a one-size-fits-all solution because too many genetic variables are involved.

Interestingly, at least one of the genes involved in metabolizing coffee also metabolizes numerous medications. Genetic differences help to explain why many people have negative reactions to prescribed drugs. *Pharmacogenomic tests* are becoming common, likely because adverse drug reactions are one of the major causes of accidental death in Western societies. Gene testing can help predict whether a medication is likely to be effective or potentially dangerous.

The same holds true for other ingestibles. Salt and alcohol consumption have very different effects on people, as does green tea. One study showed that women whose genotype produced high activity of the angiotensin-converting enzyme (ACE) had a lower risk of breast cancer if they drank green tea regularly. In contrast, drinking green tea did not reduce breast cancer risk in women with low ACE activity. In other words, the beverage's capacity to protect against cancer benefits only women with a specific genotype.

Knowledge like this allows us to target nutritional recommendations to the people they are most likely to benefit. Your genetic variations can also determine your nutrient requirements, which clarifies why distinct dietary approaches don't work for everyone.

Genes Influencing Nutrients

Have you ever wondered why some people consume calories without gaining an ounce, while others seem to expand just by looking at a french fry? Although the connection between a person's genetic makeup and their susceptibility to gaining excess weight is complex, the differences may reflect their genes, which determine their response to various nutrients and/or foods. Scientists have found, for instance, that variations in the APOA2 gene influence whether you gain weight or experience an increase in your BMI after consuming saturated fats.

Today an entirely new field of science is emerging. Nutrigenomics (often called nutrigenetics) is based on the notion that genetic variants can explain why individuals experience different outcomes in response to specific nutrients. The study of gene–nutrient interaction examines how your unique genetic variations, or *single-nucleotide polymorphisms (SNPs)*, affect how your body absorbs, stores and uses nutrients.

Nutrients Influencing Genes

Nutri-epigenomics is the study of how nutrients and food affect gene expression. It is still a murky area in terms of research, in part

YOU ARE WHAT YOUR GRANDPARENTS ATE

because we don't yet know how maternal nutrients cross over the placenta in pregnancy. However, many researchers are working to identify the various pathways.

To understand nutrient–gene interaction, it is important to know that the basic business of your body is conducted by proteins. Proteins transport oxygen through your blood and help to transform foods into the nutrients that keep you functioning. Proteins are created by processes regulated by your genes. These processes can be altered by environmental impacts, thus changing your gene expression.

Transcription is the first step of gene expression. Some nutrients, such as vitamin A, vitamin D and zinc, directly influence this stage of protein production. The timing of exposure to certain foods and nutrients (or the lack of nutrients) at critical points in development can profoundly affect the function of organ systems. One well-known example is the link between inadequate folate intake in pregnancy and neural tube defects in offspring.

Metabolic processes, including methylation, histone modification and *RNA expression*, can strongly influence the degree to which a gene is turned on or off, and these processes can be affected by nutrients. As principal author Kent Thornburg wrote in a 2010 paper, "It is becoming clear that many dietary compounds and regiments acting as methyl donors or as inhibitors of enzymatic activity can be used to regulate epigenetic modifications." We know, for instance, that in humans sulforaphane, a sulfur-rich compound found in cruciferous vegetables such as broccoli and Brussels sprouts, influences histone acetylation in colon cancer cells by enhancing genes that inhibit tumor growth. It's common knowledge that eating an abundance of cruciferous vegetables may help to reduce your risk of cancer, but now epigenetics helps to explain why.

Although we can see associations, for the most part there is no direct connection between cause and effect. We do know, however, that providing nutrients to cells impacts how genes are expressed.

Can Diet Change Your DNA?

Accepting that our metabolism is in constant communication with the outside world, often via the food we eat, the question is, are you really what you eat? Can diet change your DNA? In simple terms, the answer appears to be no. However, we have known for some time that gene expression influences metabolism.

Cells process nutrients for two basic reasons: to generate the energy that keeps you going and to support their ongoing processes related to growing, dividing and maintenance. Having an abundant supply of nutrients helps to sustain these chemical reactions. A study published in *Nature Microbiology* in 2016 indicates that nutrition may also play an important role in how some DNA sequences are expressed. The study showed that how genes behave is strongly influenced by the food we consume. Even so, we are still a long way away from the kind of personalized medicine that will furnish definitive nutritional therapies to treat a wide spectrum of conditions.

genetic factors that affected coat color, but he also realized that some variations couldn't be explained by gene transmission alone. Wright began to suspect that environmental factors might be playing a role in heredity.

In the 1950s, two French scientists, Jacques Monod, who had studied fruit flies with Thomas Morgan in the United States, and François Jacob, who had abandoned mathematics and physics for medical school, along with their occasional partner Arthur Pardee, an American geneticist, were actively exploring the possibility that genes had a dynamic component. Monod knew from his studies of *Escherichia coli* that the bacterium produced different enzymes to suit the food it was fed, and he suspected that genes had the capacity to adjust to their metabolic environment. Over time, his work with the other scientists resulted in a paradigm shift in genetics. Not only could genes be switched on or off and their volume turned up or down, but this process was coordinated and regulated by a kind of master switch.

As Monod and Jacob saw it, the genome is composed of genes that operate like a series of blueprints, along with a coordinated program and specific processes that direct how that program is executed. In 1965, along with André Lwoff, they were awarded the Nobel Prize in Physiology or Medicine for their pioneering work in what we now call *gene regulation*. There are many forms of gene regulation, and not all use the heritable mechanisms that are now clearly defined as epigenetic; rather, some use the more common process of turning genes off and on as needed from moment to moment.

A Field of Possibilities

The science of how genes regulate and express themselves has developed into a huge area of study. We now understand, for instance, the various ways in which cells realize their ultimate destinies. Think about it: all cells contain the same genetic information, yet they have unique functions. Some become brain cells; others end up in your kidneys. Genes, along with other contributors, direct the cells to where they need to be. To use an example often provided by geneticists, the caterpillar and the butterfly have an identical genome, yet one morphs into the other. How does that happen?

Genes may be "blueprints," but they are not static. In fact, scientists tell us, they are extremely unpredictable. They intersect with their environment and team up with other genes and other substances to provide instructions about developmental processes. They have been likened to playscripts and screenplays, in which the same words and stage directions can often produce very different results. They are also often compared to recipes, where they resemble the instructions that tell you what to do with a list of ingredients. However, when genes are involved, there are many more variables than any recipe method could ever produce.

In other words, it's impossible to completely predict how genes will evolve. As Nobel Prize–winning geneticist Barbara McClintock phrases it, genes will vary "according to the nature of the challenge to be met." In a paper comparing epigenetics to quantum mechanics theory, geneticist Richard A. Jorgensen reflected on this complexity: in spite of being able to learn a lot about any given gene, we will never be able to know everything about its "field of possibilities." He wrote, "It will be impossible to anticipate for every gene every circumstance that an organism may encounter."

Exactly what this means to your health and well-being is hard to say. But the science has advanced far enough to provide some clear goalposts: nurturing your genes with nutritious food and a healthy lifestyle can go a long way toward reducing your risk of developing chronic disease — and the risk for your descendants too.

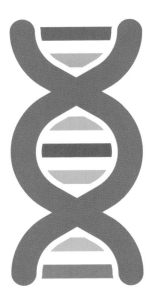

3

YOUR
FAMILY,
YOUR
GENOME,
NUTRITION
AND YOUR HEALTH

> Motor cars break down for two reasons. Either they are driven on rough roads, or they are badly put together. If they are well made they can be driven on any road. The body is no different. Chronic disease can be prevented by improving the growth and development of babies.
>
> — DAVID BARKER, *NUTRITION IN THE WOMB*

DO YOU REMEMBER YOUR grandmother? If you are lucky enough to have experienced a warm and loving granny, you probably have many fond memories of spending time with her. Her influence may have encouraged you to become a helpful person. Did she teach you, for instance, to offer your seat on public transportation to pregnant women or elderly people? To be the kind neighbor who makes up welcome baskets for new families moving to your neighborhood? Even if you didn't have much involvement with your grandmother, perhaps you are the only child in the family who inherited her vivid blue eyes. However heredity shows up, you can likely recognize physical or personality traits in yourself and your siblings that connect with the generation once removed from your own.

What you probably don't realize is that these familial connections are much deeper than identifiable physical or behavioral traits. Your grandmother is intensely embedded in your genome, and the heritage she passed on to you through genes and, perhaps more significantly, their patterns of expression, influences your health and your personality in many different ways.

It's a difficult concept to grasp, but the egg that made you — the one that mated with your father's sperm and developed into you in your mother's womb — was created in your mother's ovary while she was in your grandmother's womb. Unlike males, who don't generate sperm until after they reach puberty, females are born with their lifetime supply of eggs. Your grandmother's experiences while she was pregnant played a big role in your mother's development as a fetus. More important from your perspective, that input extended to the egg that became you, which is why it remains a significant part of your biological inheritance.

THE 100-YEAR EFFECT

If, like Kent Thornburg, you happen to be about 70 years old, you are, as he likes to say, about 100 years old in egg years. Dr. Thornburg calls this the "100-year effect." By that he means the genetic material that made you (which also includes your father's and his father's contributions) is shaped long before you were conceived in your mother's womb. In short, healthy grandchildren owe a big debt to hale and hearty grandparents.

Here's how it works. At birth, a baby girl's ovaries already contain the eggs that may one day become her children. These eggs were formed and nourished while she developed in her mother's womb. That means the egg that made you was formed and nourished in your mother's ovaries when your grandmother was pregnant with her. The foods your grandmother consumed, the air she breathed and the stress she experienced while pregnant left a lasting imprint on the egg that would merge with your father's sperm to develop into you. And, not to be forgotten, your father's sperm transported epigenetic features related to his unique history as well. Remember Lars Bygren's startling findings (See "Meanwhile," page 29)? His research showed that if boys ate too much around the time their sperm cells were being formed, their grandsons were more likely to die young.

In other words, your health does not begin with you. And if you procreate, it doesn't end with you either. In many ways your health can be viewed as a legacy. Its foundation is built upon how well your organs developed when you were in utero. In terms of your genome, it's a combination of your genes (directly inherited from both your parents) and early-life modifications, resulting from various environmental impacts, which affect how those genes express themselves. Although other factors play a role, we now know that the epigenetic changes that take place in early development have the most powerful effect on health over the long term.

And, as I've said, if you have offspring, your health doesn't end with you. Just as your health is rooted in your ancestors' experiences, so too is your grandchildren's health embedded in yours. So watch what you eat now. It will affect your grandchildren's lives.

The Barker Paradigm

Kent Thornburg is part of a team at OHSU that is among a few other world leaders in the relatively new field of life science called developmental origins of health and disease (DOHaD). This model is built around what was called the Barker hypothesis when it was first published in *The Lancet* in 1986. David Barker's key message was that what we experience in the womb stays with us for life. It programs us for good health or sets us up for the development of chronic disease later in life.

Barker's original research focused on the importance of fetal nutrition. He identified links between low birth weight and an increased risk for heart disease later in life. He also began to see that the negative effects of poor nutrition have a way of perpetuating themselves over the course of generations. An individual who was conceived, developed and born in a nutritionally deficient environment is more at risk of developing chronic disease than someone belonging to the same group from the previous generation. When you have generations of poorly nourished people (as is the case in parts of China and India, for instance), they are much more vulnerable as a group to developing conditions such as type 2 diabetes.

THE BARKER HYPOTHESIS

"As a group, people who are small at birth or during infancy remain biologically different throughout their lives. They have higher blood pressures and are more likely to develop type 2 diabetes. They have different patterns of blood lipids, reduced bone density, altered stress responses, thicker left ventricular walls, less elastic arteries, and different hormonal profiles, and they are ageing more rapidly. Out of these observations has arisen the fetal origins hypothesis, which proposes that cardiovascular disease originates through the responses of a fetus or infant to undernutrition that permanently change the structure and function of the body."

— DAVID BARKER, IN D.J. BARKER AND C. OSMOND, "INFANT MORTALITY, CHILDHOOD NUTRITION AND ISCHAEMIC HEART DISEASE IN ENGLAND AND WALES," *THE LANCET*, 1986.

Our Health Is Declining

Thanks to progress in various areas, such as medical research and public health and sanitation, between 1900 and 2000 human life expectancy increased by 30 years. The problem is, we aren't getting healthier. In fact, the opposite is true. As Kent Thornburg pointed out in a 2015 TED Talk: "Our health has been declining over the past 25 years ... [because] more people are becoming obese, more people are acquiring diabetes, more people have uncontrolled blood pressure, and these three things are the foundation for heart disease."

The statistics are alarming. In 1960 one person in a hundred had diabetes; today it's one in eight. Experts are now predicting that by 2050, one person in *three* will suffer from the condition if the trend continues. Even worse, 70 percent of people who get diabetes will also develop heart disease. Have you ever wondered why health-care costs are soaring? One reason is that heart disease is the world's most expensive disease to treat.

Worse still, these trends in public health are forcing medical scientists to confront the incredible: around the turn of the millennium they began to predict that today's young people will be the first generation to have shorter lives than their parents.

How can this be? Kent Thornburg knows exactly where to lay the blame: directly in the lap of American fast-food culture. He points out that the United States has one of the worst diets of any developed country in the world. Three generations of Americans have been raised on the so-called standard American diet (SAD), which is based on high-calorie, nutrient-deficient, overly processed foods. As a result, many Americans suffer from high-calorie malnutrition. Sadly, we are now witnessing the long-term effects of those eating patterns: runaway rates of chronic illness.

You Are What Your Grandmother Ate

These days most mothers-to-be understand that eating a nutritious diet during pregnancy helps to produce a healthy baby. They are also conscious of avoiding environmental toxins, and most heed warnings about other potential risks, such as alcohol consumption. What they may not realize is that a baby who was poorly nourished in the womb or exposed to other forms of excessive stress will, when they reach adulthood, experience heightened vulnerability to illnesses such as obesity, diabetes and heart disease. And these vulnerabilities will be part of the genetic inheritance those children will pass on to their children, and so on and so on, through the generations.

Undermining Healthy Development

A mother-to-be needs to consume enough nutrients to feed herself as well as her baby. Traditional wisdom suggests that a growing fetus receives all the nutrients it needs (along with adequate amounts of oxygen) via the placenta. However, during its development, certain impediments may prevent this from happening.

MATERNAL MALNUTRITION

Simply stated, if a pregnant woman is undernourished, she doesn't have enough nutrients to adequately provide for the fetus. We also know from studying countries such as India and China, where malnutrition is multigenerational, that a mother's nutritional status at the onset of the pregnancy will play a role in her offspring's health. In other words, what happens in pregnancy depends on what happened before.

While it's different from the ancestral malnutrition found in countries such as China and India, citizens of prosperous countries can also suffer from a form of malnutrition. Known as high-calorie malnutrition, it's characterized by an overabundance of calories and a dearth of nutrients. Mothers who experience this type of malnourishment are unlikely to be able to provide adequate nutrition to support the best developmental conditions for the fetus.

MATERNAL HEALTH

Numerous health conditions may obstruct a mother's ability to deliver nutrients to her fetus, resulting in low birth weight. If the mother has an illness such as diabetes, not only can it affect the nutrients being transported to the fetus, it may also result in surplus nutrition, spurring too much growth — the opposite problem from malnutrition, but equally challenging.

PROBLEMS WITH THE PLACENTA

The placenta is the supply line through which nutrients are delivered to the fetus. The placenta also manufactures hormones and protects the baby from harmful toxins. How well it performs its jobs determines fetal growth (too much or too little) and influences health programming.

STRESS

Epidemiological data support the idea that social stress during pregnancy can be just as detrimental to the fetus as inadequate nutrition. These two forms of stress often exist simultaneously.

Trading Off

The embryo implants itself in the wall of the uterus eight days after the egg is fertilized, thus beginning its relationship with its mother's body. As the fetus develops, myriad cells are evolving. This is a critical stage. David Barker used the word *plastic* — a scientific term used to describe the ability of developing tissue to adapt to environmental changes — to describe this period when organs, glands and tissues are being formed.

Because a fetus is (literally) connected to its mother, it is extremely vulnerable to the vicissitudes of her life. If something is amiss with her, that is problematic for the fetus because it is totally reliant on the placenta. During development, the placenta does the work for several of the fetus's organs. If, for instance, the placenta is not supplying adequate nutrition, jeopardizing its development, the fetus will begin adapting to ensure its survival. It does so by prioritizing the development of some organs over others, sacrificing functions it doesn't need.

In the early stages of pregnancy, many cell types (liver, kidney, heart and lung, to name just four) are emerging. If nutrients are scanty — that is, if there is not enough "capital" to support all aspects of this vigorous development — the fetus will begin to trade off the growth of one part of its body for another, with a view toward shielding its heart and, most importantly, its brain.

Take the kidneys. In the fetal world, kidneys are less functional than they are after birth because the mother's body takes care of their functions. So, from the fetal perspective, the kidneys are easily traded off when growth is jeopardized. If it is not receiving enough nutrition, the fetus conserves resources by producing fewer layers of nephrons. Nephrons filter the blood, and after birth, a kidney with fewer nephrons needs to punch above its weight to do its job, increasing the risk of both hypertension and kidney disease.

Epidemiological data reveal compelling connections between poor fetal nutrition and kidney-related ailments. A low nephron count is linked with low birth weight, and both are more prevalent in socially disadvantaged communities. As David Barker wrote in *Nutrition in the Womb*, not only are the rates of kidney failure in the United States highest in South Carolina (traditionally a "poor" state), they are also five times more common in African Americans than in white people.

The Stroke Belt

South Carolina is also in the middle of the Stroke Belt, a cluster of states in the south-eastern United States where stroke risk is particularly high — about 50 percent above the national average. Stroke is especially common among young African Americans, and African-American people also develop hypertension much earlier and much more severely than white people.

What is unique about the American South that can account for these discrepancies? Well, for starters, following the Civil War that region experienced profound social and economic disruption, including severe food shortages. In 1902 the first case of pellagra was diagnosed in Atlanta, Georgia. The disease caused sufferers to experience diarrhea, debilitating dermatitis and dementia. By 1920 pellagra had reached epidemic proportions and was especially high in 15 southern states. A quarter of a million cases were diagnosed annually, and 7,000 people died every year.

Eventually, thanks in large part to the work of pioneering epidemiologists, who painstakingly picked apart the erroneous assumption that pellagra was a communicable disease, scientists discovered it was caused by malnutrition. Basically, pellagra results from a deficiency of niacin, a B vitamin. One key piece of research leading to this conclusion emerged from studying clusters of the illness that appeared in institutions. An epidemic of pellagra that broke out in an Alabama institution housing mentally ill people, for example, was limited to the inmates, who were fed a nutrient-poor diet based almost entirely on corn. None of the nurses, who consumed a more nutritious diet comprising a variety of foods, was affected.

But the pellagra epidemic was just one feature of the Stroke Belt landscape. Because of its troublesome social and economic conditions, the southern United Sates has accommodated more than its share of impoverished families over an extended period of time. By virtue of their circumstances, the people in this region are particularly vulnerable not only to malnutrition but also to related stressors such as poverty and trauma. These factors similarly influence gene expression in ways that are heritable (see chapter 4). Combined, they set the stage for the epidemiological phenomenon we now describe as the Stroke Belt.

These people are not more vulnerable to stroke because of their lifestyle or genes. The Stroke Belt is very much a social phenomenon. It's a function of long cycles of poverty, social disruption, chronic stress and, of course, malnutrition. The area is also characterized by higher rates of kidney disease and hypertension. All of these conditions can be linked with poor fetal development and changes in gene expression resulting from the environmental impacts of poverty and trauma.

Refashioning Food

As an author of the *Atlas of Mortality from Selected Diseases in England and Wales*, David Barker was aware of the British statistics on stroke. The strongest predictor of stroke in any region was the death rates of women 70 years *before* the strokes actually happened. Based on this and other information, he gradually came to the conclusion that stroke risk originates before birth. Dr. Barker's research was pointing to maternal malnutrition as a key link in the chain of disease development. A fetus is not, as often assumed, "a highly successful parasite, like a tick or a leech, able to take from the mother whatever it requires and satisfy its modest needs, " he wrote in *Nutrition in the Womb*. Instead, it relies on its mother to supply it with the wide variety of nutrients it needs to develop properly.

How does the fetus get the food it needs to develop and grow? To put it simply, the mother consumes nutrients as food and these are extracted by the placenta, which channels them to the fetus. The mother's body provides the fetus with the building blocks it needs to become a healthy baby. When, for the umpteenth time, I reread Barker's thoughts on mothers' bodies as refashioning and recycling plants, I was fascinated to find references to the role the microbiota (see chapter 9) plays in these processes. Once again Dr. Barker was way ahead of his time. Beneficial bacteria do more than break down food; they also convert it to valuable substances such as vitamins, fatty acids and amino acids. He recognized that mothers need the help of those bacteria to support the work of supplying the fetus with nutrients.

However, as Barker pointed out, "A baby does not live only on what the mother eats during pregnancy. It also depends on the food stored in her body." A woman who has been malnourished throughout her life has fewer reserves to sustain a healthy pregnancy. In addition to the food its mother consumes, a fetus is constantly drawing on nutrients her body has stored: iron from her bone marrow, calcium from her bones, amino acids from her muscles and so on. Barker described this as a "flexible system" that is in a constant state of renewal. Women without adequate reserves will have an impaired ability to refashion food and are therefore less likely to meet their baby's nutritional needs.

Such a deficiency builds up in response to a woman's dietary experiences throughout her lifetime and, as David Barker came to see, the cumulative experiences of generations before her. It is a biological response to a lifetime of poverty and associated stresses. Viewed through this lens, the "stroke belt reflects the passing on through the generations of a refashioning ability that became compromised by events more than a century ago," as he wrote in *Nutrition in the Womb*.

IT'S MORE THAN LOW BIRTH WEIGHT

In one sense, David Barker's work was a paradigm shift because, probably without even realizing it, he was beginning to map the epigenetic landscape. Identifying low birth weight as a significant factor in chronic disease development was an important milestone, but it was just the starting point. As Kent Thornburg told me in an interview, "Low birth weight is a crude index of disease risk, but it has turned out to be a remarkably important one. As we learn more, our understanding of the various developmental factors affecting disease risk is expanding." These factors include epigenetic modifications that may be heritable.

We now understand that many stressors on the fetus can increase the risk of chronic disease without affecting its size at birth. Consider a 2006 study that Tessa Roseboom and David Barker authored with other researchers. They found that some adults whose mothers were in the early stages of pregnancy during the Dutch famine were born with an acceptable birth weight, but even so, they were twice as likely to have heart disease as those whose mothers had normal pregnancies.

There are numerous examples of increased risks for certain diseases that are not associated with low birth weight. Even though we don't understand the mechanisms, we know, for instance, that placental growth affects disease risk. Certain variations in the size and shape of the placenta have been linked with increased risks for hypertension, heart failure and lung cancer, even in babies born with an acceptable weight. This suggests that placental thickness and dimensions may be related to independent biological processes that affect fetal development. Similarly, certain physical characteristics of the mother, such as short stature and a high BMI, are known to increase chronic disease risk in offspring. And high birth weight is another risk factor, increasing vulnerability to obesity, type 2 diabetes and cancer.

Kent Thornburg points out that genetic background can also modify the effect of birth weight on disease development. For example, in a 2002 study, Johan Eriksson and other researchers looked at variations in certain genes in 152 elderly people. They found increased insulin resistance and elevated insulin concentrations only in individuals with certain single-nucleotide polymorphisms (SNPs) who also had a low birth weight.

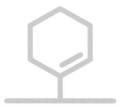

Transgenerational genetic inheritance:

The transmission of biological information from one generation to another through the genetic code embedded in the DNA of the parents' egg and sperm. By studying the occurrence of diseases across generations or in large populations, geneticists have identified hundreds of gene defects that have an impact on disease development. In addition, it is now well recognized that normal minor variations of the genetic code can make a person more or less vulnerable to acquiring a disease. Geneticists are working to identify these variations by studying large human populations.

Your Genetic Inheritance

Medical questionnaires always ask about your family history because certain illnesses run in families. While many factors contribute to clusters of disease development, a genetic component may also be at play. The strength of that connection depends upon many factors, from the type of disease and the gene involved to much broader considerations such as lifestyle, environment and, of course, the experience of previous generations.

Looking at genes in a vacuum, there are some diseases, such as sickle cell anemia and hemophilia, that result from a specific gene mutation. These are what scientists call *single gene disorders*, and the connection is strong: if you inherit the mutated gene from one or both parents, you will get some form of the disease.

Next on the intensity spectrum are genes with what is described as *high penetrance*. The BRCA1 gene, which is linked with breast and ovarian cancer, falls into this category. These days it has a very high profile because a number of well-known women with this mutation have chosen to have double mastectomies and even oophorectomies (removal of the ovaries) rather than risk developing cancer. If you inherit this gene, you have about a 60 percent lifetime risk of getting breast cancer and a 15 percent risk of developing ovarian cancer. While these rates are statistically significant, it should be noted that 40 percent of women with the gene will not get the disease.

Still, learning that you have the BRCA1 mutation is no doubt scary. Thankfully, the vast majority of genes implicated in the development of common illnesses don't operate that way. Hundreds of different genes are usually involved, each making a small contribution. Scientists call these *multifactorial diseases*. Basically, certain SNPs create vulnerability for some diseases. We have not yet identified all the connections, but we do know that some SNPs interact with the environment; in these situations, disease development depends on a combination of genes and epigenetic influences.

By the time a chronic illness becomes symptomatic, it has been percolating away in your body for quite some time. If you have coronary artery disease, for example, it developed over a period of years and may be a result of conditions such as chronic inflammation, which scientists increasingly believe is more closely linked to heart disease than high LDL cholesterol. How much your genes have to do with it is a subject of heated debate. Researchers have discovered close to 50 genetic links to heart disease. They can connect risk factors for coronary artery disease, such as hypertension and chronic inflammation, to specific variations in your genome. But when it comes to multifactorial diseases like heart disease, the "hardwired" part of your genome (your genes) is just a small part of the story. It's the programming — your *epigenome* — that really calls the shots.

People whose mothers had been pregnant during the Dutch Hunger Winter were twice as likely to have heart disease as adults. In later studies, researchers linked famine exposure with changes in the expression of several genes involved in growth and metabolism, which may ultimately pave the way to heart disease, likely via diabetes. In other words, by the time heart disease shows up, many factors have been at play over your lifetime.

Disease Development Is Complex

A predisposition to certain diseases can be linked to your genome. It may also be the result of less-than-optimal organ function because those organs were shortchanged during fetal development. Or it may be thanks to changes in gene expression that were a response to environmental stress in utero. Or a combination of all three.

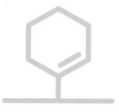

Epigenome:

The network of compounds surrounding our genes. Unlike the genome, which is fixed, the epigenome interacts with the environment, turning genes up or down, on or off, in response to external influences.

Genes and the Risk of Stroke

If your father had a stroke, you may wonder if that increases the likelihood that you will have one too. The short answer is, not much. We know from studies of identical twins, who are born with virtually identical genomes, that few diseases are genetically inheritable. Here's the longer answer: Because your father contributed half of your basic genetic material, he may have passed on variations in certain genes that increase your risk for stroke. He may also have passed on epigenetic changes resulting from the impact of experiences at sensitive points in his own development, such as exposure to toxins. However, the quality of your mother's pregnancy, and her mother's before her, is much more likely to affect your susceptibility to stroke; factors such as whether her diet was nutritious and how much stress she experienced may also influence your risk.

Strokes are the second leading cause of death worldwide. About 85 percent are ischemic, which means they happen when a blood vessel in the brain becomes blocked by a blood clot. The risk of stroke increases as you age, but it is also more common in males and people of African-American descent (see "The Stroke Belt," page 61, for more on this topic). Diabetes, obesity and hypertension have been linked with increased stroke risk, and these conditions have been on the rise in general, especially in younger people. As a result, we are now seeing higher incidence of stroke in people between the ages 15 and 49.

While some unusual abnormalities relating to single genes have been linked with stroke, from a genetic perspective, stroke risk is spread across many different genes that operate throughout your body. And how those genes express themselves may be influenced by numerous factors. Certain medical conditions — such as hypertension, diabetes, atherosclerosis and other conditions that affect the heart and blood vessels — can increase your risk for stroke. Poor growth before birth also plays a role. Underdevelopment of the liver and poor regulation of clotting factors both increase stroke risk.

An abundance of evidence links a healthy lifestyle with a reduced risk of stroke. So it's probably not surprising that consuming the standard American diet (SAD), which is high in processed foods, may increase stroke risk. Minerals such as potassium and magnesium have been specifically linked with a reduced risk of ischemic stroke, but minerals are diminished in the process of refining foods: white wheat flour has about 15 percent of the magnesium and not much more than 20 percent of the zinc, potassium and iron found in whole-grain wheat flour. Magnesium supports every major body system, yet experts tell us it is in short supply in the SAD.

The SAD isn't the only diet known to undermine health on a massive scale. For more than half the world's population, especially people living in Asia, white rice is a dietary staple. In the late 1800s a disease now known as beriberi began to show up across Asia. Depending on the type of beriberi, it affects either the heart and circulatory system or the nervous system. The numbers of affected people were significant; for instance, beriberi was identified as the national disease of Japan. Beriberi was eventually linked to a diet deficient in thiamine, a B vitamin that is lost when rice is refined.

Like refined wheat, white rice also provides far lower quantities of minerals that are associated with a reduced risk of ischemic stroke. Compared to brown rice, white rice provides about half the amount of iron and potassium, about 25 percent less zinc and almost 75 percent less magnesium. Although no studies have found a connection between stroke and the consumption of white rice, it is interesting to note that stroke is the most prevalent cardiovascular disease throughout Asia.

Many people have genetic variations that affect methylation, predisposing them to increased levels of the amino acid homocysteine. When homocysteine is elevated, there is a greater likelihood that your blood will clot, which increases your risk of ischemic stroke. Vitamins B_{12}, B_6 and folate all play an important role in metabolizing homocysteine. Good sources of folate are leafy greens, legumes, globe artichokes, broccoli and asparagus. Vitamin B_{12} is found naturally in animal foods, so vegans have difficulty obtaining adequate B_{12} unless their food is fortified with the vitamin. Vitamin B_{12} deficiencies are more common among certain groups, such as vegans and elderly people. Supplementing with folic acid is problematic when a B_{12} deficiency exists: it may mask the symptoms of anemia, an early warning of the deficiency, creating an opportunity for more serious disease development.

Another insurance policy against stroke is to eat more foods that will help decrease the chance of blood clots. These include dark leafy greens, grape juice or red wine (in moderation), pomegranate juice, tomatoes, chile peppers and berries. Foods rich in omega-3 fatty acids (most prevalent in fatty fish, such as salmon and trout) and vitamin E (such as whole-grain oats and wheat) also contribute to keeping your blood from becoming too viscous.

If you think you are at an increased risk for stroke and are serious about preventing it, a diet rich in nutritious whole foods, such as fruits, vegetables and whole grains, is an important first step. Not only do these foods provide valuable nutrients that have been shown to reduce stroke risk, but a diet high in plant foods can help to keep inflammation, which has been linked with many chronic diseases, under control. Getting off your butt is another great idea. Research shows that regular exercise can reduce your risk of stroke by about 25 percent.

If you are considering taking supplements instead of eating a more nutritious diet, you may want to think again. Nutritional supplements such as vitamin C and B-complex vitamins aren't as effective at preventing stroke as consuming those same nutrients as part of an overall healthy diet. Nature doesn't provide nutrients in isolated form, as they appear in supplements, but rather in combinations that work together to promote health and prevent disease. Plus, consuming nutrients from food creates synergy. Different nutrients interact with different organs, tissues and cells, and food components interact with each other, creating benefits that are more than the sum of their individual parts. In other words, consuming nutrients from a variety of whole foods creates a synergistic effect that boosts their benefit as individual foods.

We now know that environmental factors such as too little or too much nutrition at different developmental stages in childhood and adolescence can also influence disease risk. It's those conditions that make most people susceptible to chronic disease, much more so than gene defects or too many burgers with fries, as we previously thought. The good news is that lifestyle modifications, such as better nutrition and increased physical activity, can help to counteract this susceptibility.

Why Is Nutrition So Important?

Most of what we knew about nutrition and fetal development prior to the turn of the millennium is neatly summed up in a 1998 paper by Dr. Alan Lucas, a professor of pediatric nutrition at the University of London. Published in the *Journal of Nutrition*, his paper laid out the clinical and historical context for the developmental origins of health and disease. At that point it was becoming clear that events linked to "sensitive" stages of development could have lifelong impacts on health and longevity. Using the term *nutritional programming*, Lucas laid the groundwork for what we now recognize as key building blocks in vulnerability to disease. How well you were nourished in the womb will influence your health for the rest of your life. Or, as Dr. Lucas wrote in a 2005 paper, "the current focus of nutritional science has shifted from meeting needs to determining the biological effects that nutrition has on immediate and lifetime health." The concept of programming, the idea that "a stimulus or insult during a critical or sensitive period of development can have long-term or lifetime effects on an organism," is particularly significant.

FETAL PROGRAMMING

Summing up, here's how nutritional programming works: First, nutrition plays a key role in determining how well your organs are constructed. As noted above, if a pregnant woman doesn't obtain adequate nutrition, neither does her baby. In response, the developing fetus trades off growth in organs such as the kidneys, the pancreas and even the heart in favor of the brain. People born with "disadvantaged" organs have a predisposition to certain illnesses and will spend the rest of their lives making up for the shortcoming. This is not to say they will necessarily succumb to preordained diseases; it just means they will need to work harder to avoid them. As the old joke about Ginger Rogers and Fred Astaire put it, Ginger did everything Fred did, but backwards and in high heels.

The second major impact results from epigenetic modifications that are made in utero. These modifications influence how your genes function, and they can leave permanent marks on previously plastic cells. Over time, depending on life experience, these changes may become more pronounced. Think back to the identical twins (see "The Curious Case of Identical Twins," page 40). These individuals, who developed from the same fertilized egg, are genetically identical and yet they do not necessarily suffer from the same diseases. Research shows that their epigenomes begin to differ in utero. The changes become more striking as twins age and are most noticeable when the twins have lived apart for a long period of time.

Gene Expression

Scientists now know that when a fetus is developing, it is "plastic" — constantly adapting to its circumstances. Cells live in an extremely dynamic and complex environment, and stressors such as inadequate nutrition provoke them to adapt by altering gene expression. The changes are particularly impactful if they occur at critical periods in fetal development. This process is far more complex and difficult to predict than organ formation. However, the results can be long-lasting and have the potential to be passed on through generations.

Along with epidemiology, the science of epigenetics is helping us connect the dots between babies who seem healthy at birth, their experiences in the womb and good health or chronic illness later in life. Analysis of the Dutch Hunger Winter records revealed clear connections between malnutrition in pregnancy and the incidence of chronic disease later in life. Recent research based on those data has also linked the effect of the famine to epigenetic changes — specifically DNA methylation patterns — that can be traced back to the early stages of pregnancy.

In addition to nutrition, many other environmental factors influence gene expression, both positively and negatively. For instance, epigenetic changes in the fetus have been linked with the mother's mental health and social environment, as well as the father's exposure to toxins. Either sex can undermine fetal development by smoking or drinking alcohol. And surprisingly, the fetus maintains a biological memory of these experiences that may be passed on to future generations.

Why does this happen? Well, throughout pregnancy, as in all stages of life, the epigenome is constantly adjusting itself to keep everything running as smoothly as possible. Normally these are small adjustments, but they can accumulate over time. Also, some situations, such as the Dutch famine, can be catastrophic. Near starvation, particularly in the early stages of pregnancy, when the fetus's organs are forming, could amount to a major systemic disruption, setting in motion a cascade of events with significant effects. And as Tessa Roseboom, who works closely with the Dutch data says, not only is the epigenome probably the best archive of this prenatal experience, but "its effects can be transgenerational through both the maternal and paternal lines."

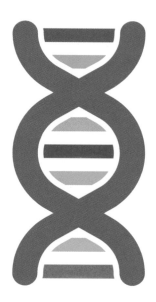

4

BEYOND NUTRITION

One of the best predictors of the health of a man or woman age 65 years is the answer to the simple question "Do you feel well?" A positive answer predicts better health for the next twenty years.

— DAVID BARKER, *NUTRITION IN THE WOMB*

HAVE YOU EVER WONDERED why certain personality traits are associated with specific nationalities? Think of Irish charm, Swedish consensus-building and German precision, to name just three. Societal norms certainly play a weighty role, and so do factors such as selective migration, whereby people with similar attributes choose to live in certain places, helping to cement their character. But other elements may also be in play — for instance, what social scientists call "social contagion," the idea that over time people become more like the people they associate with.

Not surprisingly, your life experiences also shape your personality. While we don't fully understand the mechanisms, we now know, for example, that experiences can affect brain development. Basically, your reactions to events modify your gene expression, recalibrating body systems in ways that have lifelong effects, including on personality and psychological well-being. So that raises a question: When large groups of people have common experiences over a long period of time, do they begin to share personality traits? And does this affect the health and well-being of the entire group? Recent evidence suggests the answer is yes.

ADVERSE EXPERIENCES

To backtrack, a large body of research links hardscrabble experience in early life with poor health later on. For instance, the high rates of stroke in certain areas of the southern United States can be linked with the long periods of social and economic disruption that followed the Civil War (see "The Stroke Belt," page 61). This falls into a field of research known as "the social origins of illness." The Adverse Childhood Experiences Study (2014), a major research project based in the United States, belongs to this category. Over the course of almost 20 years, investigators surveyed more than 17,000 adults, documenting their exposure to difficult experiences such as abuse, neglect and domestic violence. They found, perhaps not surprisingly, that early trauma had a major impact on both physical and mental health. They also found that the effect of such experiences is dose-dependent: the more adverse childhood experiences (ACEs) subjects had, the worse their health as adults. Many illnesses could be linked to those early experiences, from chronic obstructive pulmonary disease and hepatitis to depression and suicide. As noted, the more ACEs, the greater their impact. For instance, if a person's ACE score rose to seven or more, it tripled their lifetime risk of developing cancer or ischemic heart disease.

So, what does this have to do with population-based personality traits? Consider recent research that drilled down into data from England and Wales. Those researchers found that a prolonged experience of hardship associated with living in specific regions of those countries had a significant impact on the personality traits of the populations as a whole.

The Legacy of Coal

The seeds of the Industrial Revolution were planted in the English countryside in the early 1800s, and they grew quickly. Factories rapidly sprung up, punctuating the previously bucolic landscape with geysers of smoke and steam. With artistic prescience, the poet William Blake captured the conundrum of such progress in his poem "Jerusalem" (later to become a hymn). While interpretation of his work is hotly debated, it's highly likely that the "dark Satanic mills" mentioned in the poem referred to the burned-out shell of the Albion Flour Mill in his neighborhood. The image of that blackened hulk, a blight on the previously "lovely Lambeth," may have shaped his vision, linking the mills with hell.

In Blake's day, people were just beginning the century-long process of migration to the industrial regions in search of a better life. The problem is, they couldn't escape the meager living conditions they hoped to leave behind. Far from it, in fact. For the most part they left agrarian lives to establish communities built around a new identity: the working class. Not only was their existence still characterized by hardship, but the generations that followed also had difficult lives.

The workers who migrated to areas of Great Britain that became centers for large-scale coal-based industries set in motion a process that helped to create modern society as we know it. However, over the better part of a century, they suffered severe social and economic displacement. People migrated to those regions to work in factories. But as the coal-based industries gradually declined, they were left without employment. In time they found themselves living in what have been called "some of the most economically deprived areas in highly industrial nations," as a 2017 study published in the *Journal of Personality and Social Psychology* concluded. Sadly, that experience came with additional costs: many of their descendants still carry within themselves the residues of that experience. The authors called it "the hidden legacy of coal."

In their study "In the Shadow of Coal," the researchers were able to identify "sustained psychological consequences affecting the well-being of the populations now living in the old coal regions." They examined a wide body of research linking chronic economic hardship with well-being and health, and concluded that psychological adversity "runs deep" in these regions. That adversity, they noted, is expressed not only in the actual well-being of the people but also in personality traits linked to well-being. Broadly speaking, the people who remained in those regions over the years scored high in markers associated with negative psychological states. These markers have been linked with personality traits that psychologists use to study major dimensions of personality, such as an inability to cope (associated with a greater propensity for anxiety and depression), poor organizational skills and lower life satisfaction. In general terms, they correlate with an overall lack of psychological well-being, and they influence a wide range of socioeconomic and health outcomes, including life expectancy.

The authors of the coal study focused on regions in England and Wales because the records were available. However, they pointed out that it seems likely similar findings would result from studying industrial regions in other parts of the world, such as the Ruhr region of Germany and parts of China. While comparable historical data were not available from the United States, using other markers, they concluded that the same might be said about the so-called rust belt in America.

YOU ARE WHAT YOUR GRANDPARENTS ATE

DETERMINANTS OF HEALTH

The idea that economic and social conditions influence health has been around for decades and is now supported by a substantial body of research. We know that well-being is strongly tied to factors such as income, education, social support systems and working conditions. And let's not forget race and ethnicity or exposure to toxins. Taken together, these individual markers comprise your life experience, and they go a long way toward determining your physical and mental health. Public policy is also influential because it has a major impact on factors such as education, early childhood development, food security and access to health care.

While your lifelong experiences are certainly impactful, the recent news is that they aren't just about you. Your experiences may change how your genes behave, and those changes may be heritable — that is to say, passed on to your children. Take stress, for instance. Numerous studies of both animals and humans have shown that when mothers are stressed, their stress responses are transmitted to offspring. Results include widespread changes to gene expression and, consequently, exaggerated responses to stress in the offspring. As Kent Thornburg told me, epidemiological data now support the idea that social stress during pregnancy is just as detrimental to the fetus as nutritional stress. Unfortunately, both types of stress are often found in the same pregnant woman.

Stressed Out

Just can't "get over it"? Well, the simple truth is that you may be more vulnerable to negative experiences than your best friend, or even a sibling. Events that occurred when you were in the womb or at other susceptible periods of your life may have affected you physically by, for instance, influencing how your brain developed or how certain genes related to what experts call your *allostatic systems* are expressed. These include your nervous, endocrine and immune systems, all of which respond to stress. If these regulators are out of whack, it goes a long way toward explaining why you just can't wipe the emotional slate clean. Simply stated, some people are more resilient than others, and psychologists tell us this may be beyond your control.

Whether it's short-lived but acute, or chronic and extended over a longer period of time, stress affects certain hormones, such as cortisol. When a woman is pregnant, cortisol levels secreted by her adrenal glands pour into her blood and are transmitted to the fetus through the placenta. Increases in maternal cortisol are known to affect the developing fetus, and although the effects are not likely to be noticeable at birth, we now know they will be long-lasting. They may also be passed on to future generations.

The Effects of Traumatic Events

Over the years, scientists have mined various segments of the data from the Helsinki Birth Cohort Study (see page 24) to explore various health-related conditions, among them the effects of the 1939 winter invasion of Finland by Russian troops. The Finns fought valiantly but were greatly outnumbered, and the death toll was heavy. The researchers compared 167 children whose fathers had been killed while their mothers were pregnant with 168 children who were alive but less than a year old when their fathers were killed. They found much higher rates of schizophrenia and behavioral disorders in the children who were still in utero when their fathers died.

A similar pattern was observed in a study that looked at the effects of the 1967 Arab–Israeli Six-Day War. There, investigators found that the offspring of women who were in their second month of pregnancy were two to three times more likely to develop schizophrenia as adults. Moreover, evidence also suggests that women don't need to be pregnant to pass on the experience of trauma to their offspring. A 2017 study looked at the offspring of Finnish women who had been evacuated to Sweden as children during the Second World War. It found that their female offspring were twice as likely to suffer from a psychiatric illness and four times as likely to experience bipolar disorder or depression than a control group whose mothers had not been displaced. This study of more than 45,000 children, which was published in the *Journal of the American Medical Association* (*JAMA*), also found significant differences between the sexes. Not only did the male children of displaced mothers not experience similar psychological problems, but both the male and female children of fathers who had been evacuated as boys were similarly unaffected by the experience.

Needless to say, war is not the only cataclysmic event someone might experience. Nowadays natural disasters such as forest fires, earthquakes and hurricanes are increasingly common, and they are likely to leave a trail of devastation in their wake. In addition to personal injury and fatalities, natural disasters have been linked with a broad range of negative health effects, including pregnancy outcomes. It is well known, for instance, that the rate of premature births increases during hurricanes. At its most obvious this relates to the drop in barometric pressure, which is likely to induce labor. However, two

Nutrition and Stress

You may not be able to control everything that makes you feel overwhelmed, but you can help your body tame the negative effects of stress by consistently consuming a diet of nutritious whole foods. For starters, your gastrointestinal tract and your brain are so closely linked that your gut has been described as your second brain (see page 275). Although research is still in the rudimentary stages, we know that a healthy diet can help to keep you balanced, in part by nurturing the beneficial bacteria in your gut. We also know that certain nutrients support your body's ability to cope with stress. For instance, vitamins such as folate and certain B vitamins are necessary for methylation of DNA, which may affect the expression of certain genes related to your stress response.

Eat Regularly

If you're serious about controlling stress, don't skip meals. Enjoy a hearty breakfast of nutrient-dense whole foods to promote balanced blood sugar throughout the day. If your blood sugar is uneven, your endocrine system responds by adjusting its production of hormones such as insulin and cortisol, which initiates another vicious cycle. These elevated stress hormones may aggravate your sense of feeling pressured and decrease your resilience, making you more sensitive to new stressors.

When it comes to breakfast, simply drinking a cup (or more) of coffee on its own is probably a bad idea. Coffee contains a hefty dose of caffeine, which raises levels of cortisol and other stress hormones in sensitive people. It also stimulates acid production in the stomach and can cause irritation of the esophagus, especially when consumed on an empty stomach. If you are already dealing with raging hormones from too much stress, drinking multiple cups of coffee through the day will make the problem worse. Coffee contributes to a roller coaster of variable moods and energy levels, and its effects can carry over to nighttime, disrupting deep, restful sleep. (And sleep on its own is another stress-buster.)

You may have seen news about recent studies showing that drinking three to five cups of coffee a day can lower your risk of dying from type 2 diabetes and heart disease. This benefit may be linked with polyphenols, naturally occurring chemicals found in the coffee plant. While these substances are known to reduce inflammation (which is also linked with stress), if you are dealing with chronic stress, it makes more sense to choose beverages that provide health-promoting polyphenols but contain less caffeine, such as green or black tea or decaffeinated coffee.

Balance Nutrients to Enhance Mood

Another strategy for coping with stress is to consume protein, fat and fiber at every meal, especially breakfast. These "slow fuels" not only help keep your blood sugar balanced, but also provide nutritional building blocks that stimulate a healthy mood. Protein is composed of amino acids, which your body breaks down into components that are converted into mood-enhancing *neurotransmitters*. High-quality protein sources — such as meat, poultry, fish, eggs, legumes (including peanut butter) and dairy — are rich sources of the amino acid tyrosine, which creates dopamine, a powerful brain messenger that keeps you motivated, focused and feeling positive.

Healthy fats, especially omega-3 fatty acids, are also mood-friendly nutrients that can help you tolerate stress and keep depression at bay. Unfortunately, these fats are in short supply in the typical Western diet. The best sources of omega-3s are fatty fish, such as salmon, sardines and cod. Make a point of adding omega-3 fats to your diet. If fatty fish aren't an option, consider plant-based sources such as chia and flax seeds, which can easily be added to your morning smoothie. These days excellent vegetable-based protein powders that include omega-3-rich foods are widely available. They can be added to smoothies or baked goods to provide protein and other valuable nutrients.

Complex carbohydrates, unlike their impoverished refined relatives, have long been linked with mood enhancement. Among other benefits, they help your body create serotonin, a brain- and nervous system–friendly chemical that is perhaps best known as an antidepressive. Serotonin is often called the "good mood" neurotransmitter, promoting feelings of relaxation and calm. It is also a natural appetite suppressant. Consuming high-quality protein helps your body produce serotonin, as does the essential amino acid tryptophan.

Many whole grains are particularly good sources of tryptophan. That's one reason why starting your day with a hot bowl of whole-grain cereal or a thick slice of whole-grain toast is a good idea. To continue on this track, later in the day enjoy whole-grain pasta or stone-ground cornmeal, or nutrient-dense starchy root vegetables, such as sweet potatoes or carrots. Avoid refined grains and flours, which are found in most cookies, cakes and breads; they may provide a short-lived boost to your mood, but they come with a long-term cost.

FOOD CRAVINGS

Speaking of short-term mood enhancers, if you've been feeling stressed and are craving sweet or high-fat foods such as chocolate chip cookies or potato chips — possibly even at odd hours of the night — you are not alone. Studies have shown that distressed people (and animals) tend to prefer "hyperpalatable" foods, even if they aren't feeling hungry. Foods that are high in sugar, flour, salt and fat stimulate pleasure centers in the brain. This means they provide an accessible form of self-medication when you are feeling stressed out.

As Pulitzer Prize–winning journalist Michael Moss highlighted in his book *Salt Sugar Fat: How the Food Giants Hooked Us*, the large corporations in the business of producing processed foods are well aware of your vulnerabilities and have worked hard to exploit them. Over the past half-century, processed-food manufacturers have very deliberately manipulated their products to create what they have identified as a "bliss point": just the right combination of textures and flavors to make you want more (see "Hooked on Food," page 148, for more on this subject).

THE APPEAL OF JUNK FOOD

Chronic stress makes you more vulnerable to the attractions of junk food, and here's how it works: Acute stress is short-lived; it's an immediate response to an imminent threat. Sensing risk, your brain sends signals to your adrenal glands (the hormone-producing glands that respond to stress) to release adrenaline, which suppresses appetite (and libido). Your brain is working on your behalf, adjusting how your body allocates resources such as blood flow and energy in order to help you cope. This works as long as the stress is short-lived. The problem is, if it continues and becomes chronic, the communication between your brain and your adrenal glands becomes dysfunctional. In that case you may find yourself battling an insatiable appetite for sugary, fatty foods. Your brain is still doing its job, responding to chronic stress signals, but it has short-circuited the system by pursuing the pleasurable experiences these foods provide.

Chronic stress also alters how your brain receives serotonin and dopamine, which influence mood, motivation and pleasure. When you are stressed, it is not unusual to experience feelings of depression and anxiety. "Comfort food" is an apt term. Treats such as cakes, cookies and ice cream create genuine sensations of pleasure in the brain and offer short-term relief when you are feeling down, lonely or scared. You may also find that your sleep patterns change: you sleep poorly or wake up way too early in the morning. For many people, poor-quality sleep, or not enough sleep, can lead to a vicious cycle of cravings that conclude with overindulging in too many sugary, fatty and nutrient-deficient foods.

Nutrients and Stress

Certain micronutrients will help your body deal with both the psychological and physical effects of chronic stress. For instance, studies show that a high intake of vitamin C (at least 1,000 mg a day) improves stress tolerance. If you're aiming to consume this amount of vitamin C, you will likely need to supplement, in which case seek the guidance of a health-care provider. Try a natural source of vitamin C, such as camu camu berries, which also contain a panoply of nutrients that work together to support good health.

The connection between folate deficiency and depression is well-established within the psychiatric community. While it is not known whether folate deficiency leads to depression or vice versa, maintaining a folate-rich diet or supplementing with folic acid (around 400 mcg daily) can help you stave off or cope with depression. (If you have a vitamin B_{12} deficiency, be aware that supplementing with folic acid may be harmful.) In some jurisdictions, foods such as breads, cereals and pastas are fortified with folic acid. However, it's likely those products are made with refined grains, which are not recommended. If necessary, take folic acid or, better still, consciously add folate-rich foods to your diet. Good dietary sources of folate include dark leafy greens, citrus fruits, legumes, nuts and seeds. Low zinc levels are also associated with depression. Pumpkin seeds, red meat and oysters can provide daily doses of food-based zinc.

Magnesium is another nutrient that is particularly valuable if you are trying to cope with stress. Stress burns up the magnesium in your body (as does drinking alcohol). Studies repeatedly link magnesium intake with improvements in a wide variety of mood disorder problems ranging from depression and anxiety to poor sleep. Magnesium also helps to relax the tense muscles associated with chronic stress. Magnesium-rich foods include dark spinach, Swiss chard, pumpkin seeds, almonds, black beans, avocados and dark chocolate (which also provides cocoa flavonols that can improve mental functioning during times of stress).

Whole grains, such as brown rice, buckwheat and "ancient grains" (including amaranth, millet and quinoa), are always a good option when battling stress. In addition to magnesium, they provide other stress-busting nutrients, such as folate and zinc, and many other helpful nutrients, all of which work together synergistically to promote well-being. Consuming a diet based on a wide variety of nutrient-dense foods will ensure that your nutritional needs are met over the long term.

studies that examined the effect of separate earthquakes established a clear link between the stress of the event and premature delivery. Both also confirmed that the women most likely to delivery prematurely were those who were in their first trimester at the time of the earthquake, and one found that they were slightly more likely to have babies with a low birth weight even when carried to full term.

SEVERITY INFLUENCES EFFECT

Clearly it is stressful to experience extreme weather. But as one 2008 study found — echoing the research that found the "dose" of adverse experiences influenced the degree of impact — the severity of the storm experience was a key factor in how much it affected an individual's health. The study defined "high hurricane exposure" as including three or more grueling experiences, which included feeling that your life might be in danger or dealing with significant damage to your home. After adjusting for many variables, the researchers concluded that women who were pregnant during Hurricane Katrina or became pregnant immediately after the storm, and who experienced high hurricane exposure, were at increased risk for giving birth preterm and of having infants with a low birth weight. The women with high hurricane exposure were also much more likely to suffer from post-traumatic stress disorder (PTSD) than were women whose experience was less distressing (13.8% compared to 1.3%), and the frequency of low-birth-weight babies was higher in women with PTSD (23.1%) than in women without PTSD (9.1%).

Another study, which examined the effects of Hurricane Sandy, confirmed these findings. It, too, found that long-term health effects were related to how intensely individuals experienced the storm. Those whose experience was intense were more likely to develop depression, anxiety and PTSD. In that study, displacement was a key indicator of whether survivors would suffer long-term effects. People who could find refuge with friends or family were far less likely to develop PTSD than those who were accommodated in public shelters.

Post-Traumatic Stress Disorder

Rachel Yehuda, a professor of psychiatry and neuroscience at Mount Sinai Medical Center in New York City, is an expert in PTSD, an interest that was inspired by her work with Holocaust survivors. As a graduate student she became intrigued by research that identified connections between stress hormones and brain development. With a view to taking her research out of the lab and into the community, in the early 1990s she set up a clinic to treat Holocaust survivors. Imagine her surprise when some of their adult children showed up. Like their parents, many presented with symptoms of PTSD, such as disturbed sleep and recurring nightmares.

That experience piqued her curiosity. Dr. Yehuda began to wonder whether PTSD could be·inherited. Are biological changes in traumatized parents somehow passed on to their children? Does the body have a capacity to remember trauma? On September 11, 2001, when the Twin Towers were attacked by terrorists, Dr. Yehuda was in charge of the Traumatic Stress Studies Division at Mount Sinai. After the attack, the clinic was inundated with phone calls, some of which came from pregnant women. She recruited 38 mothers-to-be so she could study the effects they had experienced after the attack.

INCONSISTENT RESPONSES

Her findings were in some ways surprising. First, not all of her subjects developed PTSD; some were more resilient than others. Second, the cortisol levels in the group that developed PTSD were unexpected. As previously noted, cortisol is a stress hormone, and in stressful situations cortisol levels are expected to increase. However, the women who developed PTSD had lower, rather than higher, levels of cortisol. Identifying the link between cortisol levels and PTSD was an important breakthrough in understanding the condition.

A year later, the researchers measured cortisol levels in the babies of the PTSD sufferers, and once again they found intriguing differences. If the mothers were in their second or third trimester when the attacks took place, the babies had lower levels of cortisol. Somehow the memory of that traumatic experience had been transmitted to the fetus. The question was, how? Yehuda is currently working on answering that question. In general terms, her research suggests that trauma may have permanent biological effects. Trauma alters gene expression, and traumatized parents may pass on these changes to their offspring. The process aligns with the transgenerational inheritance that Marcus Pembrey documented (see "Epigenetic Inheritance," page 38), but in this case it's the memory of trauma that is being passed on through the generations.

THE EFFECTS ARE SYSTEMIC

It should be noted that while cortisol levels in people with PTSD are consistently lower than average, they are not wildly out of the normal range, which limits their potential as a diagnostic tool. But Yehuda has also shown that, in addition to lower cortisol levels after the trauma is over, people with PTSD have lower levels of the enzyme that breaks down cortisol. This adaptation effectively helps to keep cortisol circulating in the body. It may be a biological adaptation: the body's way of dealing with situations of prolonged threat.

BULLYING

Sadly, being bullied is not an uncommon experience. These days cyberbullying in particular has become a serious concern. More than 40 percent of adolescents report being bullied online, the effects of which include low self-esteem, anxiety, depression and tragically even suicide.

Not surprisingly, one 2013 study linked the chronic stress of being bullied with long-term effects that resemble PTSD. Researchers from Canada and the United Kingdom focused on 28 pairs of identical twins, part of a group that had been followed since the age of five. Within this subset, one twin from each pair had subsequently been bullied. When the researchers revisited the bullied twins, now 10 years old, they found significant changes in their gene expression. These twins had higher serotonin transporter gene (SERT) methylation, a process that dials down the activity of the SERT gene. They also had lower cortisol levels when exposed to stress. Like the children Rachel Yehuda studied, their epigenomes were adapting, working to protect them from the effects of bullying by dulling their response to persistent stress.

Interestingly, the cortisol-busting enzyme is also involved in certain aspects of metabolism that help the body deal with long-standing starvation. The problem is that over the long term this biological strategy is maladaptive. The low levels of cortisol in the blood of PTSD offspring make them more susceptible to stress, including their ability to survive famine. In an environment where food is plentiful rather than scarce, it may also put them at greater risk for conditions such as obesity. Studies have shown that people with PTSD are more likely to become obese, and researchers are now exploring the common pathways that may link the conditions.

DIFFERENT STRESS, DIFFERENT OUTCOMES

While the science is extremely complex and scientists don't yet understand the underlying mechanisms, maternal stress during pregnancy will have different outcomes for offspring depending on what might broadly be described as *degree*. Women (and men) who have PTSD will produce offspring who throughout their lives have lower-than-normal levels of cortisol and are more vulnerable to developing PTSD when faced with adversity.

On the other hand, women who are chronically stressed but not suffering from PTSD will typically have elevated cortisol levels. Their children will have compromised organs and exaggerated responses to stress. If the mother's stress levels are too high, the power of the cortisol-busting enzyme in the placenta will be overwhelmed, and cortisol will cross into the baby without being deactivated. The problem is worsened by conditions, such as malnutrition, that suppress the formation of the deactivating enzyme in the placenta.

The mechanisms underlying these processes are extremely complex, but there is little doubt that changes to gene expression play a significant role. Yehuda suspects there is also a genetic component: certain common alleles may increase susceptibility. And she is looking at what experts describe as *allostatic overload*, the physical and mental wear and tear that are the long-term effects of chronic stress. In simple terms, bearing too much for too long erodes resistance.

People's lives are complex and dynamic; over time, the interactions among numerous factors affect how the body responds to stress, influencing resilience or susceptibility to the effects of trauma. The good news is, research is showing that many relatively simple lifestyle changes, ranging from better nutrition to mindfulness and exercise, can improve or even reverse some of these epigenetic changes.

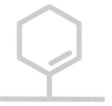

Allostatic systems:

Allostasis is the process of achieving stability through change. Body systems that work to keep your body on an even keel in response to environmental impacts such as stress are often called allostatic systems.

Allostatic overload:

The long-term physical cost of adapting to negative experiences, such as chronic stress, predisposing an individual to developing chronic illness.

Broken Social Scene

Broken Social Scene is the clever name of a Canadian indie band, but it also works as a metaphor for the adverse childhood experiences that may continue to affect you for your entire lifetime. Studies show that certain aspects of a difficult childhood reach beyond the psyche and well into your physical being. The higher you are on the socioeconomic ladder, the better your health — both physical and mental. People on the lower rungs of the ladder die younger and experience more sickness throughout their lives. They are also more likely to have what social scientists call "poor social outcomes." Among other things, they have fewer friendships, less social interaction and less involvement in community life. A wide variety of explanations for this disparity have been suggested, ranging from poor nutrition and education to unstable employment and insufficient access to medical care.

Socioeconomic status (SES) is defined as a widespread measure of your life situation, including occupation, education and economic and social position. Researchers have been able to link SES directly with the incidence of certain diseases. For instance, using information from the Helsinki Birth Cohort Study, researchers examined the history of a group of children who were born in public maternity hospitals in Helsinki between 1934 and 1944. These data showed links between low SES and heart disease, a connection that has been confirmed in other studies.

It has been suggested that the link between low SES and poor health is restricted access to medical care. But in Canada, where publicly funded health care ensures relatively good access to medical care, Canadians with lower incomes have been shown to be more vulnerable to cardiovascular disease and more likely to die earlier because of it. This disparity is common to countries with governmental health-care systems around the world. In the United States, money diverted from Medicare to providing social support for low-SES people has been shown to reduce the incidence of chronic disease more than spending comparable amounts on medical care. It's a compelling reaffirmation of the old saying "An ounce of prevention is worth a pound of cure."

A 2006 study done at Johns Hopkins Hospital in Baltimore added an interesting spin to data linking SES and heart disease. Over a period of 40 years, it tracked a group of medical students enrolled at Johns Hopkins University. Those students, who came from a variety of backgrounds, became an elite group of physicians. They were well-educated and affluent, but by the time they reached 50, their childhood experiences were showing up in their health. Those who were impoverished in childhood were 2.4 times more likely to have heart disease than those who had been raised in more affluent circumstances.

Experience Influences Biology

Neuroscientist Tomas Paus, now based at the University of Toronto, is one of a growing number of scientists studying the ways that experience influences biology. His special interest lies in the relationship between adolescent brain development and social status. In 2017 he published a study in the journal *Scientific Reports* that looked at the social and economic status of nearly 1,000 girls, relating their position in this hierarchy to the neighborhoods they lived in. The girls were assigned to two groups: low-income and high-income households. Basically, Paus found differences in how the girls' brains developed, depending on their economic status.

The girls most affected were those whose families were poor but who lived in neighborhoods also occupied by more affluent families (not uncommon in large cities). They demonstrated increased cortical thinning, a measure associated with brain development that has been linked with an increased risk for depression, among other conditions. Living in a neighborhood with a large disparity in household income constantly exposed the girls to contemporaries who were much better off, and this awareness of their low position in the social hierarchy affected how their brains developed. It's a compelling statement about the high costs of income inequality, which most experts agree is one of our most pressing social concerns.

Dr. Paus's team then went on to test whether stress and sex hormones played a role. In the group of low-income girls with cortical thinning, they found strong associations with the expression of two genes: the glucocorticoid receptor NR3C1 and the androgen receptor (AR), both of which are linked with certain stress-related hormones. The researchers also identified connections between this gene activity and cortical thickness. They concluded that the girls' experience and its effect on how their brains developed potentially placed them at higher risk for mental illness as adults. Interestingly, exposure to income inequality didn't affect males the same way. A possible explanation is that their higher levels of testosterone may have a "ceiling effect" on the hormones activated by social stress.

Although all this work is in the early stages, a clear message is emerging: the daily grind of a psychologically taxing life can muddy biological pathways. In 2017 researchers at Duke University in North Carolina established that adolescents with even modestly impoverished backgrounds were at greater risk for depression as a result of epigenetic changes. They identified a connection between social status and differences in how a gene associated with serotonin production is methylated. Other studies have also connected the dots between social stress, genetic expression and the risk of mental illness. For instance, Gunther Meinlschmidt, a German neuroscientist, found that stress can alter methylation of the oxytocin receptor gene, which has been linked with self-esteem and coping skills. On a positive note, scientists such as Dr. Meinlschmidt are exploring the idea that social support can mitigate the biological effects of stress, and evidence is emerging that this may be the case.

Behavioral Epigenetics

The indelible mark that experience leaves on your epigenome defines the emerging field of *behavioral epigenetics*. Two Canadian scientists based at Montreal's McGill University have been at the forefront of some of this research. In 1992 Michael Meaney, a neuroscientist, and Moshe Szyf, a geneticist, met at a conference in Madrid and discovered they had similar interests in exploring how genes react to experience. They were both intrigued by the then-radical notion that these reactions might be passed on to offspring. They knew diet and toxins could affect the epigenome, but they were interested in establishing a link between "softer" experiences, such as parental neglect and nurturing.

The scientists formed a research partnership and in 1999 conducted an experiment on rats that demonstrated a link between maternal care and the offspring's physiological ability to deal with stress. In rats, nurturing is determined by the amount of licking and grooming mothers bestow on their offspring. Researchers used two groups of mother rats; the first was high-strung and inattentive, while the second was calm and affectionate. And there was, indeed, a link between maternal care and epigenetic changes. When the mother rats licked and groomed their offspring infrequently, the babies were more anxious than those whose mothers had been more affectionate. Investigating more deeply, the researchers found differences in DNA methylation between the baby rats with nurturing mothers and those whose mothers were aloof. Specifically, inadequate nurturing suppressed the activity of a particular gene. But with one simple step — giving the neglected pups to an affectionate mother — the researchers were able to reset the program. Once they were adopted by a caring mother, the previously unloved babies settled down, and when they became mothers, they were nurturing. Later studies showed that a caring temperament was also passed on to their descendants.

Air Quality and Your Health

Do you sometimes step outdoors, take a deep breath and wonder if the air you are breathing might be hazardous to your health? Worse still, that it might be having detrimental long-term effects that could be passed on to your children? Depending on where you live, your concern might be justified. Several studies, based on data collected in diverse locations — Lanzhou (China), California's San Joaquin Valley and northern England, to name just three — have linked air pollution with higher rates of birth defects.

Polluted air can irritate your eyes, throat and lungs, but more seriously, exhaust fumes and other outdoor pollutants have been connected to a wide range of illnesses, from asthma and other respiratory diseases to stroke, heart attacks and Alzheimer's disease. Long-term exposure to benzene, found in gasoline, has been associated with cancer. Moreover, you don't need big exposures to experience some of these effects. A paper published in *JAMA* in 2017 connected "acceptable" levels of exposure to air pollution with increased rates of death in elderly people. And the consequences extend beyond physical ailments. At least one study has tied pollution exposure to depressive-like behaviors and impaired cognitive function in elderly people.

Research is beginning to link inhaling polluted air with epigenetic changes. One example is a 2018 paper published in the journal *Nature Communications*. Researchers looked at 1,000 people of French-Canadian heritage, the majority of whom were descended from a small group of settlers who colonized Quebec beginning in 1608. After separating the subjects into three groups based on their geographical isolation, the researchers sequenced their genomes and subsequently investigated their *RNA modulation*, a process related to gene expression. The scientists started with the assumption that the subjects' genomes would determine which genes were expressed, but they found something very different. Although the researchers noted that genetic modifications can modulate the response to inhaling polluted air, they found that differences in gene expression related most strongly to the quantity of exhaust fumes the subjects inhaled. Their conclusion: environmental impact overpowered genetic ancestry.

Studies have also found connections between changes in gene expression and exposure to air pollution during sensitive stages of development. For instance, in one review of children with asthma, researchers were able to connect pollution exposure during the first year of life with changes in the methylation of a specific gene and a diagnosis of asthma at age seven. Another analysis identified that women who lived near highways while pregnant were more likely to have children with asthma. Other research supporting the association between traffic-related air pollution and childhood asthma has linked the changes in gene expression with specific environmental impacts, such as chronic stress. For example, children with low social and economic status are more vulnerable to developing asthma when exposed to air pollution.

A Toxic Brew

In addition to polluted air, a wide range of toxic substances that are well integrated into everyday life, such as pharmaceuticals and certain chemicals, can also have long-lasting effects on human development. Many people think of the word *toxins* and imagine a

THANK YOU FOR NOT SMOKING

The connections between cigarette smoking and poor health have been well documented. Cigarette smoking increases your risk for numerous types of cancer, including lung, pancreatic, ovarian and bladder cancer. However, because we didn't have tools to connect the dots until recently, some of the processes underlying these outcomes were poorly understood. Smoking is the single greatest risk factor associated with lung cancer, but not everyone who smokes gets the disease. Why doesn't smoking affect everyone the same way? Your genes and, perhaps more significantly, your epigenome go a long way toward explaining these differences.

Today we can connect specific genes with the likelihood you will get lung cancer and, if you do, how long you might expect to survive with the disease. Such research focuses on your genome, the genetic hand you were dealt at birth. But other studies, such as a 2010 paper by David Barker, Kent Thornburg and Johan Eriksson, published in the *American Journal of Human Biology*, have looked at the links between fetal development and lung cancer. Using Finnish data, they found that body size at birth and maternal body size, in combination with the weight and shape of the placenta, could predict the development of lung cancer in both smokers and nonsmokers. They suggested that oxidative stress (a component of inflammation) is the likely culprit.

Other research has shown that smoking paves the way for lung cancer by triggering certain epigenetic changes. A Swedish study published in 2013 tied cigarette smoking with changes in gene expression. Not only did it identify 95 sites in the genome of smokers that were methylated differently from those of a control group who didn't smoke, it also connected some of those processes with the development of numerous diseases, including lung cancer (which isn't surprising) as well as other, unexpected conditions such as diabetes, poor immune system function and infertility. (Interestingly, the nonsmokers group included people who inhaled snuff, indicating that it is the harmful substances created by burning tobacco that are problematic, a conclusion that aligns with some current thinking on chronic inflammation. See "Inflammation: A Common Thread," page 211, for more.)

Various studies have shown that when either parent smokes, their children are at increased risk for a variety of health problems. Parental smoking (and exposure to tobacco smoke in general) has long been associated with respiratory problems in children, including a poor rate of lung development and chronic obstructive pulmonary disease in adulthood. Smoking has also been shown to damage DNA in male sperm. Recall Marcus Pembrey and Lars Bygren's research on the long-term effects of smoking at an early age (see "It's More Than Genes," page 36): when young males smoke, it increases the risk of obesity in their offspring.

Some researchers have zeroed in on the effects smoking has on pregnant women and the fetus. They have connected smoking during pregnancy with a wide range of negative birth outcomes, from premature delivery and low birth weight to increased risk of certain birth defects. Moreover, if you were exposed to cigarette smoke when your mother was pregnant, you are more likely to be obese and/or to develop heart disease, asthma or certain types of cancer later in life. Laboratory studies indicate that exposure to nicotine in utero is likely to result in higher blood levels of harmful fatty acids in adulthood. Methylation is one of the processes that likely underlie this increased risk. It has been shown, for instance, that when pregnant women smoke, the methylation patterns in their babies are affected.

Neuroscientist Tomas Paus discovered that exposure to cigarette smoke in the womb also affects how the brain develops in adolescence, and that this difference affects behavior. He found that one part of the brain, the orbital frontal cortex, was thinner in children whose mothers had smoked while pregnant. In later life, these children were also more likely to experiment with drugs.

distant industrial waste site or people in hazmat suits. But toxins are found much closer to home. They are in our food, cosmetics and personal-care and cleaning products, on our lawns and in our parks, in the air we breathe and the water we drink. We are bombarded with chemical toxins every day. You may find it shocking to learn that babies arrive in the world bearing a toxic load. Newborns have been found to have up to 200 chemicals in their umbilical cord blood at the time of birth, including bisphenol A (BPA), an endocrine disruptor that increases the risk for some types of cancer and type 2 diabetes, among other adverse conditions.

A toxin is a chemical that can harm the body. Toxins can interfere with how organs function, and their negative effects can impact the health of our offspring long after exposures have occurred. Unfortunately, they may be heritable. The work of Michael Skinner, an American biologist, provides a case in point. In laboratory studies he showed that exposing pregnant rats to a variety of chemicals in common products, ranging from pesticides to plastics, resulted in ovarian disease, not only in their immediate offspring but also in two subsequent generations of female descendants.

Endocrine Disruptors

The group of toxins known as *endocrine disruptors*, which turn up in prescription drugs as well as in common household products, are particularly troubling. Diethylstilbestrol (DES) is a good example. As discussed later (see "The DES Story," page 236), it's a synthetic form of estrogen that was widely prescribed to pregnant women for many years, and it had dire consequences for the daughters of those who took the drug. Numerous studies have shown that DES alters the expression of many genes associated with the reproductive tract, and that those changes affect both male and female offspring.

Unfortunately, you don't need a prescription to come in contact with endocrine disruptors. Some chemicals found in familiar household products, such as polychlorinated biphenyls (PCBs) and bisphenol A (BPA), also disrupt hormones. BPA, a component of plastic water bottles, has been found to affect DNA methylation in agouti mice. And a study of rats in utero linked exposure to low doses of BPA with increased cancer risk and changes in DNA methylation that the researchers suggest could be inheritable. Phthalates, which often turn up in personal-care products such as body lotion, have also been shown to disrupt genetic pathways in rats, resulting in abnormal testicular development.

Parabens and Low Sperm Counts

For decades men's sperm counts have been falling. In parts of the developed world, they have declined by about 60 percent over the past 40 years. At this point there are few human studies, but like those taking place in laboratories, the ones that exist are producing alarming results. Parabens, chemicals widely used in products such as toilet soap, shampoo and makeup, have been associated with DNA damage to male sperm. A Polish study published in 2017 found that high concentrations of parabens in male urine samples were linked with changes to sperm robustness that contributed to male infertility. In 2017 *New York Times* columnist Nicholas Kristof extrapolated from current data on lower sperm counts to propose that, if present trends continue, by 2060 a majority of the men living in Europe and North America might be infertile.

Pesticides and More

Other common chemicals, such as pesticides and fungicides, and exposure to heavy metals can also disrupt your genes. The chemical chlorpyrifos is a nerve agent used in some

ONE PILL MAKES YOU LARGER, THE SAME PILL MAKES ME SMALL

We know that individuals can exhibit a range of responses to the same drug and that some reactions can be serious — even fatal. In the United States, for instance, almost 300 people a day die from taking a drug prescribed by their doctors. Traditionally, doctors have taken a trial-and-error approach to prescribing drugs, but recent advances in genomic testing are opening the door to an era of personalized medicine that should reduce the risk of bad reactions. The relatively new field of *pharmacogenomics* uses your genetic makeup to predict how you will respond to a wide variety of medications.

While your genome certainly plays a role in how your body responds to environmental factors such as pharmaceuticals, in a 2015 paper published in the journal *Acta Pharmaceutica Sinica B*, researchers suggested that it accounts for only 10 to 30 percent of the differences. As they pointed out, even identical twins respond differently to drugs. Changes to epigenetic processes — such as DNA methylation, histone acetylation and some types of RNA signaling — also affect how your body metabolizes drugs. And researchers are looking into the bacteria in your gut as well. These microbes play important roles in how you break down ingestibles, which means they affect how you metabolize many medications. For instance, a 2018 review of more than 100 studies of diabetes medications, published in the journal *EBioMedicine*, found that the patients' microbiota determined whether the drugs were effective, ineffective or even toxic.

There is also a growing realization that prescription drugs, like chemicals, may initiate epigenetic changes that persist long after the patient has stopped taking the drug. For instance, one 2015 mouse study looked at the long-term consequences of treating newborns with a specific drug. The researchers found that the effects on gene expression were dose- and time-dependent. Basically, they concluded that gene expression in adults would be altered if the drug treatment was administered within a "sensitive window" in early life.

pesticides, including Roundup, an herbicide often sprayed on large grassy spaces (like golf courses) and on "Roundup ready" genetically modified crops. Chlorpyrifos has been linked with brain damage and lower IQ in children, as well as Parkinson's disease and lung cancer in adults. In a memorandum dated November 3, 2016, the United States

Toxins, Your Body and Nutrition

Children and adults are drinking, eating, breathing and absorbing chemicals every day. The more we are exposed to these chemicals, the higher the toxic load, which challenges our ability to detoxify. Fortunately, certain strategies, including nutrition, can help your body to manage toxins.

Your Body's Detoxification System

Your liver is your second-largest organ (after your skin) and it is your body's main detoxification tool. Liver detoxification is a complex two-step physiological process that helps to neutralize and eliminate toxins from your body. It renders toxins safe so they can be eliminated through your kidneys (via urine) and digestive tract (via stool).

PHASE 1

Phase 1 detoxification involves enzymes produced by the cytochrome P450 family of genes. During this phase, your liver makes fat-soluble toxins water-soluble, rendering them less toxic and easier to eliminate. If this phase functions inefficiently or your liver is overwhelmed by toxic load, the fat-soluble toxins aren't converted properly and can accumulate in fat cells and cell membranes. Toxins stored in fat cells are sometimes called *obesogens*. These chemicals negatively affect various body processes, potentially leading to metabolic changes that hinder your ability to lose weight and increase your risk of obesity, diabetes and heart disease.

Genetic variations in the CYP450 enzyme system can influence how you metabolize certain compounds, including coffee and many common pharmaceutical drugs. Caffeine is metabolized primarily through the CYP1A2 gene during phase 1 detox, and secondarily through the acetylation pathway in phase 2. Genetic variants in each pathway can alter how your body processes caffeine. Specific foods can also modify the activity of the CYP450 enzymes. For example, grapefruit juice inhibits an enzyme that metabolizes certain pharmaceutical drugs, which is why pharmacists advise against drinking grapefruit juice when taking some medications.

Efficient phase 1 detoxification requires adequate nutrition, including the antioxidant glutathione, found in a variety of foods rich in protein and sulfur (such as cruciferous vegetables), and flavonoids such as quercetin, found in fruits and vegetables. The B vitamins — B_2, B_3, B_6, B_{12} and folate — are particularly useful. With the exception of vitamin B_{12}, they are found in leafy dark green vegetables, fruits, whole grains and legumes. Vitamin B_{12} is found naturally only in meat, poultry, fish, eggs and dairy.

Sometimes, in the process of rendering chemicals water-soluble, phase 1 detoxification makes them more toxic, producing free radicals, which can cause oxidative damage to liver cells. To ensure that this natural process doesn't have lasting effects, consume antioxidant-rich fruits and vegetables, such as dark-colored berries and vegetables, as well as green tea.

PHASE 2

Phase 2 detoxification involves the conjugation pathways: methylation, sulfation, acetylation, glucuronidation, amino acid conjugation or glutathione conjugation. These pathways neutralize toxins, making them safe for elimination through the kidneys (in the urine) or through bile (in the stool). Their effectiveness depends not only on genetic variations — some people have single-nucleotide polymorphisms (SNPs) in their DNA that undermine the process — but also on the degree to which metabolic genes are epigenetically modified, as well as overall toxic load.

Supporting Your Detox System

Much of the groundbreaking work in nutrigenomics (see "Nutritional Epigenetics: An Emerging Science," page 50) involves investigating nutritional support for genetic pathways. With more research, we may be able to target genetic variants that affect detoxification using individualized food and nutrient strategies that support more efficient functioning of those pathways. Until then, an overall healthy diet and lifestyle can reduce toxic exposure and help to support your detoxification pathways.

- **Avoid processed foods.** Processed foods are loaded with additives. These manufactured chemicals contribute to toxic load and increase stress on your liver.

- **Buy organic food.** Unfortunately, many of the pesticides used on fruits and vegetables have been implicated as risk factors for various diseases. They are also known to be harmful to the environment. Consuming organic produce will reduce your intake of pesticides. Research also shows that organically grown produce is higher in antioxidants, which support detoxification.

- **Eat more plant foods.** It's a good idea to consume a diet that is rich in a wide variety of fruits, vegetables and whole grains. These foods provide the nutrients (including fiber) that support your detoxification system. Some foods do double duty. Flax seeds, for example, are more than a good source of fiber; they can also bind to toxins in your digestive tract, assisting your body with elimination. Other foods contain specific compounds that help the body detoxify. Cruciferous vegetables (such as cauliflower, collard greens, kale and Brussels sprouts) and those from the allium family (such as garlic, leeks and onions) are high in sulfur-rich compounds. These substances stimulate the production of enzymes that support detoxification. Beets also have detoxifying power: they contain phytonutrients called betalains, which increase enzyme activity in phase 2 detoxification. Artichokes contain the phytonutrients silymarin, an effective liver-support compound, and cynarin, which is both a choleretic (it increases bile production) and a cholagogue (it increases bile flow). Bile transports toxins to the digestive tract, where they can be eliminated in stool. In general, bitter greens, such as dandelion greens, also support bile flow. Fresh cilantro is traditionally used as a gentle chelator, which means it can bind to heavy metals and help your body eliminate those toxins.

- **Consume adequate protein.** Protein provides the essential amino acids needed during phase 2 detoxification.

- **Invest in a water filter.** A good-quality filter (carbon block or reverse osmosis) can remove heavy metals and pesticides from drinking water, helping your large intestines and kidneys eliminate waste products regularly and efficiently.

Environmental Protection Agency (EPA) warned about potential negative effects on the brain development of children when they are exposed to the pesticide in utero.

Even in situations where it is not sprayed directly on agricultural land, chlorpyrifos is known to disperse in the air and possibly end up on food crops at unsafe levels. In 2018 a groundskeeper in California was awarded $289 million by a jury that accepted he had developed cancer as a result of exposure to the chemical. However, companies such as Monsanto, which are heavily invested in the use of chlorpyrifos and other pesticides, have been aggressively defending its safety and use.

In 2000 a research project known as Chamacos was established to look at the long-term effects of pesticide exposure on the children of California farmworkers. Although it will take time for many of the results to develop, so far it has found associations with respiratory problems and developmental disabilities, including lower IQ.

BEWARE OF LEAD

Lead turns up in old paint and in water, among other places. The World Health Organization (WHO) warns that lead affects multiple body systems and is particularly harmful to young children. If a woman harbors excessive levels of the heavy metal, it is released from her bones during pregnancy and could affect the fetus. Lead's effects are cumulative and in high doses can be fatal.

Safe Until Proven Harmful

In a fascinating 2012 paper about environmental epigenetics and disease risk, cancer researcher Shuk-Mei Ho and a team of other experts reviewed the literature connecting environmental toxins with changes in genetic behavior and subsequent disease risk. They focused on diseases that could be linked to factors in the external environment, and what they found is pretty scary, particularly since, as they themselves said, their review was "by no means exhaustive in details."

As the researchers pointed out, one fundamental problem with regulatory approaches is that chemicals are generally regarded as safe until they are proven to be harmful. The question is, how is harm determined? Traditional approaches use a formula to determine the acceptable daily intake of a substance — for instance, BPA. This method has been challenged for a number of reasons; for starters, it fails to capture the actual experience of daily living. BPA is just one of many toxins you are likely to come in contact with during the day. Contaminants are experienced not as isolated substances but as something of a toxic brew. During a typical 24-hour period, you may inhale polluted air, consume food that has been treated with pesticides and/or fungicides, use household cleaning and/or personal-care products that contain endocrine disruptors, be exposed to heavy metals such as mercury or lead ... and so on and on. Over time, these exposures accumulate, filling up the "tolerance tub" like a leaky tap, slowly but surely, drop by drop.

In 2018 the American Academy of Pediatrics (AAP), an organization of more than 45,000 board-certified pediatricians, issued a policy statement that aligned with these thoughts. In their report, published in the journal *Pediatrics*, they noted that in the United States more than 10,000 chemicals may be added to or come in contact with food. A fundamental problem is that the Food and Drug Administration (FDA) "is unable to ensure all of those chemicals are safe," in part because the "regulation and oversight of many food additives is inadequate." Among the chemicals the pediatricians highlighted are BPA, phthalates and nitrites, which are often added to processed meats. They were clear that these chemicals may contribute to disease and disability. They noted not only that people with low incomes and/or those belonging to minority groups may experience "disproportionate" exposure to these compounds, but also that children may be more susceptible to their effects.

Both the AAP and Dr. Ho's paper emphasized the fact that there are developmental windows of heightened sensitivity to epigenetic programming. Exposure to toxins during these periods may have a disproportionate effect later in life. Overall, your first thousand days of life — which includes your nine months in the womb — have been identified as the most significant developmental period that will influence your health status as an adult.

5

THE
FIRST
THOUSAND
DAYS

People talk about children growing to their "genetic potential," when the reality is that children grow according to their circumstances ... Development and growth are not like musical symphonies, commanded by a single set of detailed instructions; they are like jazz, dynamic processes with improvisations and elaborations that depend on circumstances.

— DAVID BARKER, *NUTRITION IN THE WOMB*

WHEN YOU STOP TO think about it, the moment the male sperm and female egg meet up in a fallopian tube, nothing short of a miracle takes place. In that instant, a baby's sex and its genes, the fixed constituents of its being, are determined. And slightly later, its epigenome, the more dynamic component of development, is established. The early embryo is launched into its continuous process of growth, actively dividing and replicating its cells as it develops from embryo to fetus to baby and child, eventually becoming an adult. In the best of times, this path is smooth and easily traversed; in the worst, it is rutted and risky to navigate.

A baby arrives in the world not in "utter nakedness," to borrow from the poet Wordsworth, but "trailing clouds" of past experience in the form of programming, some of which took place even before it was conceived. Nutrition played a key role in creating you, not only while you were a fetus, but also well after you were born. And while you were in the womb, a wide variety of other factors contributed to your development. They include the lifestyles of both your parents, even before you were conceived, and events that were beyond their control, such as flu epidemics, war, famine and natural disasters — even terrorist attacks.

How much did these various factors influence the person you became? We don't have definitive cause-and-effect answers to that question, but we do know that the quality of your prenatal life had a major influence on your health and well-being as an adult.

So, too, did your first two years of life. This is a period characterized by equal amounts of potential and risk. Key body systems, such as the immune system — as well as the brain — are still in full development mode. Overall, how you grew and developed during this time will impact your health for decades to come. So it's not surprising that the experts agree: the most critical period in human development is the first thousand days after conception.

PRECONCEPTION

We now know that the time to begin thinking about having a baby is well before you actually try to become pregnant. The fetus is most vulnerable to environmental factors such as inadequate nutrition, emotional or physical stress or trauma, and exposure to environmental toxins during the first eight weeks after conception. Unfortunately, most women don't know they are pregnant for at least part of that period. If the intrauterine environment isn't ideal, the fetus will start making adjustments to ensure its immediate survival. Some of them may compromise how its organs develop; others may shape hormonal and metabolic responses. All will have an impact on its health and well-being throughout life. This means that parents-to-be should be preparing long before conception actually occurs.

Those in the know advise allowing for at least three months of preparation (ideally a year) before attempting pregnancy. One reason is that it takes about that long for new sperm to develop and fully mature. As our knowledge of epigenetics grows, it's becoming increasingly clear that paternal health plays an important part in fertility and pregnancy outcomes, even though the woman's body assumes the starring role once conception occurs. The quality of her eggs has already been determined by her mother and grandmother (remember, women are born with all their eggs), but from the moment of conception it's the mother's role to provide the best environment possible to support the embryo's development.

Clearly, good nutrition plays a key role in this process. When researching this book, however, I was astounded to discover that official bodies in the United States provided no official dietary guidelines related to pregnancy. Worldwide, experts agree that poorly nourished women give birth to poorly nourished babies, perpetuating a cycle of poor health. Once economists entered the picture, they could calculate the economic burden associated with such long-term intergenerational malnourishment. Although the figures vary depending on the source, in general terms they are alarming.

In his role as director of the Moore Institute, Kent Thornburg is spearheading movement toward developing official US dietary guidelines for pregnant women, which appear to be somewhat in flux at the time of this writing. In the meantime, an abundance of solid nutritional information on what to eat when you are pregnant or planning to get pregnant is available. In preparing the dietary recommendations relating to preconception and pregnancy for this book, I worked closely with two naturopathic doctors, Julie Briley and Courtney Jackson, co-authors of the excellent book *Food as Medicine Everyday: Reclaim Your Health with Whole Foods*. I am confident that the information is solid.

Diet Makes a Difference

Good nutrition is vital for the developing fetus throughout pregnancy, but, as noted, it's particularly crucial during the first weeks following conception. Experts tell us this is a critical developmental window, a period when the embryo is particularly vulnerable to the impact of environmental exposures. The problem is, as mentioned, that a woman often doesn't know she is pregnant during all or much of that time.

That's why, if you are thinking about getting pregnant, you should immediately start making any healthy lifestyle changes you've been contemplating. Eliminate fast food: rodent studies have linked a maternal diet of high-calorie, highly processed food with overweight offspring that demonstrate a taste for junk food as adolescents. Make a point of consuming a nutrient-dense diet of whole foods to ensure an adequate intake of necessary nutrients, including iodine, vitamin B_{12}, choline, omega-3 fatty acids, vitamin D, iron and folate. Laboratory studies show that during the first few weeks of embryo development, deficiencies in these nutrients can increase the risk that the babies will suffer developmental disorders. Spinal cord abnormalities are perhaps the best-known of the conditions that can be avoided by nutrient therapy. Studies show that when a woman takes 400 micrograms (mcg) of folic acid daily before pregnancy and up until 6 to 12 weeks postconception, her chances of delivering a baby with a neural tube defect are reduced by 75 percent. (For more about specific dietary strategies for the preconception period, see "Planning for Pregnancy," page 102.)

Sperm and Epigenetic Inheritance

In biological terms, the paternal role in pregnancy is most significant in the preconception period. Sperm quality plays a major role in fertility, as well as in the epigenetic imprinting that sperm transmit. More and more evidence is linking environmental factors such as diet, toxin exposures (particularly smoking) and lifestyle with epigenetic changes to sperm that can be passed on to offspring.

It's long been known that your father contributed half your genes. Now we are learning that, thanks to heritable epigenetic changes, the father's sperm have the potential to influence other aspects of his offspring's development. Since a fetus develops in the mother's body, the father's role in pregnancy outcomes has usually been overlooked, but new evidence suggests that his role is more significant than we previously thought. It may even contribute to whether the fetus develops to term. The paternal impact on his offspring's health has recently become an active area of research, so much so that the authors of a 2017 review study suggested a new area for focused research: the paternal origins of health and disease (POHaD).

The idea that a father's diet, experience and lifestyle can influence the adult health of his offspring is based on the knowledge that sperm carry information with the potential to affect various mechanisms in the developing organism. Although scientists don't fully understand how these processes work, it appears that sperm can be epigenetically altered and that these changes to gene expression can be passed on at fertilization. We know that sperm influences how the placenta develops, which may help to explain the results of one 2004 study that linked a father's drinking during the preconception period (10 or more drinks a week) with an increased risk of miscarriage.

More and more research is showing not only that a father's input can influence the health of his own offspring, but also that it can contribute to disease development in successive generations. Here are some examples of how this plays out in real life:

- A 2018 study of more than 40 million births, published in *BMJ*, found that when fathers were older than 45, their babies were 14 percent more likely to be born prematurely and to have a low birth weight. Perhaps surprisingly, it also found that conceiving a child with an older father raised the mother's risk of developing gestational diabetes by 28 percent.

- Older fathers are also more likely to produce children with neurological disorders such as schizophrenia and autism spectrum disorder. Research suggests that changes in methylation patterns due to aging may help to explain these links.

- The research of Marcus Pembrey and Lars Bygren (see "It's More Than Genes," page 36) showed that when young boys overindulged in food just before puberty, their grandsons were more likely to die young. Pembrey and Bygren's work also showed that the sons of men who started smoking at an early age were more likely to be overweight, beginning in adolescence.

- Animal studies show that if a father eats a low-protein diet, it will alter how his offspring metabolize lipids and cholesterol, increasing their risk of hypertension.

- When male rats are fed high-fat diets, their female offspring are more likely to suffer from early-onset impaired insulin secretion and glucose intolerance.

- The sperm of mice fed low-protein diets has been shown to be hypomethylated; offspring of such mice had characteristics associated with metabolic syndrome and nonalcoholic fatty liver disease, including glucose intolerance and altered gut bacteria profiles.

- Studies link paternal obesity with an increased risk that offspring will be obese, likely because of epigenetic changes in DNA.

- Research shows that when fathers drink too much alcohol around the time of conception, their offspring are at increased risk for behavioral problems, including poor performance in school and attention deficit hyperactivity disorder.

- Evidence suggests that when men smoke, the resulting damage to their DNA may increase the risk that their offspring will develop cancer.

Planning for Pregnancy

Planning for pregnancy involves both of the parents-to-be. Among its objectives are optimizing fertility, promoting health for the mother and creating the healthiest environment possible for the developing fetus. The following strategies are key components of a preconception plan.

Eat a Nutrient-Dense Diet

Prospective parents can boost their fertility by adopting the same healthy eating patterns. That means committing to a balanced diet consisting mostly of vegetables (especially leafy greens), whole fruits (not just juice), whole grains, legumes, nuts and seeds, and healthy fats from plant foods such as olives and avocados.

Emphasize Healthy Fats

The quality of dietary fat is important for both boosting fertility and sustaining a healthy pregnancy. Avoid all trans fats and increase your consumption of foods rich in omega-3s, specifically those that provide docosahexaenoic acid (DHA). Intake of omega-3 fatty acids has been linked with improved fertility in women and better-quality sperm in men.

The best sources of DHA are oily fish, such as salmon, mackerel and sardines, algae and fish oil supplements. Unfortunately, fear of mercury has prompted many women to avoid eating fish, leading to omega-3 deficiencies. The simple truth is that mercury poisoning is rare, even among fish eaters, whereas omega-3 deficiencies are quite common. However, it is wise to avoid fish that are high in this neurotoxin. Larger fish are likely to have accumulated significant amounts of toxic mercury; these include shark, swordfish and most tuna (the smaller skipjack tuna are fine). Salmon, anchovies, sardines and mackerel are all good choices. Check out the Natural Resources Defense Council's guide to the mercury levels in different types of fish (www.nrdc.org/stories/mercury-guide). Their specific recommendations based on body weight for limiting mercury exposure are also worth considering.

There is also clear evidence that increasing your consumption of seafood can be helpful if you are trying to conceive. While it doesn't separate out the specific impact of omega-3 fats, one 2018 study published in the *Journal of Clinical Endocrinology & Metabolism* found that couples who were trying to get pregnant significantly increased their chances of success if they ate a 4-ounce (125 g) serving of seafood at least twice a week (92 percent, compared to 79 percent in the couples who consumed fish less frequently). Perhaps incidentally, couples who consumed higher quantities of seafood also enjoyed sexual intercourse more often.

For information on other food sources of omega-3 fatty acids, see page 134. To ensure adequate intake, women who are following strict vegetarian or vegan diets should take omega-3 supplements.

Support Fertility with a Healthy Body Weight

If you are planning to get pregnant, maintaining or achieving a healthy weight is one of the best strategies for both sexes, because fertility is compromised if either partner is overweight or obese. It is thought that toxins from fat create inflammation in the sperm, the egg and the lining of the womb, which undermines fertility.

Insulin resistance is another concern. While not all obese people are insulin resistant, those who are may experience fertility issues. In females, insulin resistance disrupts communication between the brain and the ovaries, which can lead to irregular ovulation patterns or even no ovulation at all. When men are overweight or obese, extra body fat and insulin resistance can decrease testosterone and increase estrogen, reducing sperm count and diminishing fertility.

One of the leading causes of female infertility is polycystic ovary syndrome (PCOS), a condition characterized by weight gain, irregular menstrual cycles and a high level of male hormones. PCOS affects up to 10 percent of women of childbearing age. Women with PCOS who are overweight can restore potentially compromised fertility by losing 10 percent of their body weight.

On the flip side, being underweight also jeopardizes fertility in both sexes. Having a low body mass can reduce the production of sex hormones, lowering the incidence of ovulation in women and reducing men's sperm count.

Consume Adequate Zinc

Maintain the recommended dietary allowance of zinc (15 mg a day). Zinc supports fertility in both sexes. It encourages healthy semen and testosterone production in men, and ovulation and fertility in women. It also reduces insulin resistance. Generally, animal foods such as meat and oysters (the highest food source) are the best sources of zinc. But pumpkin seeds, nuts, dark chocolate and many whole grains also provide varying amounts.

Check Your Vitamin D Levels

Human studies looking at the impact of vitamin D on fertility are limited by their small size; they have determined association but not cause. PCOS, a common cause of female infertility, may suggest a connection. Low vitamin D levels in women with PCOS are known to exacerbate symptoms that impact fertility, such as menstrual and ovulatory irregularity, as well as insulin resistance. That's why it's a good idea to test your vitamin D level before you become pregnant; if it's not optimal, work toward improvement as part of your preconception planning. For more information on vitamin D, see page 120.

Check Your Thyroid

Your thyroid is a major player in your endocrine system. It is important that it functions effectively at all stages of reproduction, from preconception to the birth of your baby. To learn more about this gland, see "Your Thyroid," page 107.

Reduce Exposure to Environmental Toxins

Certain toxic agents have known epigenetic consequences. These toxins include organochlorine pesticides, air pollution, arsenic, mercury and endocrine-disrupting chemicals such as bisphenol A (BPA), all of which can affect fertility and harm a developing fetus. Endocrine disruptors are concerning at all stages, including preconception, as they affect hormone levels, which can impact the quality of semen and/or make it difficult for women to conceive.

Your liver helps your body detoxify, cleansing it of environmental toxins and common chemicals, such as those found in medications — including the synthetic hormones in birth control pills. You can support your body's detox pathways by eating more foods that support detoxification (see "Toxins, Your Body and Nutrition," page 92) for a few months before conception. This is a great strategy for reducing your toxic load.

Choose Organic Foods If Possible

According to a 2017 study published in *JAMA*, consuming large amounts of residue from common pesticides significantly reduces a woman's chances of becoming pregnant. Choosing organic food is one way to reduce exposure to pesticides. If that isn't an easy option, avoiding conventionally grown fruits and vegetables known to contain high levels of pesticides, such as strawberries, peppers, spinach and tomatoes, can reduce your body's toxic load, as can thoroughly washing all produce. Use the Environmental Working Group's Clean 15/Dirty Dozen list as a guide to help you reduce dietary exposure to pesticides. Adopting this lifestyle for at least three months prior to conception will reduce your exposure to toxins and hormone-disrupting chemicals that may influence the developing fetus.

Don't Smoke

Abstaining from smoking is one of the best health decisions anyone can make, not only for personal health benefits but also for the health of future generations. Cigarette smoke, which is a known carcinogen, is dangerous and it should be actively avoided if you are planning to get pregnant and while you are pregnant. If a father-to-be is a smoker, smoking can damage DNA in his sperm, which has a negative effect on his fertility. It may also increase his offspring's risk of developing childhood cancer. And, if he started to smoke around the time he was entering puberty, his sons will be at greater risk for obesity and type 2 diabetes.

Limit Consumption of Alcohol

All major medical organizations recommend complete abstinence from alcohol, even during the preconception period. However, if you are a woman trying to get pregnant, enjoying an occasional alcoholic drink (equivalent to one or less serving a day) will likely not impair your fertility. The real problem is heavy drinking. One prospective study looked at 6,120 Danish females, 21 to 45 years old, who were in a stable relationship with a male partner. They were trying to conceive and not receiving fertility treatment. Researchers found that consumption of the largest amount of alcohol (more than 14 servings a week) was associated with an 18 percent decrease in fertility compared with no alcohol consumption.

If you are male, moderate alcohol intake (approximately two drinks a day) does not negatively affect fertility, but drinking heavily can impair sperm quality and count. And, as noted, when a father drinks excessively around the time of conception, it has a negative impact on fetal development.

Monitor Intake of Caffeine and High-Fructose Corn Syrup

Alcohol is not the only beverage with potentially negative effects on fertility and pregnancy. While caffeine in moderation is okay, excessive caffeine intake (three cups or more of black coffee per day) can affect fertility in some women. Beverages sweetened with high-fructose corn syrup are even more problematic. A 2016 study published in *Scientific Reports* looked at both mice and women and showed that consuming too much high-fructose corn syrup during early pregnancy may cause defects in the placenta and restrict fetal growth, potentially increasing a baby's risk for metabolic problems later in life. Preconception is a great time to wean yourself off all sweetened drinks, and especially high-fructose beverages, such as soda. Drinking plain water and herbal teas while limiting caffeine and alcohol seems to be the best course of action to improve your chances of becoming pregnant.

Diet and Sperm Quality

The male role in reproduction has traditionally focused on fertility, which is becoming a major concern because of precipitously declining sperm counts in Western nations. In practical terms, male fertility is influenced by factors such as the shape and robustness of sperm. We have reason to believe that a healthy diet can improve sperm quality. It has been shown, for instance, that men who consume too much saturated fat have less robust sperm. So it makes sense that men can boost the quality of their sperm by concentrating on a diet that is low in saturated fat while, as other evidence suggests, providing moderate levels of protein.

Nutrients that support cell division also support sperm quality, a result of their role in creating DNA. They include folate and other nutrients involved in metabolizing methyl donors, such as vitamins B_6 and B_{12}. Dietary factors can also impact the structure of sperm. The sperm membrane has a fatty-acid composition that differs from other cells: it has a much higher concentration of polyunsaturated fatty acids (PUFAs), which are particularly important for membrane fluidity and flexibility.

Research on the relationship between diet and sperm quality led one researcher to study walnuts, which are rich in omega-3 fatty acids, folate and selenium, all of which have been associated with sperm quality. A 2012 study published in the journal *Biology of Reproduction* found that adding a daily serving of $2^1/_2$ ounces (75 g) of walnuts to a typical Western-style diet improved sperm vitality, motility and morphology.

IN THE WOMB

How a fetus develops and grows depends on many factors. In biological terms, any effects caused by the father are likely to result from epigenetic modifications of DNA transmitted via his sperm. On the other hand, the fetus responds to the mother's input in numerous ways, almost from the moment of conception. During pregnancy, particularly in the early stages, environmental impacts such as stress, exposure to toxins and poor nutrition spark developmental changes that will affect health and well-being throughout life.

About four weeks after conception, a mass of embryonic cells implants itself in the uterine wall. Even before implantation, the developing embryo has two primary cell types. One type goes on to form the fetal body, while the other becomes the placenta. This disk-shaped organ shares the same genes as the fetus, and they are connected via the umbilical cord. The placenta is an active partner in pregnancy, responding to signals from both the mother and the fetus in a complex system meant to ensure that their mutual needs are met.

Thanks to the work of David Barker and others, we know that developing body systems in utero are very "plastic" — they are vulnerable to environmental impacts, the effects of which the placenta tries to regulate. The placenta is a kind of metabolic trainmaster. It manages available resources and, when supplies are inadequate, it protects some organs at the expense of others. For instance, if the fetus receives inadequate supplies of oxygen or nutrients, the placenta directs its blood flow to ensure that the heart and brain suffer less from the deficit than other organs lower down in the developmental hierarchy.

Past Forward

The quality of a mother's experience while pregnant is probably the most significant factor shaping the health and well-being of her offspring. However, the behind-the-scenes participation of the father, through the sperm that fertilized the mother's egg, and of the grandmother, who provided that egg while she was pregnant with her daughter, also play weighty roles. And research tells us that grandfathers stay in the picture too. The sum of these various contributions has a major impact on pregnancy outcomes — in some cases, even more than was originally thought. By the time you become an adult, your health largely reflects influences from previous generations and your experience in your mother's womb from the time of conception until you were born.

Take your school smarts, for instance. Until recently it was assumed that a child's environment after birth determined their ability to learn. However, we now know that low-birth-weight children are more likely to have poor cognitive function than those who fall within the normal range. Thanks to epigenetics, we have insight into biological mechanisms that are linked with this result. A 2015 study conducted under the auspices of the EpiGen Global Research Consortium used umbilical cord tissue collected at birth to examine epigenetic marks related to brain development. The researchers could link these marks to cognitive performance and learning ability in two groups of British children aged four and seven. In a related study of another group of children in Singapore that also studied umbilical cord tissue, the scientists could connect similar epigenetic changes generated in utero to poor performance in school and socially disruptive behavior.

YOUR THYROID

The thyroid gland has a strong influence on fertility, as well as the ability to enjoy a healthy pregnancy. Hypothyroidism, which occurs when the thyroid gland is not producing adequate amounts of thyroid hormone, affects 2 to 4 percent of reproductive-age women. Low levels of thyroid hormone can interfere with the release of eggs from the ovary, which impairs fertility. Even if a woman with hypothyroidism successfully conceives, she is at increased risk of miscarriage, premature delivery, postpartum bleeding, anemia and postpartum depression, so it's important to correct the condition as soon as possible.

Congenital hypothyroidism, the most common neonatal endocrine disorder, occurs when a newborn doesn't produce enough thyroid hormone. It is most often caused by an iodine deficiency in the mother's diet. It may also be due to developmental problems with the baby's thyroid gland or an error in its thyroid metabolism. Whatever the cause, it puts the baby at risk for a number of problems, including a failure to grow and permanent intellectual disabilities. In developed countries, all newborns are screened at birth for hypothyroidism.

An overactive thyroid gland is known as hyperthyroidism. Although much less common than hypothyroidism, this condition can impact fertility by causing irregular menstrual cycles. Maternal hyperthyroidism may stunt development of a fetus's pancreatic beta cells (which make insulin) and heart muscle cells.

Although thyroid problems are much less common in males, hypothyroidism can affect male fertility by reducing testosterone levels and libido.

Iodine for a Healthy Thyroid Gland

For optimum functioning, the thyroid gland depends on adequate amounts of iron, zinc and dietary protein. However, in many ways iodine plays the most significant role in keeping your thyroid healthy; deficiency in this essential mineral is the leading cause of hypothyroidism and the development of congenital hypothyroidism. The recommended daily intake for adults is 150 to 200 mcg. Analyses of National Health and Nutrition Examination Survey (NHANES) data sets from 2001 to 2008 indicate that up to 57 percent of pregnant woman in the United States have insufficient levels of this mineral.

Most prenatal vitamins contain an adequate amount of iodine. Seaweed and cod remain some of the richest food sources, but shrimp, eggs, prunes and lima beans also provide notable amounts. Using iodized salt is another option; in the United States it contains 45 mcg of iodine per gram.

And, of course, if your mother was poorly nourished while pregnant with you, your risk of developing chronic disease shoots up. This knowledge raises questions about processed food, which is widely available and notoriously lacking in nutrients. While we don't have human studies that directly link junk food consumption with pregnancy outcomes, research on rats confirms what may seem obvious. In a 2006 study published in the *British Journal of Nutrition*, researchers fed pregnant and lactating rats a diet of highly processed, *energy-dense* but nutrient-deficient foods containing high amounts of sugar, salt and/or fat. The mothers produced pups that were overweight and prone to overeating. Another study was published the same year in the *Journal of Physiology*. Those pups, whose mothers were also fed junk food while pregnant, demonstrated poor muscle development and indications of insulin resistance, some by the time they were three weeks old. Worse still, the mother's diet programmed offspring to enjoy junk food. As the pups grew, it became clear that they preferred the taste of highly processed foods. Their early-life experiences had set them up for poor eating habits, increasing their risk of obesity and related conditions such as type 2 diabetes and heart disease later in life.

The Placenta

When I was pregnant, I doubt that I devoted a single thought to what was happening with my placenta. Sure, I knew it existed, but beyond that my knowledge was spotty, to say the least. Now I know better — the placenta was my partner in pregnancy. Like me, it was committed to ensuring that my fetus prospered and survived, and to producing the healthiest baby possible.

The placenta is a remarkable organ. It serves as lungs and kidneys for the fetus and provides every nutrient the growing baby receives. It also makes hormones that regulate the way the mother maintains her pregnancy, and it acts as a protective barrier against many toxins and most bacteria. However, we now know that certain toxins and some infections cross the placenta, as do dietary carcinogens, alcohol, nicotine and other drugs.

As Kent Thornburg and Nicole Marshall noted in a 2015 paper published in the *American Journal of Obstetrics & Gynecology*, toward the end of human gestation, levels of a type of hormone known as glucocorticoids increase in the mother. One of their jobs is to finalize the development of significant organs, including the lungs and the heart. But under certain circumstances, such as when the mother is experiencing unusually high levels of stress, the levels of these hormones become excessive. For example, the placenta can usually inactivate cortisol. However, if the mother's cortisol level increases beyond the capacity of the placenta to neutralize it, cortisol "spills over" into the fetus, harming it in many ways. Excess cortisol may even stunt the baby's growth, increasing the risk for certain chronic diseases. Shortened telomeres (see "Telomeres," page 227) are another result.

Providing adequate nutrition for the fetus is one of the placenta's many jobs. Generally speaking, if a pregnant woman has not been well nourished, her placenta will not develop properly, and this will have a negative impact on the long-term health of her baby. The placenta has been described as a "nutrient sensor." But while it can sense and respond to changes in nutrient levels in the mother's blood, it can't rectify nutrient deficiencies in her body. However, when nutrients are in short supply, it will attempt to compensate. For instance, if there aren't enough nutrients during the first half of gestation, the placenta will grow larger. Simply put, the larger the placenta, the more food the baby receives.

Pregnant Ewes

We know from observing sheep that pregnant ewes that move to poor pasture early in gestation then return to rich pasture later on produce larger lambs than those whose mothers remain well fed throughout their pregnancies. Why does this happen? Because in the early stages of pregnancy, the placenta is in full growth mode. When nutrients are in short supply, the placenta in a healthy ewe grows, enhancing its ability to acquire more nutrients from the mother's blood. It grabs nutrition and develops rapidly, with a view to creating reserves for the developing lamb in case the scarcity continues.

Farmers have long known that they can produce heavier lambs by stimulating placental growth early in gestation. We don't yet know how this works in humans, although researchers suspect that during certain periods the placenta may have the ability to respond to peripheral demands. However, they also suspect that this plasticity may subsequently disappear. The truth is, we know shockingly little about this organ. As Thornburg and Marshall noted, most of our knowledge of the placenta is derived from animal studies. However, we do have a growing body of information on humans that directly links the placenta with disease development later in life.

Size, Shape and Weight Matter

How much the placenta weighs, as well as its shape and size, influence how the fetus matures and grows. Smaller placentas, which are more likely to result in smaller babies, have been linked to conditions such as hypertension and obesity. However, in terms of placental development, the greatest risk for chronic disease can be traced back to small babies with big placentas and large babies with small placentas.

Although we don't yet understand how this actually works, we do know that the size and shape of a mother's placenta may increase her offspring's risk of developing heart failure, hypertension and lung cancer as an adult. In fact, as Thornburg and Marshall pointed out, epidemiological studies focused on the placenta have provided particularly accurate forecasts of disease development later in life. Research that recorded the mothers' physical characteristics and linked them with specific placental characteristics has proven, in their words, to "predict disease with much more precision than does birthweight alone."

Additional Factors

Placental inflammation is another influence on fetal programming, as Thornburg and Marshall pointed out. Along with various types of infection, maternal conditions such as diabetes and obesity may create inflammation in the placenta, which has been associated with premature birth and even fetal mortality. A 2016 study published in *Circulation Research* looked at preeclampsia — a condition that researchers admit is remarkably lacking in factual data — and linked it with inflammatory factors in the placenta. Specifically, they found that levels of a certain receptor protein, CD74, were lower in women who suffered from preeclampsia because they had fewer CD74 receptors in the placenta, triggering the release of more substances that promote placental inflammation.

Although we don't know much about the epigenetic landscape of the placenta, some researchers have shown that it is hypomethylated compared to other healthy human tissue. It also appears that placental methylation increases as pregnancy progresses and that the degree of methylation may influence pregnancy outcomes. Australian expert Tina Bianco-Miotto identified differences in methylation between placentas that supported healthy pregnancies and those that were preeclamptic.

Nowadays, experts are questioning why we know so little about this organ. The Eunice Kennedy Shriver National Institute of Child Health and Human Development in the United States has called the placenta "arguably one of the more important [organs], not only for the health of a woman and her fetus during pregnancy but also for the lifelong health of both." Studying the placenta in births that go wrong has already provided specialists with insights into why pregnancies go off the rails. In some cases this awareness has prompted positive changes and improved results. The links between the placenta, fetal growth and rates of chronic disease suggest that public policy initiatives supporting programs that generate healthy placentas should be a priority for improving long-term health.

THE PLACENTA AS CULTURAL ARTIFACT AND MORE

In Westernized societies, the placenta is usually regarded as waste and discarded after the birth, but in many locations this life-sustaining organ is highly regarded and surrounded by mystery. It's possible that primitive people intuitively understood what we now know scientifically: the baby and placenta share the same gene pool.

Understandably, the placenta is shrouded in superstition. Many groups believe that a baby's placenta must be protected and treated with respect or they will lead an unfortunate life. In some societies, complex rituals exist to ensure that the no-longer-useful organ is safeguarded from scavengers and evil spirits. These include laying the placenta to rest with full funeral rites. In North America, some Indigenous peoples bury the placenta under a tree; not only does its decaying matter provide nourishment for the soil, as it did for the baby, but proximity ensures that the tree maintains a supernatural connection to the person throughout their lifetime.

The Ibo people of West Africa view the placenta as the dead twin of the living baby, and, as such, it receives a ceremonial burial. The Hmong, a Laotian people whose word for placenta means "jacket," bury the organ with a view toward future utility: when a person dies, their spirit can return and don the jacket to wear during the next stage of existence.

Because the placenta is such a rich resource of substances such as hormones, it's only logical that some people have realized its potential for commercialization. Placental extracts, usually derived from sheep, have long been used in the cosmetics industry. In Britain, placentas were routinely collected in hospitals (without the donor's knowledge) and sold to pharmaceutical firms until the practice was challenged and stopped. Products using placental material ended up in treatments for burns and enzymes to treat genetic disorders. Some pharmaceutical companies still use "pharmaceutical-grade" placental extract, although the practice is controversial.

Boys Grow Differently

Boys will be boys — impatient from the beginning. As a fertilized egg makes its journey to the uterus, those that carry a Y chromosome are already dividing their cells more rapidly in a push to speed up their development, even before the mother is actually pregnant, technically speaking. They are hungrier too, snatching up nutrients to sustain this strategy of rapid growth throughout their life in the womb. Somehow, male fetuses even "convince" their mothers to consume more calories while pregnant to feed their voracious appetites. Studies show that mothers who are carrying boys gain more weight because they consume more nutrients, especially fats, than a girl fetus demands.

Thankfully, the mother isn't in this alone; the placenta is looking out for *her* needs too, and it responds to the ravenous male appetite by developing less rapidly and staying smaller than if she were carrying a girl. Or it could be that the male fetus itself limits placental growth because it doesn't want to share nutrients with the placenta. As Kent Thornburg framed it in an article called "Boys Grow Dangerously in the Womb": "Nutrients are difficult to acquire when you are a fetus and males don't make it easy on themselves because, contrary to logic, they make the smallest placenta possible. Why waste precious nutrients by investing in building a placenta when your strategy is simply to grow as fast as possible?"

Naturally, this strategy comes with a cost. Thanks to the work of researchers who have studied the placenta, including David Barker, Kent Thornburg and Johan Eriksson, we know that smaller placentas have less reserve capacity, which makes boys more vulnerable when nutrition is scant. That helps to explain why more male fetuses die in utero and fewer male preemies survive. Evidence from the Great Leap Forward famine in China indicates that when food was extremely scarce, more girls were born than boys.

Looking at a group of men and women born in Helsinki between 1934 and 1944, when there were food shortages, Barker, Thornburg, Eriksson and their colleagues learned that, in some situations, male fetuses responded to nutrient shortfalls by enlarging the placenta in the later stages of gestation. The problem was, unless the mother was well nourished before pregnancy, she was unable to transfer additional nutrients to feed the larger placenta, and the growth of organs such as the kidneys was more likely to be compromised. Those male babies had higher rates of hypertension and heart disease later in life.

Following up on research suggesting that males are more vulnerable to the effects of prenatal stress, scientists at the University of Maryland decided to look at whether epigenetic changes in the placenta might play a role in this gender difference. Their 2018 study, published in the journal *Nature Communications*, found that it does. Sex-based differences in an enzyme produced by the placenta influence the effects of prenatal stress on neurodevelopment. Basically, higher levels of expression of the gene that encodes this enzyme help female fetuses to be more resistant to stress.

The gender differences continue even after babies are born. Scientists believe that mothers produce different nutrients in breast milk for male babies. Studies of rhesus monkeys show that mother's milk produced for male babies has 35 percent more fat and protein. Milk for female offspring has less fat and more calcium, possibly because female skeletons grow faster.

Navigating Nutrition during Pregnancy

In general terms, dietary recommendations for pregnancy are very similar to those for the preconception period: make a practice of consuming nutrient-dense foods and increase their intake during the second and third trimesters. During this time, the rapid growth of fetal tissues requires additional calories, particularly from protein and fat. These macronutrients are the fundamental building blocks of cells, including in the developing brain.

The First Trimester

In terms of diet, the initial weeks of pregnancy can be tricky. Many women face serious challenges managing the complex hormonal changes associated with the early stages. As a result, their appetite and energy levels may be affected. Nausea and fatigue are common during the first trimester, which makes it challenging to consume three balanced meals a day. There is often a wide fluctuation in what seems appetizing (or repulsive) to a pregnant woman. This is totally normal, but it means the best strategy is to eat the best, most nutritious food you can. You often won't feel like eating something you feel you should consume. Prioritize foods that are nutrient-dense rather than those that increase caloric intake, to ensure that the developing baby gets the essential building blocks it needs at this critical time.

While the mom-to-be is adapting to numerous hormonal changes, the fetus is busy too. Four weeks after conception, the neural tube, which develops into the brain and spinal cord, closes. At eight weeks the kidneys, eyes and heart are taking shape; these organs will be completely formed at 12 weeks. Proper organ formation depends on good nutrition. If the fetus doesn't get the full range of nutrients it needs, it will trade off the development of some organs to protect others that are more critical to its survival.

Nutrition During Pregnancy

Consuming a nutrient-dense diet prior to becoming pregnant goes a long way toward ensuring a healthy pregnancy. But once you know you've successfully conceived, it's even more important to make sure your diet is top-notch. While sound nutrition helps to ensure that your baby will develop into a healthy adult, it also provides essential support for you. A mother's body must constantly change to meet the demands of constructing and developing a human being. By any assessment, this is a momentous job.

If you are struggling to choose healthy foods, ask your doctor or a dietitian with special training in pregnancy nutrition for additional support, and enlist your spouse or partner to help make your home a center for wholesome food. They can, for instance, help you keep the house stocked with nutritious whole foods and ensure that minimal amounts of refined food cross the threshold.

Dietary Recommendations

While it's always important to consume a wide range of nutrients, when you're pregnant, some are vital, including protein and healthy fats, in particular omega-3 fatty acids. Crucial micronutrients include folate, vitamins B_6 and B_{12}, iron, zinc, iodine, vitamin A, vitamin D, calcium and choline. These nutrients can be obtained from a balanced diet consisting of nutrient-dense whole foods, as well as protein-rich foods from healthy animals and fish. But while it is theoretically possible to obtain the required nutrients by eating a wholesome diet, in practical terms it is very challenging. That's why pregnant women are advised to take a prenatal supplement.

Nutrients that play a particularly significant role throughout pregnancy include:

FOLATE

Folate plays a key role in preventing spinal cord abnormalities and other organ defects. Fortifying flour with folic acid has been a public-health success in a number of countries. A meal consisting of 1 cup (250 mL) of cooked lentils and 1 cup of leafy greens (such as chard, spinach or kale) provides more than 400 mcg of folate, which puts you within striking distance of the daily requirement during pregnancy (600 to 800 mcg). See "Folate: The Tip of an Epigenetic Iceberg," page 44, for more on folate.

VITAMIN D

Vitamin D activates more than 3,000 genes. Given its pervasiveness in the human body, it's not surprising that experts are connecting a deficiency in vitamin D with a number of pregnancy-related conditions. In early pregnancy, vitamin D deficiency has been associated with an increased risk of developing gestational diabetes. Insufficient levels have also been linked with an increased risk for adverse pregnancy outcomes, including high rates of caesarean delivery, spontaneous preterm births and preeclampsia.

Low levels of vitamin D have also been shown to affect fetal development. The Southampton Women's Survey found links between low vitamin D levels during pregnancy and lower bone and mineral density in offspring, when measured at birth and at four and nine years. Lower bone density in childhood is associated with an increased risk of osteoporosis later in life.

Many women do not have adequate supplies of vitamin D. In the United States, for instance, 28 percent of pregnant women were found to have insufficient levels, and one 2015 study found that even in sun-soaked Mediterranean countries, deficiency levels ranged between 50 and 65 percent, possibly because of prevailing concern about sun exposure.

Pregnant women should supplement with vitamin D, but for various reasons, experts can't agree on ideal levels of the nutrient. Vitamin D is fat-soluble, which means your body stores any excess, so it's important not to take too much — 4,000 IUs (international units) is the safe upper limit, according to the Institute of Medicine, which is associated with the National Academy of Science. Overdosing can lead to toxicity in the form of too much calcium in your blood and possibly even hypertension. Foods such as vitamin D–enriched dairy products and canned fish with the bones help to increase intake of both calcium and vitamin D.

IRON
Anemia occurs when you don't have enough red blood cells to carry adequate oxygen to your body's cells. Iron deficiency is the most common cause of anemia, affecting 15 to 25 percent of pregnant women. Pregnant women are at a higher risk for iron-deficiency anemia because, in order to supply nutrients for the fetus, the volume of blood in their bodies increases, as does the need to make more blood cells.

Pregnant women need about 30 mg of iron daily, compared to the normal requirement of 18 mg, so it's wise to increase consumption of iron-rich foods when you are pregnant. See page 119 for more information on food sources of iron. Nutritionists recommend also taking a prenatal supplement.

HEALTHY FATS
An adequate intake of healthy fats, particularly omega-3 fatty acids, is important for women during pregnancy and lactation, and at every stage of fetal development, from preconception through delivery. The research on the benefits of omega-3 supplementation during pregnancy is very robust. Numerous studies have shown that it reduces the risk of premature birth and of delivering a low-birth-weight baby. It also lowers the risk of preeclampsia and postpartum mood disorders. Omega-3s are especially important during the last trimester, when the baby's brain and nervous system are forming, a point at which the mother's reserves are likely to become depleted. Because an adequate supply of these fatty acids has been linked with healthy fetal development of the brain, eyes and immune system, a mother should consume more of these nutrients in the second and third trimester to shore up her reserves.

Once the baby is born, the mother's body continues to need omega-3s to make breast milk. Foods such as fatty fish, algae supplements and foods fortified with these nutrients, including eggs produced by chickens fed flax seeds, will support healthy development not only in utero, but after the baby is born, when its immune system and organs such as the brain are still very plastic.

Nutrients that are particularly important at this stage include folate, vitamins A, B_6 and B_{12}, iron, zinc, iodine and omega-3 fatty acids, as well as adequate protein. Because these nutrients are so important for proper organ development, a prenatal supplement that includes the full basket is strongly recommended.

Research shows that a low-carb diet should not be followed during pregnancy. One 2011 study linked a low-carb diet in early pregnancy with higher rates of obesity by the time the children turned nine. By examining DNA from the umbilical cord, the researchers were able to link methylation of a gene called RXRa, which plays a role in how fat cells develop, with the mothers' low-carb diets and their children's obesity.

In early pregnancy, some women find it particularly difficult to eat breakfast, because this is the time of day they are most likely to feel nauseated. If eating a full breakfast is unappealing, try beginning the day with a smaller bite or two that still provides a good amount of nutrients. How about whole-grain or seed crackers and a fruit smoothie, ideally with added leafy greens? Rather than eating an entire hamburger for dinner, add a few spoonfuls of ground chicken or beef to something that sounds appetizing, such as noodles or brown rice.

Keeping well hydrated is very important. A mother-to-be's blood volume rises

VITAMIN A

While vitamin A is necessary for normal fetal development, excessive vitamin A can be toxic to a developing baby and may lead to birth defects. The best way to obtain vitamin A is via beta-carotene, which the body converts to vitamin A. This phytonutrient is abundant in brightly colored red, orange and yellow vegetables. The recommended daily intake (RDI) of vitamin A for pregnant women is 770 mcg, and the tolerable upper limit is 3,000 mcg. Liver and cod liver oil (also an excellent source of omega-3s) are rich in vitamin A. One teaspoon (5 mL) of cod liver oil may contain 275 mcg of vitamin A, close to half the RDI. An ounce (30 g) of chicken liver may contain more than 1,000 mcg, and the same amount of beef liver may provide twice that amount, so be careful. Overindulging in these foods could easily push you over the tolerable limit (3,000 mcg). Read the labels on nutritional supplements carefully to ensure that they do not contain too much preformed vitamin A.

throughout her pregnancy, and hydration supports this increase. If necessary, add a splash of pure fruit juice to make your water more pleasing. With regard to alcohol, the advice for preconception stands: all medical organizations advise avoiding alcoholic beverages. High-fructose beverages such as soda, energy drinks and large servings of sweetened fruit juice should be avoided because they can negatively affect an offspring's long-term metabolic health. Caffeine should be limited to less than 200 mg a day; although the caffeine content of coffee varies, this works out to about one cup.

The Second Trimester

By the second trimester, most women happily report that their appetite and energy have returned, and some may be ready to "eat for two." While pregnant women do need to increase their nutrient and caloric intake, this does not mean eating double portions or double the calories. To support healthy weight gain, most pregnant women need to increase their caloric intake by only about 300 calories a day during the second and third trimesters. This can easily be accomplished. Nutritious additions that will do the job include two hard-boiled eggs and an apple, a turkey sandwich on whole-grain bread, or a bowl of plain full-fat yogurt with fruit and a dash of honey.

At this point most of the critical organ development is finished. The fetus is now focused on growing tissues such as skin, hair, muscles and bones. Brain development is continuing. Adequate dietary protein and healthy fats become even more critical during this growth phase. Aim to get 60 grams of protein daily from foods such as meat, fish, yogurt and cheese, and consume healthy fats such as olive oil, avocados, nuts and seeds.

With regard to bone development, the placenta is incredibly efficient at transferring calcium and vitamin D from the mother's nutrient stores to the fetus during the second trimester. Keep an eye on your vitamin D levels at this stage, and aim for around 1,300 mg of calcium a day. Dark green leafy vegetables are rich in calcium and are also high in folate, another critical nutrient in pregnancy.

The hormonal changes of pregnancy and the demands of the growing baby often place stress on the mother's digestive system. This may lead to constipation, so it's wise to increase your fiber intake to 30 to 35 grams daily. Eating more fruits (the whole fruit, not just juice), vegetables, whole grains, nuts and seeds will help you achieve this goal.

In addition, the risk of anemia increases in both the second and third trimesters, so continue to focus on consuming iron-rich foods. Remember, if plant foods are your primary source of iron, you will need to help your body absorb this mineral by eating them alongside foods that are rich in vitamin C.

GESTATIONAL DIABETES

Toward the end of the second trimester, a mother-to-be will be checked for gestational diabetes (see page 182). This condition affects about 7 percent of pregnancies, and if it develops, it's usually after the 20th week of pregnancy. At that point the placenta is producing more hormones that interfere with the mother's ability to regulate insulin. Because insulin plays a key role in managing blood sugar levels, the mother-to-be may temporarily develop diabetes. Although blood sugar levels typically return to normal after delivery, gestational diabetes has been associated with a number of future disease states for both mother and child. The fetus adjusts to the overabundance of blood sugar available from its mother, which increases its risk of being overweight at birth, and of type 2 diabetes and other health problems as an adult.

One of the best strategies for reducing the risk of gestational diabetes is to have your blood sugar checked before you become pregnant. This will alert you to any risks and enable you to take steps to manage them before you conceive. Any predisposition to insulin resistance will be heightened during pregnancy. The standard of care for pregnancy calls for glucose tolerance testing between 24 and 28 weeks. If you have diabetes or a past history of gestational diabetes, it will probably be done sooner.

To keep your blood sugar stable, a balanced diet with protein, fat and fiber at every meal is important. Eating a low-carb diet during pregnancy leads to obesity in offspring and increases their risk of birth defects. When it comes to carbs, the key is to consume those that qualify as complex — for instance, whole grains, legumes, nuts and seeds — and avoid the processed versions, especially those found in nutrient-deficient snack foods like pastries and sugary drinks. This will help to keep your blood sugar on an even keel.

The Third Trimester

As they head into their final trimester, it's common for pregnant women to feel awkward ("I move like a beached whale" is how some describe it). Eating with a small human-to-be pressing on your digestive tract may also interfere with your desire to eat full meals. By the third trimester, most major organs in the fetus are fully developed. The baby is putting on weight to build muscles to support movement, and fat to keep them warm after delivery, so their mother needs to consume the calories required to sustain this development. Once again, her focus should be on consuming adequate amounts of protein and healthy fat. The fetus has special needs during this time because the brain and the immune system are actively developing and the eyes are maturing. Its bones need an ever-increasing supply of calcium, and growing muscles need an ample amount of amino acids. Eating smaller meals throughout the day may be helpful with achieving dietary goals.

During the third trimester, the mother's risk of anemia increases. Her blood volume continues to expand, and to protect the baby from postnatal anemia, she transfers a large amount of iron to the fetus. To avoid becoming anemic herself, she needs to replenish her iron stores. Consuming red meat from well-raised animals should help her meet these additional needs, not only for iron but also for protein. For vegetarians, whole grains, legumes, nuts, seeds and soybean products are good sources of these nutrients.

Vitamin D continues to be important because it boosts the mother's ability to absorb calcium, which is being actively transferred to the baby to support bone development. Adequate consumption of vitamin D throughout this term will also help to ensure that the mother continues to provide this nutrient in her breast milk. Because sun exposure will be limited, after birth the baby will receive almost all of their vitamin D from Mom's breast milk.

A WORD ABOUT IRON

Iron plays an important role in metabolism. While this mineral is abundant in many foods, your body can't use all of the sources with equal effectiveness. Heme iron, found in animal foods such as meat, poultry and fish, is easily absorbed. Nonheme iron, found in plant foods such as dark leafy greens, legumes and whole grains, is not as easily used by the body. If your primary dietary source of iron is plant foods, make sure to eat foods that are rich in vitamin C at the same time, because vitamin C improves the absorption of nonheme iron. Vitamin C–rich foods include citrus fruits, kiwis, bell peppers and broccoli. Some nutritionists recommend soaking (and even sprouting) legumes and whole grains before cooking, to make nutrients, including iron, more accessible to the body.

VITAMIN D

Vitamin D is a fat-soluble vitamin that plays many significant roles throughout life, from influencing fertility to helping to prevent osteoporosis and maintain muscle strength in old age. It is stored in tissues, where it acts like a hormone supporting health in various ways. Many people are deficient in vitamin D. While experts disagree on ideal blood levels of the compound, it is generally accepted that a significant number of people suffer from vitamin D deficiency. If you live in a cloudy climate, be sure to have your plasma vitamin D measured.

Vitamin D is not widely available in foods. The best way to increase your levels of vitamin D is through sun exposure, which stimulates cholesterol in the skin to create the vitamin. However, dermatologists raise serious concerns about the elevated risks of melanoma caused by ultraviolet (UV) radiation in sunlight. Many doctors now recommend taking vitamin D supplements or consuming cod liver oil, a rich source of the vitamin.

Living in the Real World

A woman is likely to feel stressed simply because she is pregnant. Not only does she need to adjust emotionally to the idea of becoming a mother, which includes the challenges involved in caring for a baby, but massive variations in her hormones predispose her to nausea, mood swings and fatigue. She needs plenty of rest and emotional support. We know that stress, particularly during the first trimester, has negative effects on pregnancy outcomes. In addition, environmental exposures can have significant impacts on development.

Cigarette Smoke

Tobacco smoke continues to be one of the most recognized toxins that affect pregnant women. It is loaded with dangerous chemicals that have been linked with a wide range of pregnancy complications, from miscarriage to stillbirth. Studies show that secondhand exposure to cigarette smoke may be as harmful to a fetus as if the pregnant woman were a smoker herself. Prenatal exposure to either active or passive maternal tobacco smoke has been associated with increased risk of low birth weight and subsequent development of asthma, obesity, cancer and type 2 diabetes. One 2016 study published in the journal

PLoS One, based on a meta-analysis of the literature, connected maternal smoking with cancers of the nervous system in offspring. The US Centers for Disease Control and Prevention (CDC) link maternal smoking with *placental insufficiency*, premature birth and low birth weight, among other problems. Smoking has also been identified as a risk factor for sudden infant death syndrome (SIDS).

Alcohol

Once conception occurs, all major medical organizations recommend complete abstinence from alcohol. Not only can the toxic effects of alcohol affect the baby's developing brain, but drinking when pregnant can burn up nutrients, reducing the nutrition available to the fetus. For instance, alcohol depletes folate in the mother's body, an effect that is heightened if her diet is already nutrient-poor. Interestingly, according to the CDC, about 10 percent of women consume alcohol while pregnant. Binge drinking is not uncommon among younger women, who may accidentally become pregnant during an episode.

Exposure to Toxins

Unfortunately, toxins are all around us and it is probably impossible to navigate contemporary life without coming into contact with hazardous substances. While they are harmful to everyone, toxins are particularly dangerous to a fetus because fetal organs are so sensitive to environmental stressors. Experts now tell us that most environmental chemicals can cross the placenta, where they initiate a variety of fetal responses that increase that baby's risk for chronic disease later in life.

Relevant toxins range from the air we breathe to prescription drugs — thalidomide and DES (see "The DES Story," page 236) are two of the most compelling examples. A 2018 study published in the journal *Hypertension* found that exposure to air pollution in utero increased the risk that offspring would develop hypertension, which showed up as early as three years of age. Not surprisingly, the greater the exposure, the higher the risk. Another study originating in London, England, linked exposure to air pollution and low birth weight. A 2018 study published in the *American Journal of Epidemiology* linked air pollution, specifically from coal- and oil-fired power plants, with preterm births. Researchers found that when such plants were closed (between 2001 and 2011), the air pollution levels fell significantly, as did the incidence of preterm births in the surrounding areas.

Endocrine-disrupting chemicals (EDCs) are also a concern, not only because their use is widespread, but also because they behave like hormones and are, therefore, likely to have a particularly profound effect on a developing fetus. One of the most studied of this

CHILDHOOD CANCER

Cancer is a disease of aging (see pages 231–243). In the broadest terms, it results from a series of changes that may be programmed in the womb and take place over a long period of time. So how do you explain childhood cancer? Although cancer in children is rare, its incidence rates are gradually increasing, which suggests that environmental factors are at play. Perhaps not surprisingly, a growing body of research is now linking various toxic exposures in utero to cancer in children.

In a 2003 review paper published in the journal *Environmental Health Perspectives*, researchers noted a number of factors associated with experiences in the womb that are risk factors for childhood cancer. These include low doses of ionizing radiation, especially during the mother's last trimester; parental exposure to occupational chemicals; and maternal exposure to "solvents, paints or paint thinners from preconception to birth." Parental use of pesticides has also been linked with increased risk of cancer in offspring, a particular concern for agricultural workers. And exposure to pesticides, both in utero and in early childhood, has been on the epidemiological radar since at least 1982, when a cluster of children with cancer whose parents were farmworkers was identified in McFarland, a small California town. Moreover, some evidence connects exposure to traffic-related air pollution with a small increase in the risk of childhood cancers.

Interestingly, the links between cigarette smoking and childhood cancer are not as strong as some others, although evidence does suggest that when fathers smoke, it institutes epigenetic changes that may increase cancer risk in their offspring. One Chinese study found a "significantly elevated risk of childhood cancers, particularly acute leukemia and lymphoma," but only when the male parent had been a long-time smoker before his child was conceived. On the other hand, the United Kingdom Childhood Cancer Study concluded that there was no "significant evidence that parental smoking is a risk factor for any of the major groups of childhood cancers." However, in addition to being present in the breast milk of mothers who smoke, by-products of tobacco have been detected in the placenta, in fetal blood and in the urine of newborns. Although there are questions as to whether parental smoking has an impact on the development of childhood cancer, it has certainly been associated with other chronic diseases later in life.

From an epidemiological perspective, studying childhood cancers is challenging because they are so uncommon. To look at populations and determine whether toxic exposures in utero are linked with early disease development would require a very large sample size. As a result, one group of European researchers decided to take a look at the problem from the perspective of biomarkers. A summary of their research was published in the *British Medical Journal* (*BMJ*) in 2015. First they measured the presence of dietary carcinogens such as acrylamide (deep-fried potato products, biscuits and crackers are big offenders) and nitrosamines (high amounts are found in processed meats and fish) in the umbilical cord blood of a sample of newborns. Then they linked these substances with biomarkers associated with cancer risk in adults.

The researchers found "significant" associations between the two. The higher the exposure to the carcinogen, the higher the level of the biomarker in the cord blood. Moreover, when they looked at certain gene expression levels, they found that when boys had high levels of exposure to dioxin (found in fatty meat, fatty fish and full-fat dairy products), processes linked with uncontrolled cell growth were activated. They concluded: "Overall, fetal exposure to selected dietary carcinogens seems to induce molecular events that indicate increased cancer risks." They also noted that these risks were particularly significant in relation to boys and the development of leukemia.

Why are some children more susceptible to developing cancer following exposure to carcinogens in utero? After additional investigation, the authors of the *BMJ* study concluded that gene variants may be at fault. Using *genome-wide association studies* (GWAS), they were able to identify the presence of certain single-nucleotide polymorphisms (SNPs) in cord-blood DNA that are linked with biological processes that may make the fetal organs more sensitive to carcinogens. The researchers believe these SNPs have a genetic predisposition that increases a child's risk of developing cancer when exposed to dietary carcinogens in utero. If this is the case, it's possible that other carcinogens, such as toxins and air pollution, could have a similar impact on such children.

group is BPA, present in a wide range of household products such as plastic water bottles and baby bottles. We now know that BPA can reach a human fetus, where it can alter DNA methylation and the growth of fetal organs. Studies of sheep have shown that prenatal exposure to BPA interferes with their endocrine system and influences how genes behave in a number of important physiological pathways.

Worse still, our food supply is affected by environmental toxins. One study published in *JAMA* in 2018 found that women undergoing fertility treatments who ate the most pesticide-laced produce were 26 percent less likely to produce a live birth compared to women who ate fruits and vegetables with the least pesticide exposure.

How Much Weight Should You Gain?

It goes without saying that weight gain is part of a healthy pregnancy. Doctors generally advise women to gain 28 to 40 pounds (13 to 18 kg) if they are underweight, 25 to 35 pounds (11 to 16 kg) if their weight is normal, 15 to 25 pounds (7 to 11 kg) if they are overweight and 11 to 20 pounds (5 to 9 kg) if they are obese.

The good news is, even if you are underweight or obese while pregnant, you can still have a healthy pregnancy. A commitment to regular prenatal care and an increased focus on consuming nutrient-dense foods and committing to reasonable levels of exercise during your pregnancy can help to ensure a healthy outcome.

If You're Overweight

Obesity is a complicating factor in pregnancy. A 2017 study found that the risk of serious birth defects increased in step with the degree of the mother's obesity. Although traditional advice has urged even obese women to gain weight during pregnancy, recent research suggests otherwise. Current thinking is that an obese woman should attempt to lose as much excess weight as possible before she conceives and limit the amount of weight she gains while pregnant.

A study conducted in 2009 followed more than 200 obese pregnant women. One group of participants followed a balanced diet intended to limit weight gain and kept a daily diet journal. In comparison to the control group of equally obese women who were advised to gain a standard amount of weight, the monitored group gained less weight, had fewer caesarean deliveries, were less likely to develop gestational diabetes and retained less weight after the baby was born. The average weight gain in the control group was 31 pounds (14 kg), compared to an 11-pound (5 kg) weight gain in the monitored group.

The takeaway from this study is that, at the very least, obese pregnant women should talk to their doctors or midwives about the impact of increasing calories during pregnancy.

If You're Underweight

Being underweight is usually not an issue in developed countries: only 2 to 5 percent of women in the United States and even France (where women are thought to be elegantly svelte) qualify as underweight. However, it has been identified as a problem in Japan, where being slender has traditionally been highly valued. In addition, the medical guidelines in that country encourage women, many of whom are already thin, to keep their weight low while pregnant. Emerging evidence is linking this adulation of slimness with markers for increased health risks. The average height of a Japanese adult has declined every year since 1980, and statistics also show a particularly high rate of babies with low birth weights. According to a 2018 article in *Science* magazine, a trend toward heavier babies that began after the Second World War likely started to shift in the late 1970s, when Japanese obstetricians began to recommend lower-calorie diets, a concept that was incorporated into official guidelines in 1981. By 2010 the percentage of low-birth-weight babies had increased to 9.6 percent from 5.5 percent in 1978. This remains a serious problem in Japan.

Being underweight can also be linked with involuntary malnourishment, a problem in places that are economically underdeveloped. For instance, 60 percent of women in South Asia are underweight. In this case the problem is often due to nutritional deficiencies and may be related to poverty.

In economically developed parts of the world, societal pressures equating beauty with thinness may drive some women to purposefully restrict calories to unhealthy levels. In America, as many as 1.5 percent of women are affected by eating disorders. These include anorexia nervosa, an emotional disorder characterized by food avoidance, and bulimia nervosa, which involves recurrent episodes of binge eating followed by purging or fasting. These conditions increase the risk that a woman will not only be underweight prior to pregnancy but will also not gain enough weight while pregnant. Women who suffer from eating disorders and who want to have a healthy pregnancy can team up with a dietitian and a mental health professional before pregnancy, or as soon as possible once they are pregnant, to help them overcome their condition.

Women who are underweight face additional challenges during pregnancy and are at increased risk for complications. Studies have shown that mothers who were underweight before they became pregnant and didn't gain enough weight during pregnancy had six times the normal risk of infant mortality within the first year after the baby's birth. Underweight moms are also more likely to give birth prematurely and/or to produce a low-birth-weight baby. Pregnant women who are severely underweight have a low turnover of protein in muscle and are less able to provide amino acids to the fetus. They are also likely to have an inflamed placenta.

Because being underweight is a risk factor for both iron-deficiency anemia and osteoporosis, underweight pregnant women need to not only consume more calories to gain weight, but also focus specifically on nutrient-dense foods that supply abundant amounts of iron and calcium. These include meat, legumes and dark green leafy vegetables. Although whole grains are not a good source of calcium, most do provide iron, and serving them with a dairy product (oatmeal with milk for breakfast, creamy polenta spiked with cheese at dinner) can help to provide adequate amounts of these nutrients.

THE FIRST TWO YEARS

The first two years of life is when the environment outside the womb has the greatest impact on future health. How infants develop and grow during this time affects their chances of developing chronic disease later in life. Research based on the Finnish and Hertfordshire data indicates that an infant who gains weight too slowly during this period, appearing thin or stunted by age two, is more likely to develop hypertension, heart disease, stroke and diabetes as an adult. Other studies have linked rapid weight gain in the first four months of life with an increased risk of obesity. Dr. Alan Lucas, an expert on childhood nutrition who some credit with coining the term "the first thousand days," attributes the development of insulin resistance and raised blood pressure in children specifically to a diet that accelerates growth during this crucial period.

Babies gain weight in the months after birth faster than at any other time in their lives. Nutrition plays a key role. As Dr. Lucas notes, not only does nutrition meet the baby's immediate needs for energy and development, it also establishes the basis for health and wellness in the years to come. For instance, infant nutrition affects intellectual development and educational attainment. Studies show that babies fed more nutritious enriched formula or breast milk had improved IQ scores (as much as 12 to 15 points higher) than those fed regular formula. They also exhibited an overall reduction in cardiovascular risk factors. Other studies have demonstrated that children identified as undernourished at age two are 16 percent more likely to fail at least one grade in school. Data from the United Nations Standing Committee on Nutrition have linked even moderately poor nutrition with poor academic performance and reduced mental capacity.

Early infancy is a critical period because that is when your child's growth is most rapid. By their second birthday, the pace slows. An infant uses about a quarter of their energy for growth, but by the time they turn two, that rate has declined to about 6 percent. As David Barker writes in *Nutrition in the Womb*, at about two years of age a child's "growth rates become 'set' by the internal environment and are less sensitive to the day-to-day supply of food." Obviously, there's a delicate balance in a diet that avoids thinness while ensuring that the infant doesn't become overweight. Infants with a normal appetite and adequate nutrition grow at a normal rate. Mothers who breastfeed and supplement with wholesome foods will have a normally growing child so long as the child does not have a disorder.

Premature Birth

Preterm delivery occurs when a baby arrives prior to 37 weeks of gestation. In the United States it occurs in about one out of every 10 births. Factors that may contribute to premature birth include poor prenatal care, age, tobacco smoke and stress. It has also been linked with preeclampsia, placental position and a maternal history of hypertension.

Babies born prematurely are at increased risk for various health-related issues. They are more likely to have cognition deficits; problems with vision, such as vision loss and increased rates of nearsightedness; and delays in reaching developmental milestones such as sitting without support, walking without help and getting their first teeth.

Low Birth Weight

Low birth weight resulting from *intrauterine growth restriction* (IGR) provides the basis for David Barker's work on the developmental origins of health and disease. In general terms, *low birth weight* describes babies who weigh less than 5 pounds 8 ounces (2,500 g) at birth. There are two basic reasons for low birth weight: premature birth and IGR, which occurs when growth is impeded for various reasons, such as placental insufficiency, environmental impacts and/or a poorly nourished mother. When babies are born prematurely, they are naturally smaller and will require hospital care until they gain an appropriate amount of weight. Babies whose low birth weight results from IGR are often (but not always) carried to full term. There are numerous factors, discussed throughout this book, that may have contributed to them not growing properly in utero.

Premature birth and low birth weight are often related and overlap on many levels. For instance, both premature babies and those with a low birth weight experience feeding issues, difficulty regulating their body temperature and an increased risk of infection.

Breast Milk Is Best

Much of our knowledge about the influence of nutrition on infant health comes from studies involving breast milk. Breastfeeding has been described as the gold standard of infant nutrition. Studies show that breastfed infants have lower risk factors for cardiovascular disease, obesity, high cholesterol, type 2 diabetes and hypertension. As little as one month of breastfeeding has been linked with positive effects, but studies confirm a clear relationship between the overall amount of breast milk and the reduction of disease risk. When researchers looked at a group of adolescents between 13 and 16 years old, they found that the more breast milk they had consumed as infants, the less likely they were to show signs of chronic illness or conditions such as metabolic syndrome by the time they became teenagers.

Transitioning to Solid Food

While breast milk is the perfect food for babies, around the age of four months your baby may start to show signs of wanting to expand their diet. At this point their gastrointestinal system is sufficiently developed that they can handle solid food if it is properly introduced. Expanding the range of nutrients they consume will support healthy growth and development. A balanced diet that includes lean proteins, whole grains, fruits, vegetables and healthy fats should provide all the nutrients they need. Introducing solid food in the form of nutrient-poor junk food is not advisable.

Developing healthy brains and bodies requires a good balance among the macronutrients: protein, carbohydrates and fats. These provide energy and support growth. Protein also builds, maintains and repairs body tissues. In addition, a wide range of micronutrients and other substances, such as amino acids, play a significant role in establishing robust body systems.

It's important to provide children with a balanced diet, a point that was brought home by a 2014 Australian study. The researchers noted that many parents who followed low-carb diets were providing their children with a narrow selection of foods. This lack of variety meant that the children weren't obtaining all the nutrients they needed, and that their intake of essential nutrients, such as fiber, was limited. In short, the researchers found that low-carb diets are harmful to children.

While it's advisable to limit children's intake of nutrient-deficient refined carbs, as part of a balanced diet of whole foods, complex carbs such as legumes and whole grains have been linked with many health benefits. The nutrients in these foods feed gut bacteria, directly benefitting your child's immune system. They also support cognitive development and performance, keep energy levels up and prevent feelings of sluggishness. They have also been linked with production of serotonin, which supports a positive mood, helping to prevent irritability.

The most common nutritional deficiency in young children is iron, because they're burning up significant amounts of iron to support rapid growth and healthy cognitive development. The best (most absorbable) food sources are poultry, fish, meat and eggs. Plant sources, which are not as readily absorbed, include most whole grains and legumes.

A Finnish study published in 2017 found that higher levels of omega-3 fatty acids reduced the risk that children at genetic risk would develop type 1 diabetes. The researchers linked the infants' favorable fatty acid status with breastfeeding, which is a good source of these essential fats. Those who were not breastfed had lower levels. Type 1 diabetes often develops in infancy, and the first year of life is a good time to take preventive steps. If a genetic predisposition to diabetes runs in your family, in addition to breastfeeding, consider adding oily fish, such as salmon, to your baby's diet once they begin to eat solid food.

In recent years the thinking on introducing potentially allergenic foods while weaning your baby off breast milk or formula has changed dramatically. In the past, parents were advised to avoid foods, such as cow's milk, peanuts or eggs, that are associated with higher rates of allergic reactions. However, studies now show that introducing such foods before a baby has its first birthday reduces the risk of an allergic response to these foods later in life.

The benefits of breastfeeding extend to babies born prematurely as well as those birthed at full term. One study found that preemies fed human breast milk, particularly those born at 30 weeks of gestation or later, showed significantly lower rates of necrotizing enterocolitis (NEC), a very serious intestinal disease.

An important takeaway from this research is that bigger is not necessarily better during infancy. Breastfed babies grow more slowly than those fed formula, but breast milk provides an infant's best nutritional start. For instance, it contains oligosaccharides, complex carbohydrates that encourage the development of a healthy gut microbiota (see chapter 9), which among other benefits supports a healthy immune system.

Supporting Mom's Health

Mothers who are breastfeeding must keep close tabs on their own nutritional needs as well as their baby's. Producing milk involves a considerable amount of energy: exclusive breastfeeding requires 400 to 500 additional calories per day. A good portion of that intake should consist of healthy fats (such as those provided by oily fish, whole grains and seeds), since it's important for breast milk to be rich in this nutrient. Ensuring an adequate intake of iron-rich legumes, dark green leafy vegetables and whole grains, which provide a natural source of folate, is also recommended. These fiber-rich plant foods also encourage the growth of healthy gut bacteria, which have many benefits for both mother and child.

Although vegan mothers will reap the nutritional rewards of consuming abundant amounts of plant foods, they need to make sure they have an adequate intake of certain nutrients. These include zinc, iron (because they are obtaining it from less absorbable sources) and especially vitamin B_{12}, which is difficult to obtain from a plant-based diet. They will also need to supplement with omega 3s, because this essential fatty acid supports brain and eye development in their child.

It may be worth noting that breastfeeding is not a one-way street in terms of its benefits. Studies show that, while nursing, a woman may lose some weight and find that her blood pressure and cholesterol are lower than her previous norm, all of which support cardiovascular health. The link with metabolic improvements was highlighted in a 2018 study published in the *Journal of Hepatology*. Researchers followed more than 800 women for 25 years and found that women who breastfed for a minimum of six months were 52 percent less likely to develop nonalcoholic fatty liver disease (see page 176) than those whose babies were breastfed for less than a month. And mothers who breastfeed also reduce their risk of developing breast cancer. A study published in *The Lancet* in 2002 found that the risk of breast cancer declined by 4.3 percent for every year a woman breast-fed (which could be spread over multiple children).

The Immune System

Once rare, allergic diseases are becoming increasingly common, particularly in more developed countries. Fundamentally, allergies are the immune system's inappropriate response to the environment. The stage is set for their development very early in life. Dr. Susan Prescott, an expert in the immune system, notes in her book *Origins: Early-Life Solutions to the Modern Health Crisis* that more than 25 percent of infants develop eczema and 20 percent show some sensitivity to common foods by their first birthday. Allergic responses apparently evolved as protection against irritants and toxins, and Prescott suggests that the increase in their incidence may have its origins in the relatively rapid life-style changes associated with contemporary life.

The immune system is very complex, but there is little doubt that bacteria play a significant role in its development. The food a baby eats, the air they breathe and the surfaces they touch are all populated by bacteria, some beneficial, and others potential *pathogens*. These bacteria take up residence throughout the body, but particularly in the gut, and they play a significant role in determining health.

David Barker described a baby's gut as an "incubation chamber" colonized by the bacteria they encounter, likely first in tiny amounts while still in the womb and then in more substantial quantities after arriving in the world. These microbes play a helpful role in recycling food waste into valuable nutrients, including vitamins, *short-chain fatty acids* and amino acids. Breast milk is so beneficial for babies in part because it contains complex carbohydrates that encourage the growth of healthy bacteria in the gut. Among other benefits, these bacteria support the development of a healthy immune system. Studies of infants have shown that early introduction of *prebiotics* — in the form of oligosaccharides, which are found in breast milk as well as in foods including wheat, milk, legumes and soft cheeses — reduce the incidence of infections and allergic diseases such as asthma-like symptoms and hives.

So it's probably not surprising that researchers have identified differences in the gut bacteria of infants who are allergic and those who aren't. In general terms, children with the most abundant and diverse bacteria are the least likely to suffer from allergies. In Eastern Europe the rates of allergic disease are extremely low, so the question is why? One study, which looked at almost 14,000 children in Belarus, found that children who had pets, had regular contact with farm animals and younger siblings, and lived in a rural area were far less likely to suffer from allergic diseases. This and other studies support what is known as the "hygiene hypothesis," the theory that children raised in environments that are "too clean" are more likely to develop allergies (see "The Hygiene Hypothesis," page 272). It is believed that early and extensive exposure to a wide range of bacteria and infectious agents strengthens the immune system, encouraging it to develop in a healthy fashion (see also "The Immune System," page 141).

Unfortunately, of all the body's systems, the immune system is the least studied in terms of early-life environment and later-onset disease. But recent research is linking fetal development with immune system problems. Allergic responses such as eczema often manifest in the first few months of life. In a paper published in *The Lancet* in 1999, Susan Prescott noted that some babies show signs of allergies at birth, which suggests they have been programmed for allergic disease while in the womb. Thomas McDade, a biological anthropologist, has found that babies who are small for their gestational age and those who grew poorly as infants are more likely to have immune system deficiencies in later life.

Today the word *epidemic* is often associated with increased rates of potentially life-threatening food allergies. In Dr. Prescott's opinion, many environmental factors — including nutrition, air pollution and exposure to microbes, to name just three — are driving this upsurge. The roots of some of these changes extend to the baby's epigenome. In response to various situations, genes associated with the immune system change how they express themselves. These modifications are most active during the periods of greatest developmental plasticity: in utero and during the first two years of life.

The immune system of infants is particularly vulnerable to the effects of air pollution, exposure to microbes and potential allergens in food. Another potential disruptor to immune system development is antibiotics. While these drugs have saved millions of lives, when prescribed to children, particularly those younger than two, they may have lifelong consequences because they undermine bacterial diversity in their gut at a critical developmental period. The research into antibiotic use in infancy and increased disease risk later in life is seen as controversial because there is so little of it. Nevertheless, a 2016 study published in the journal *Genome Medicine* linked antibiotic use during infancy and early childhood with an increased risk of childhood obesity, infections, asthma, allergies and both type 1 and type 2 diabetes.

The Brain

The delicate infant brain has an enormous capacity to develop and is constantly adapting to experiences. Between birth and six months, a baby's busy little brain is forming 700 neural connections a minute. That's very vigorous activity. As a parent, you want to make sure all this energy is heading in a positive direction. Fortunately, because the environment plays such a starring role in how your baby's brain and central nervous system mature, there are many steps you can take to encourage positive development.

Experts all agree that constructive stimulation, such as music, colorful toys and art (think mobiles hung over the crib) and talking and even reading to your baby (which helps them develop language skills), fosters their natural curiosity. When it comes to toys, simpler is better. Your baby should be able to get what they're about. There's a reason rattles have been around forever: they are about noise, colors and shapes — fascinating concepts to an infant's brain.

On the other hand, if the environmental influences are adverse, the developing brain's responses may, over the long term, prove to be maladaptive, leaving permanent scars. The brain is most susceptible to environmental impacts, including toxins, during its period of greatest growth. Exposure to potentially hazardous substances like heavy metals and common household and environmental chemicals can disrupt processes that build the brain's circuitry. One 2017 report from UNICEF sounded the alarm about the effects of air pollution on brain development. The effects of these exposures may not become apparent until later in life, when they show up in symptoms such as learning difficulties, attention deficits or emotional problems.

Nutrition and Cognitive Development

What and how much food a newborn is fed is probably the single greatest influence on its cognitive development. As noted, breast milk is the nutritional gold standard. Healthy brain development requires specific nutrients: protein; healthy fats, such as omega-3 fatty acids; the minerals iron, zinc, copper and selenium; vitamin A and folate; and the amino acid choline.

We know that inadequate nutrition detrimentally affects cognition and behavior. Even moderate shortfalls in nutrition have been linked with poor academic performance. Poor nutrition has also been associated with emotional problems, such as depression and anxiety, and behavioral problems, such as hyperactivity. One study showed that children who were not well nourished in their first two years tended to be socially inadequate and withdrawn.

OMEGA-3 FATTY ACIDS

Docosahexaenoic acid (DHA) and eicosapentaenoic acid (EPA) are omega-3 fatty acids that have numerous health benefits, from supporting fertility and healthy fetal development to keeping your brain healthy in old age. The best sources of these fats are oily fish, such as salmon, mackerel and sardines, and fish oil supplements. If you are an omnivore, moderate or regular consumption of meat from healthy animals (pasture-raised beef, lamb, pork and poultry), and eggs from yard-roaming chickens, can also help to boost omega-3 levels.

Obtaining adequate amounts of omega-3s is more complex for vegetarians and vegans. Plant sources (flax seeds and walnuts are among the best) provide alpha-linolenic acid (ALA), a precursor to both DHA and EPA. The trouble is, ALA is not easily converted to active omega-3 fatty acids in the body. Studies do show, however, that people who don't eat fish may have an improved ability to convert ALA to DHA and EPA — their blood levels of these fatty acids are comparable to those in people who consume fish. Even so, nutritionists recommend that people following a plant-based diet take omega-3 supplements.

Happy Children Grow Better

While good nutrition is probably the most important building block to support healthy development during this period, other "softer" factors, such as the child's physical environment and socioeconomic status, play increasingly significant roles. It's common knowledge that happy children grow better. Childhood growth is controlled by hormones — insulin at first, then growth hormone, which takes over around a child's first birthday. The release of these substances is controlled by the brain, which means that psychological distress may undermine healthy growth even when an infant is appropriately nourished.

Based on a review of the literature published in 2011, psychologist Gregory Miller suggested that various stressors, such as poverty and abuse during early childhood, could modify certain types of brain cells and affect brain development. Miller speculated that stress likely gets programmed into a type of white blood cell known as a macrophage via epigenetic marking. This programming predisposes the cells toward inflammation. In addition, the life circumstances of socially disadvantaged or poorly treated children make them more prone to poor lifestyle choices (including a nutrient-deficient diet) and possibly vulnerable to more serious behavioral problems. Early stress also permanently affects the metabolism, particularly hormonal patterns. All these effects create a cascade of changes that work together to support the development of chronic disease at a later age.

At this stage of development, the most important things to a baby are interactions with their significant others. Children need to feel protected and loved. If they don't feel secure, their neural pathways will develop in ways that emphasize survival rather than learning. Many of these factors are beyond parental control. For instance, poverty can initiate a cascade of negative impacts. As Frank Oberklaid, a pediatrician and expert on child development, commented in the research paper "The First Thousand Days," children need more than a loving and supportive environment at home. They also need "safe communities, secure housing, access to green spaces, environments free from toxins and access to affordable nutritious foods."

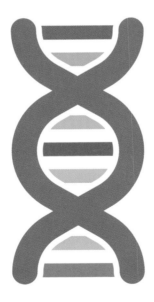

6

CHILDHOOD

— AND —

ADOLESCENCE

People who develop chronic disease grow differently as children.

— DAVID BARKER, *NUTRITION IN THE WOMB*

T HERE'S LITTLE DOUBT THAT the first thousand days of life, from the moment of conception until your child's second birthday, is a particularly important period of development because that's when organs are being formed and their functions are established. Thanks to what experts call "developmental plasticity," even small adjustments made during that time can have significant consequences later in life. However, all body systems remain plastic throughout puberty, and the brain continues to develop into the twenties.

Although childhood is a different stage than the first thousand days, it is no less important for the health and well-being of children. That means there's a lot parents can do to foster healthy development after a child passes the age of two. Good nutrition continues to play a meaningful role in how children develop and grow throughout their childhood and adolescence. So, too, do their life experiences. Not all of these factors are within parental control, but how they weave together are threads in the fabric of children's health and well-being for the rest of their lives.

CHILDHOOD

After celebrating their second birthday, your child is likely walking steadily, carefully climbing and descending stairs, and chattering in simple sentences, among other accomplishments. It's exciting to watch them develop on so many different levels: physically (growing taller and putting on weight), emotionally (beginning to show signs of empathy and concern for others) and cognitively (developing capabilities such as eye/hand coordination and problem-solving skills). While all advancements aren't necessarily welcome — for instance, a tendency to become impatient and more prone to temper tantrums — these phases are definable stages of development. Although every child is unique, in general terms experts can determine how well your child is doing by when they meet certain milestones, such as the rate at which they grow, how their gross motor, language and thinking skills are developing, and their ability to successfully interact in social situations.

Milestones

Milestones are important, in part, because how a child grows and develops influences their risk of chronic disease later in life. For instance, children who are born small but whose BMI increases rapidly between the ages of three and fifteen are more vulnerable to developing hypertension as adults (see "The Developmental Origins of Hypertension," page 199). And, in a 2007 study published in the journal *Stroke*, David Barker and his colleagues showed that those who are short and thin at two years old and remain small are more likely to have a stroke later in life.

One problem is that it's not usually noticeable when children grow differently from the norm. Unless their growth is recorded from birth, their risk of developing chronic disease may fly under the radar. Hence, the value of milestones. When milestones aren't met, experts can look for causes and begin to take preventive steps.

Good nutrition is one tool for helping keep children on the proper growth trajectory, and its benefits begin early. Researchers tell us that a healthy diet in early childhood can modulate some of the negative effects resulting from epigenetic changes triggered in utero. For instance, studies based on information from the Helsinki Birth Cohort Study suggest that when children with birth weights that fall into the normal range for their population are subjected to appropriate interventions to keep childhood BMI in check between the ages of three and eleven, the incidence of later type 2 diabetes in the population is reduced by half.

A nutrient-dense diet will also help to ensure that those body systems that are still quite plastic in children, such as the brain, liver and immune system, will develop properly. Because all parts of their bodies are still developing, children have a vital need for the nutrients that a healthy, balanced diet provides. Those who do not receive adequate nutrition become nutrient-depleted and malnourished.

The Musculoskeletal System

Young children are actively engaged in developing numerous body systems, including muscles and bone. The strength of your child's bones is established in the womb and early in life. By the time they reach adolescence, their bone mineral density has been established; this occurs between the ages of 11 and 14 for girls and after puberty for boys.

Bone mineral density determines the risk for certain conditions later in life (osteoporosis being the most obvious) and it is highly dependent on how a child grows. Studies show that children who grow slowly in early life and more rapidly later on are more likely to suffer from osteoporosis and hip fractures as adults. As David Barker pointed out, bones need to grow at a slow, steady pace. This allows adequate time for calcium salts to be properly set down. If proper mineralization doesn't occur, when minerals begin to dissipate in old age, as they naturally do, weak bones and fractures are a likely result.

Permanent teeth (with the exception of so-called wisdom teeth) are also formed early in life. You may not think teeth are significant in the grand scheme of overall wellness, but experts tell us that dental health is about much more than cosmetics. Teeth are good indicators of physical well-being; for example, stressors such as poor nutrition show up in teeth — the link between too much sugar and dental cavities is well known. Aspects of poor oral health have been linked with conditions such as heart disease and shorter life expectancy.

Fortunately, we have a good idea of the nutrients it takes to build strong bones and teeth. Calcium, found in foods such as dairy products and leafy greens, and vitamin D, which comes from sunshine as well as oily fish and egg yolks, are particularly valuable. Magnesium, which is abundant in whole grains, nuts and seeds, works closely with both those nutrients to strengthen bones and teeth.

Obesity

One in three children (and two in three adults) in the United States are either overweight or obese. That's an alarming statistic. Obesity is a complex condition (see page 165), and although we don't understand all the mechanisms, in general terms obesity seems to be related to the body's systems for regulating energy. Babies born at both the low and high ends of the birth-weight scale tend to be at greater risk for obesity. Another risk factor for children who grew poorly in the womb is rapid weight gain after the age of two.

So-called catch-up growth is a common part of children's development. When they are ill, for instance, it's normal for their growth to slow, but their bodies make up for the setback after recovery. However, when catch-up growth is driven by slow growth extending back to the womb, a precipitous rise in a child's BMI is especially problematic. It can, for instance, interfere with muscle development. David Barker noted that the time in utero and the first year of life are the critical period for muscle growth. Sometime around their first birthday, a baby stops making new muscle. If they start to gain weight rapidly after the age of two, fat will accumulate and their ratio of fat to muscle will be thrown out of whack. This means that as an adult, they will have a high proportion of fat in relation to muscle. This unfavorable ratio leads to insulin resistance, which is linked not only to obesity but also to diabetes and heart disease, among other conditions.

Surprisingly, research based on data from the Dutch Hunger Winter established that malnutrition in early life also increases the risk of being overweight as an adult. When researchers studied more than 8,000 women affected by that famine, they found that those who were most severely exposed to hunger between birth and nine years of age were 25 percent more likely to have an elevated BMI as adults.

Metabolic Networking

Metabolic abnormalities are one factor that influences obesity. Susan Prescott noted numerous connections between a child's metabolism and their immune system in her book *Origins*. Not only is the immune system constantly engaged with a child's metabolism, but both systems are regulated by the same hormones — those that control appetite and fat storage. According to Dr. Prescott, when children are obese, they are also more likely to develop asthma and food allergies. Once allergies develop, leptin, the appetite hormone (see "What Is Leptin and Why Should You Care about It?" page 172), may come into play. Leptin levels are higher in people with allergies, and leptin influences metabolism. Leptin may also fan the flames of an allergic response, which, in turn, provokes the release of more leptin from fat stores. As Dr. Prescott sees it, the relationship between allergy and obesity is likely a two-way street, with obesity affecting allergy and vice versa.

Diet may be another link between the immune system and obesity. Diets that are low in fiber and high in unhealthy fat (features of processed foods) reduce the richness of the microbiota, the bacteria in your gut (see chapter 9). Obese people have been shown to have low levels of certain beneficial bacteria. Feeding your child a diet of nutritious whole foods that are high in fiber will help to promote a healthy weight and support the growth of supportive bacteria in their gut.

The Immune System

Allergic responses are very common in young children, and these days their prevalence seems to be on the rise. While infants and children have always been particularly vulnerable to allergies because their immune systems aren't fully developed, many experts now believe that environmental factors play a significant role in their increasing incidence. The basic theory is that young children in industrialized societies aren't exposed to a wide enough assortment of germs. For starters, consider the vast number of antibacterial soaps, shampoos and so on in common use. Like nutrient-deficient diets, these environmental influences limit children's exposure to beneficial microbes, undermining how their immune systems develop.

One study that looked at the *gut flora* of 757 infants (published in the *Canadian Medical Association Journal* in 2018) buttressed the links between allergy, obesity and the microbiota. The researchers found that commonly used household disinfectants altered the gut flora of infants and toddlers. The more the products were used, the greater the increase in Lachnospiraceae, a family of bacteria thought to contribute to metabolic dysfunctions such as obesity. The offending products had the greatest effect on the youngest subjects, babies three to four months old. By the time they were three years old, their BMI was higher than in children who had not been exposed to high levels of these cleaners. The study also found that children who lived in households that used standard detergents or eco-friendly cleaners had more favorable gut bacteria and were less likely to be overweight.

Your child's gut is a vital component of their immune system, and you can actively support it by nourishing their *microbial diversity* even before they are born. Although research is in the early stages, some studies are showing that when pregnant women take *probiotics* (beneficial bacteria), their offspring are less likely to be allergic. So, too, when they consume a nutritious diet that includes supplementation with fish oil. But once your child begins to eat solid food, a wholesome, fiber-rich diet is an important tool for supporting development of their immune system.

Various components in whole foods are known to promote a healthy gut. Children have a particular need for fiber — found in fruits, vegetables, whole grains and legumes — because fiber is one of the best foods for promoting the growth of beneficial bacteria. Researchers have identified links between high-fiber foods and strong immune systems. For instance, one 2006 Dutch study found that children who ate whole grains were 54 percent less likely to develop asthma and 45 percent less likely to develop wheezing than those whose diets did not provide whole grains. Other nutrients that support immune system development include vitamin C (found in high amounts in citrus fruits and vegetables such as bell peppers and leafy greens) and the mineral zinc (found in seafood, legumes and whole grains).

Autism and the Immune System

The benefits of a robust *microbiome* aren't limited to physical health. Some experts are now looking into the links between gut health and conditions such as autism, which may be connected via the immune system. We know, for instance, that the guts of autistic children have what experts describe as a "distinct bacterial signature," and that the risk of autism in the offspring may increase if a woman has an allergic reaction while pregnant. Research has also shown that certain genes involved in immune responses are methylated differently in children with autism. Piecing these various factors together, a 2016 paper published in *Frontiers in Neuroscience* concluded that when the mother has an allergic reaction, a genetically predisposed fetus may respond with epigenetic changes that affect its own immune system. An autism disorder is a possible result. Research is in the early stages, but studies are examining the use of probiotics to treat autism; the results, although mixed, appear to show some promise.

Genes, the Gut and the Immune System

Genes, the environment and epigenetic changes influence immune system development, both in the womb and in early life. Consider, for example, the results of a Dutch study. When researchers examined a group of children who were allergic to cow's milk, they found that, compared to a control group, the allergic children had several genes that were differently methylated. These genes are known to be involved in immunological pathways associated with other allergies. Another study, published in 2015 in the *ISME Journal*, found differences in the gut bacteria of children who were allergic to cow's milk, compared to healthy controls. After being treated with probiotics, some of the previously allergic children were able to tolerate cow's milk. When the researchers looked a little deeper, they found that this new tolerance could be linked not only to the treatment but also to the species of bacteria that already inhabited the children's guts. Those who improved after taking the probiotics had more beneficial gut bacteria to start with — specifically, higher levels of species that produce a particular short-chain fatty acid. Those who didn't become tolerant had a very different microbial profile.

The Brain

The period before your child starts school is a time of rapid cognitive development. Like their immune systems, children's brains are still quite plastic and, therefore, especially sensitive to environmental influences, including emotional experiences (both positive and negative) and nutrition. Researchers have linked poor nutrition with delayed development of intellectual and motor skills, and have found that good nutrition supports cognitive development. One Finnish study that monitored the academic performance of children in the first to third grades found that those whose diets emphasized fruits, vegetables, fish, whole grains and nuts could read better and more effectively than those whose daily dietary intake was less nutritious.

Children's Brains Are Ravenous

Children's brains burn up about 20 percent of their caloric intake, so they require a significant amount of energy in the form of nutritious food. They also need energy to support their robust physical activity, which, in turn, stimulates brain development. Their emotions are developing rapidly too. Experts tell us that children who consume a nutritious diet can cope with stress and are better equipped to control their emotions.

Because so much of their behavior can't be controlled, toddlers and preschoolers are difficult to study. As a result, research has focused on measuring milestones of cognitive development, such as the ability to pay attention and retain memories. The brain requires a wide range of nutrients to support these developmental processes, which are extremely complex. Necessary nutrients include choline, folate, iron, zinc and certain fats.

Early childhood is a critical time to ensure adequate supplies of DHA, the omega-3 fatty acid found in fish oil. DHA has been found to enhance children's ability to solve problems and to improve how their nervous systems function. Recent science supports the traditional wisdom that fish is brain food, likely thanks to its omega-3 content. A 2017 study of 541 twelve-year-old Chinese schoolchildren, published in *Scientific Reports*, found that children who ate fish frequently scored significantly higher on IQ tests than those who never or seldom consumed fish. In addition, the study found that the children who ate more fish also enjoyed better-quality sleep, a potential benefit for how well they function cognitively over the long term.

Iron also supports cognitive development. Iron supplementation (carefully undertaken, as iron poisoning is common in children) for longer than four months has been shown to improve mental performance and motor-skill functions in children younger

Attention Deficit Hyperactivity Disorder

Attention deficit hyperactivity disorder (ADHD) is one of the most common neurobehavioral disorders diagnosed in childhood. It affects about 5 percent of children worldwide. ADHD is a complex condition (some experts believe it is a cluster of symptoms rather than a disease in itself) that develops in childhood or adolescence. It is characterized by hyperactivity, inability to concentrate, temper tantrums and/or impulsivity. It may also be linked with short-term memory problems, insomnia, mood swings and even depression.

Studies conducted in the United States suggest that up to 11 percent of children in that country aged 4 to 17 are affected by the condition. Some experts believe that ADHD is being overdiagnosed. Gender disparity is another concern: the male-female ratio may be as high as 10:1, possibly because boys exhibit disruptive behavior more often than girls. In the United States ADHD appears to be increasing dramatically in children from low-income families. Between 2003 and 2007 the incidence of ADHD in kids raised in poverty rose by 60 percent, compared to a 10-percent rise among those from higher-income groups.

No single cause has been linked to ADHD, but one 2008 Finnish study, published in the *American Journal of Psychiatry*, found that babies who had a very low birth weight (less than 1,500 grams) were at increased risk. Maternal smoking during pregnancy is also a strong risk factor. While studies are mixed about the effects of maternal alcohol consumption, we know that alcohol reduces the availability of folate to the developing fetus.

Folate deficiency undermines the function of neurotransmitters such as dopamine and serotonin, which have been implicated in the development of ADHD. An epigenetic connection is likely, because methylation affects the functioning of genes related to these neurotransmitters. Adequate amounts of folate, as well as vitamins B_{12} and B_6, are critical during pregnancy. These nutrients directly impact DNA methylation patterns that are being established in the brain of the developing fetus.

If left untreated, ADHD can continue into adulthood. About 5 percent of the adult population and as many as 20 percent of those with a mental health disorder are affected by ADHD. Adults who live with it say it undermines every area of their lives.

Treating ADHD

Drugs are often the first line of treatment for ADHD. Between 2004 and 2011, 6 percent of children in the United States between the ages of 4 and 17 were taking medication. Whether these pharmaceuticals are being overprescribed is a topic of active debate among the medical community. While some effectively manage symptoms, all have been associated with a range of risk factors.

Avoid Environmental Toxins

Exposure during pregnancy to environmental toxins such as organophosphates (pesticides) and phthalates (used to make soft plastics) has been associated with increased risk that a child will develop ADHD. There is also a strong link between elevated lead levels in children and the development of the condition. The Flint, Michigan, water crisis, which dominated the North American news throughout 2016, highlighted the problem with "legacy lead." Since the virtual elimination of lead from gasoline and other consumer products in the United States, lead-based paint in homes remains the major source of exposure among US children.

There also appears to be a link between ADHD and exposure to industrial chemicals. Research conducted in New Bedford, Massachusetts, an area that was industrialized early in US history, identified that boys who were exposed to higher levels of polychlorinated biphenyls (PCBs) in utero had poorer concentration, which is a predictor of ADHD.

While environmental exposures are inevitable, their negative effect can be checked by taking extra care, particularly during pregnancy, infancy and a child's first years. For instance, choosing organic foods when possible and drinking out of glass or metal containers limits exposures to pesticides, BPA and phthalates (both found in plastic), all of which have been associated with hyperactivity.

Parents who have easy access to medical care should have their children's blood levels of lead checked at one and two years of age, because exposure will show up during the first two years of life, peaking between 18 and 24 months.

Provide a Nutritious Diet Based on Whole Foods

Childhood ADHD has been linked to typical nutrient-deficient dietary patterns associated with developed countries — in other words, a high percentage of processed foods. Key components include foods high in fat, refined sugars and sodium, and low in fiber, folate and omega-3 fatty acids. And although the United States Department of Agriculture (USDA) maintains that artificial food colorings are safe, studies have linked food dyes with ADHD.

Various mineral deficiencies have been specifically implicated in the condition. A 2002 study found that 84 percent of a group of children with ADHD had abnormally low levels of iron. It also concluded that the greater the deficiency, the more severe their symptoms. Numerous studies have linked ADHD with zinc deficiency. Again, the lower the levels of zinc, the more hyperactive the children. Zinc is necessary for synthesizing neurotransmitters such as dopamine and serotonin. We know that certain environmental toxins, such as BPA and phthalates, bind to zinc and deplete it from the body. Foods rich in both zinc and iron include beef, turkey, sesame and pumpkin seeds, lentils, chickpeas (garbanzo beans) and quinoa.

A small study of children with ADHD found that 72 percent were deficient in magnesium. Magnesium is known as a calming and relaxing mineral that helps the body cope with stress. Increasing dietary magnesium can reduce irritability and improve attention span. Obtaining adequate magnesium can be challenging. Levels of the mineral have been depleted in soil, and refined foods are notoriously low in it. Refined grains are among the worst offenders: refining grains removes as much as 80 percent of their magnesium. On the other hand, most whole grains provide magnesium, as do pumpkin and sesame seeds, Swiss chard, spinach, cashews and legumes (beans and lentils).

than three. It's also worth noting that children's bodies are actively manufacturing myelin, a layer of protective insulation that surrounds some nerves, and that iron is one of the nutrients required for its development.

Fast-Food Nightmare

At a certain stage, children begin to select their own foods, and as everyone knows, kids love junk food, especially candy and other sugary treats. You don't need a background in science to see the effect sugar has on kids. For starters, it causes their blood sugar to soar, and although studies don't support this conclusion, most people feel that too much sugar really gets kids wired up. What parent hasn't experienced birthday parties with a horde of kids running wild? But sugar isn't the only suspect linked with such out-of-control behavior. Processed foods also contain additives, such as food coloring and preservatives, that are likely to trigger chemical and physiological changes in children's brains. These substances can affect how children behave, sparking mood swings, temper tantrums and an inability to sleep.

It's easy to blame families (especially mothers) for kids' addiction to processed foods, but truth be told, we are all being victimized by a wide range of forces beyond our control. I vividly remember when my almost-two-year-old daughter returned from an outing with her playgroup friends chanting, "Donald's, Donald's, fries, fries." I immediately realized that, although I'd done a good job of outlawing junk food from our house, unless I wanted to destroy her social life, bad food choices were destined to creep in. (On a positive note, I also remember her as a baby sitting in her high chair, banging her spoon and demanding "'cado, 'cado" — the mashed avocado I'd introduced her to early in her solid-food regime.)

For more than half a century food companies have been seducing children with the joys of processed foods, using TV advertising to lead the way. I remember discovering sugary breakfast cereals — in my case Sugar Frosted Flakes, pitched by Tony the Tiger — by watching ads on TV. I asked my mother, who, bless her heart, was very old-fashioned when it came to food, to buy them for me. Until then I had always enjoyed a bowl of freshly cooked old-fashioned rolled oats for breakfast, which my mother, who worked at home, had time to prepare every morning.

Now I know she knew best. Hundreds, if not thousands, of studies have linked the consumption of whole grains with a panoply of health benefits because they are loaded with nutrients, many (if not all) of which work together to promote health. For instance, one serving of oatmeal provides about 4 grams of dietary fiber, a range of B vitamins, and minerals such as manganese, iron, phosphorus and magnesium, in addition to a cascade of beneficial phytonutrients. It also contains just 1 gram of sugar. Although it's difficult to make exact nutritional comparisons between the two, Tony the Tiger's breakfast offering isn't nearly as nutritious, even when I was lapping it up decades ago. For starters, it provides less than 1 gram of fiber and almost 12 grams of sugar, which, of course, was a significant part of its appeal.

Sugarland

I'm old enough to have missed the processed food companies' full-frontal marketing assault on children, which really geared up in the 1980s. However, deceptive advertising is just part of the problem. An abundance of evidence suggests that packaged food companies are deliberately revving up the content of crave-worthy substances like sugar in order to hook consumers, especially children, on their products.

Consider a 2017 article by journalist Danny Hakim, published in the *New York Times*, which explored the evolution of Honey Nut Cheerios. At that point it was America's best-selling breakfast cereal. The product was introduced in 1979 as a spin-off from Cheerios, an oat cereal launched in 1941. As Hakim pointed out, not only does Honey Nut Cheerios contain about nine times as much sugar as the original Cheerios, but the cereal's name is misleading. The product has more sugar than honey and not one fragment of nuts, unless you allow almond flavoring to make the cut.

THE CASE AGAINST SUGAR

In his thoughtful and well-researched book *The Case Against Sugar*, science journalist Gary Taubes linked the overconsumption of sugar with the epidemics of obesity, metabolic syndrome, type 2 diabetes and heart disease. While it's not uncommon to come across these associations, you might be surprised to learn that sugar may also be a dietary trigger for Alzheimer's disease. Taubes suggested that the route is insulin resistance, which some experts believe can be caused by the sugars we consume. As much as 20 years ago, researchers were seeing that, in Taubes's words, "direct or indirect effects of insulin could contribute to the risk of dementia." Studies show that people with type 2 diabetes are almost twice as likely to develop Alzheimer's as those without the disease. Today the connections between the two diseases are so strong that some researchers are now referring to Alzheimer's as "type 3 diabetes" (see "Risk Factors for Dementia and Alzheimer's Disease," page 255.)

HOOKED ON FOOD

As a society, our health has been declining over the past 25 years, and medical scientists are now predicting the unthinkable: today's young people will be the first generation to live shorter lives than their parents. The reason? To a large extent, three generations of consuming the so-called standard American diet, which is high in processed food. Although the numbers vary depending on the source, experts agree that North Americans consume about 70 percent of their calories in processed foods.

Sugar is just one of the tools that food companies use to encourage dependence on their products. Sugar helps to make us, in the words of investigative journalist Michael Moss, "heavy users" of processed foods. In his blistering book *Salt Sugar Fat: How the Food Giants Hooked Us*, Moss presented a frightening case, documenting the tactics processed-food purveyors use to exploit not only vulnerable children but also socially and economically disadvantaged people. Subtly (and not so subtly), industry scientists and marketers condition customers to consume nutrient-deficient, calorie-dense foods by enticing them with not only the "bliss point" of sugar, but also the pleasurable "mouthfeel" of fat and the hugely addictive power of salt. Make no mistake, said Moss, processed food companies invest significant amounts of money in creating foods that make you feel happy and, as a result, will turn you into a heavy user — their ultimate goal.

Is it any surprise that in the fast-food universe the word *addiction* frequently crops up? In 2017 Dr. Richard A. Friedman, a professor of clinical psychiatry at Cornell University, published an article in the *New York Times* that sketched out connections between certain pleasure centers in the brain and fast food. Like sex and recreational drugs, food triggers the release of dopamine, a neurotransmitter linked with the experience of pleasure. Your likelihood of becoming addicted to that pleasurable experience is influenced by your natural supplies of certain dopamine receptors known as D2s. The basic gist is that some people have fewer D2s in the reward circuits of the brain — those who are chronically stressed, for instance. These people are, therefore, more likely to become addicted to the gratification provided by processed foods.

Another problem with processed food is that the more you eat, the more you want. Every bite of chemically altered food takes you farther down the fast-food rabbit hole, gradually decreasing D2 receptor levels. The more processed foods you eat, the lower your D2 levels, and the lower your D2 levels, the more likely you are to crave processed foods. As Dr. Friedman wrote, "It's a vicious cycle in which more exposure begets more craving."

The good news is that the cycle can be broken. Laboratory studies tell us that making positive changes to an animal's environment increases the number of D2 receptors in its brain. One implication for humans is that limiting access to cheap, calorie-dense foods will reduce their consumption. Community interventions to improve the food environment by, for example, making healthier options more available, have produced positive results (see "Food Insecurity," page 152).

Convenience is another issue. Part of the appeal of fast food is that it requires little effort: just open the package and eat. Making sure your house is not stocked with junk food and having easy-to-access healthier options on hand — such as fresh fruit, presliced veggies, unsweetened yogurt, nuts, granola and whole-grain bread — will go a long way toward helping children develop healthier eating habits.

As we learn more about the role beneficial gut bacteria play in health and well-being (see chapter 9), emerging research shows that the high levels of sugar consumed in a typical Western-style diet negatively affect bacterial diversity. A 2018 mouse study published in the journal *Proceedings of the National Academy of Sciences of the USA* found that a diet high in sugar blocked production of a protein (Roc) that enables a specific species of beneficial bacteria to colonize the gut. These bacteria, *Bacteroides thetaiotaomicron*, are usually found in the microbiomes of lean and healthy people.

The problem is, unless you cook everything from scratch, using only whole foods, it's extremely difficult to escape refined sugar in the contemporary food chain. These days sugar is routinely added to prepared foods such as soups and sauces. It even turns up in "health foods" like yogurt. Sugar is one of the weapons food scientists routinely use to manipulate our taste buds. They may start by getting kids hooked on sugary cereals, but they actively continue their marketing of processed foods throughout our lives, pitching foods like sodas, potato chips, ready-to-eat meals and so on to all of us at every turn.

Junk Food Propagates

Simply stated, our addiction to junk food is ruining our health — and the health of generations to come. Thanks to shrewd marketing and sophisticated food science, our society has become hooked on the kinds of junk food that kids learn to love from an early age. We now know that indulging these appetites has long-term negative effects because, as Kent Thornburg points out, junk foods are harmful in several different ways. First, they provide excessive amounts of sugar, salt, harmful fats and calories, while providing few, if any, nutrients. People who regularly consume highly processed food eventually gain excess body fat. Because they don't get enough nutrients, they also become malnourished, leading to the condition known as high-calorie malnutrition.

Dr. Thornburg also notes that the effects of malnourishment can be passed on to the next generation and beyond. Basically, wholesome foods contain nutrients that promote healthy epigenetic changes in the body's cells, including the sperm and eggs that generate offspring. When crucial nutrients are missing, genes are not properly regulated. Those negative messages are recorded and may be passed on to future generations.

The Big Picture

Experts tell us that it is challenging to study the effects of poor nutrition on its own because a child's diet is usually part of a bigger package. How and what they eat is determined by their unique circumstances. Family stress (which may include low social and economic status) and poor nutrition often exist simultaneously, and they are tightly interwoven. For instance, poor nutrition influences how well we cope with stress, and stress affects neuro-endocrine mechanisms, which among other functions support energy balance.

Chronic Stress

Chronic stress profoundly affects health, beginning in the womb and continuing through infancy and childhood. If a mother is depressed when her child is an infant (sadly, not an uncommon situation), her emotional state influences her ability to form strong attachment bonds with her baby. Poor attachment has been linked with a wide range of psychological problems later in life. Babies of depressed mothers are likely to have increased levels of stress hormones, such as cortisol. As preschoolers, they are more likely to be anxious and socially withdrawn.

Some of the effects of family stress show up as changes in gene expression. For instance, infants whose mothers are highly stressed have higher levels of methylation (although DNA methylation levels change over the course of a lifetime). A mother's influence is strongest in infancy. A father's contributions (or lack thereof) show up later, and they tend to have a greater impact on daughters. When fathers are highly stressed, their daughters are more likely to demonstrate altered methylation patterns in their preschool years. A father's absence or low commitment to parenting has been linked with the earlier onset of puberty and a difficult temperament in his female offspring.

Among other physical conditions, early-life adversity has been associated with the development of gastrointestinal problems such as irritable bowel syndrome and inflammatory bowel disease. A 2017 study published in the journal *Neurogastroenterology & Motility* found that chronic stress triggered increased sensitivity to pain in areas associated with the gut, which, in turn, initiated changes in gene expression.

Poverty Is All-Encompassing

In addition to being malnourished, children who grow up in poverty may be more likely to experience unsettling family disruptions. They may not receive adequate affirmative attention from their parents, who may (necessarily) be more focused on surviving the trials and tribulations of daily life. They are also less likely to have access to enriching resources like books and travel. For various reasons, including access to transportation and the expense involved in participating, their involvement in extracurricular activities such as sports, which promote physical and mental health, is probably reduced. Instead, they are likely to spend more time being sedentary. Among other risks, sedentary behavior sparks changes in gene expression that contribute to metabolic disorders such as obesity.

Poor children are also likely to be poorly housed — perhaps even homeless. Inadequate housing is associated with a wide range of problems. These include physical effects like overcrowding and increased exposure to air pollution and other toxins, such as mold. Not surprisingly, a greater incidence of respiratory illnesses has been linked to poor living conditions. Children's mental health is likely to be affected as well. Deteriorating or poorly maintained buildings may be fire and safety hazards. Because it is less likely to be safe, living in a low-income neighborhood increases the fear of being victimized by crime. It's not surprising that growing up in substandard housing has been found to have a pervasive effect on health and well-being that lasts throughout life. To paraphrase Winston Churchill, we create our architecture, then our architecture creates us.

Growing up in poverty is much more than a single experience. It is systemic. The experience exposes a child to ongoing risks on a constant basis. The accumulation of those impacts has a pervasive influence on mental and physical health later in life. Psychiatrist Gustavo Turecki, a Canadian expert on suicide who has linked early-life adversity to a significant association with suicide and suicidal behavior, has tied this association to epigenetic changes that may affect physiological development.

FOOD INSECURITY

Good nutrition is the foundation of healthy growth, but not all children have access to a consistent supply of nutritious food, even if they live in a developed country. Studies have shown that many children in North America — even some who get enough calories — are nutrient-deprived. This situation is most likely to affect but is not always restricted to low-income families, and is known as food insecurity.

Food insecurity exists when an individual or family:

- Cannot afford to purchase nutritious whole foods. In these situations, less expensive, energy-dense (high in calories but low in nutrients) food is the basis of their diet.

- Limits their quantity of food because they cannot afford to provide adequate portions. In these cases, they may have a tendency to overeat when food is plentiful.

- Lives in a "food desert" — a geographic area that is distant enough (usually about a mile in urban areas, 10 miles in rural) from a source of fresh foods, such as fruits, vegetables and whole grains, to limit regular access.

The concept of food insecurity recognizes that eating behavior is influenced by the environment. Food insecurity is associated with increased consumption of processed foods that are high in calories, as well as ingredients such as salt, sugar and unhealthy fats. Various studies have connected the dots between food insecurity and health problems such as obesity and related conditions, including cardiovascular disease and type 2 diabetes.

The effects of food insecurity on young children are particularly devastating. Researchers have termed aspects of this problem the *hunger/obesity paradox*, a term that was first coined in 1995 by Dr. William Dietz in the journal *Pediatrics*. He included a case study of a seven-year-old girl who was more than 200 percent heavier than her ideal weight. Her family was on welfare and often consumed processed foods because they couldn't afford healthier options. Since then other studies have confirmed that a key driver of obesity is the overconsumption of calories that lack nutrients.

By the time a child turns four, they may be showing signs of obesity related to experience of food insecurity as an infant and toddler. Connections between food insecurity and other nutrition-related conditions have also been established. For instance, one study of low-income children younger than three linked food insecurity with iron-deficiency anemia. Another associated it with learning and developmental problems, such as emotional difficulties and low achievement in school.

Solutions to food insecurity include a variety of social and community programs to ensure not only that nutritious food is available but also that it is accessible. Well-designed school meal programs have been shown to be extremely beneficial, particularly for children at risk, both in terms of improving their performance at school and also in helping to counteract the risk of chronic disease later in life. Improving access to nutritious food through community outreach, with projects such as community gardens and setting up farmers' markets in food deserts, has also been beneficial. Recently, programs to support selling fresh fruits and vegetables in corner stores have been established in many locations.

ADOLESCENCE

The word *adolescence*, which defines the period between childhood and adulthood (from 10 to 19 years of age) is derived from the Latin word *adolescere*, which means "to grow up." It is a rapid phase of human development. In addition to physical growth, it includes brain development and sexual maturation. Adolescents are no longer children, but they are certainly not adults. This is the time when young women are building up their bodies in preparation for reproduction. To develop properly, they need a healthy diet, lots of exercise and a supportive environment that is low in stress. Adolescence is also when both sexes become more independent from their parents and are particularly vulnerable to peer group pressure. Understandably, navigating this period of transition is challenging — not only for teens, but also for their parents and everyone involved with them.

Although the research is still in its early stages, evidence suggests that young adulthood may be a time when fault lines linked to future health first appear. For instance, adolescent girls are particularly susceptible to the pressures of social stress. Studies have shown that this vulnerability may affect how their brains develop and might predispose them to mental illness as adults (see "Experience Influences Biology," page 84).

In males, the rifts may show up in puberty, when sperm are forming. When boys smoke around this time, the toxic exposure induces epigenetic changes that can be passed on to their offspring (see "It's More Than Genes," page 36).

Other problems that show up in adolescence can be traced back to early development. Researchers have linked certain epigenetic changes and hormonal variations originating in utero with teenage impulsivity and risk-taking behavior. Another study shows that adolescents who had a low birth weight are more likely to have hypertension, particularly in response to social stress. They are also predisposed to being socially withdrawn. Adolescent girls who had a low birth weight are more prone to depression and, if they become pregnant, are more likely to give birth to babies with a low birth weight.

We are far from having all the answers, but we do know that early-life experiences, including a child's socioeconomic environment, become biologically embedded via gene expression. The consequences of these alterations may begin to show up in adolescence. The good news is that positive lifestyle changes can influence whether and to what degree genes are expressed. For instance, we know from laboratory studies that physical exercise can benefit adolescent brain development by improving gene expression. Good nutrition is another stimulus for positive change.

Big Soda

Adolescence is a time of accelerated growth. Young people need the benefits of a nutritious diet more than ever just to keep them on top of their pressure-cooker lives. At the same time, teens are making even more independent food choices than they did as children. They have greater access to unhealthy foods and are influenced by advertising and, most significantly, their peers.

Do you remember the song "I'd Like to Teach the World to Sing"? It has a catchy tune and delightfully inclusive lyrics about apple trees and honeybees and love and harmony. But the song didn't originate as a paean to togetherness. It was born as an advertising jingle, the first words of which were "I'd like to buy the world a Coke." It was launched in 1971 as a TV ad and is now recognized as one of the most effective commercials of all time.

Although the power of TV advertising has declined since those golden years, it still wields a hefty clout. A study done in 2013 by the Yale Rudd Center for Food Policy and Obesity showed that, at that point, manufacturers were spending almost a billion dollars (US $866 million) annually on marketing sugary drinks. And from their perspective, it seems to be money well spent. Like it or not, adolescents obtain a significant portion of their daily calories from soda, energy drinks and sports drinks. Twenty percent of high school students drink at least one soda every day, and some drink significantly more. Research from the United Kingdom indicates that its young people between the ages of 11 and 18 drink just over 234 cans of soft drinks per year. That's a lot of added sugar — empty calories that have repeatedly been linked with obesity, which may cascade into type 2 diabetes and eventually heart disease.

Using global data, a 2015 study published in the journal *Circulation* specifically linked the consumption of sugar-sweetened beverages (SSBs) not only with obesity, but also with type 2 diabetes that develops independent of being overweight. In addition, it connected SSBs with cancer and heart disease. Sounding the alarm about the high intake among young adults, who as a group consume far more SSBs than older people, the authors wrote, "The burdens attributable to SSBs are also relatively unique because of their predominant proportional impact on the young." They highlighted the enormous global economic cost related to SSB consumption, estimating that, in people younger than 44, about one in every 20 disability-adjusted life years (the number of years of health and life lost because of ill health, in this case as a result of *adiposity*-related diseases) can be attributed to SSB intake.

Puberty Doesn't Follow a Clock

One problem with trying to plot a course through the stormy seas of adolescence is that puberty, the root cause of most of the *Sturm und Drang*, does not follow a chronological clock. The time frame for sexual maturation varies dramatically among individuals. Generally, it's from 9 to 14 in girls and 12 to 16 in boys. Moreover, the changes associated with puberty occur bit by bit and over an extended period of time. Even experts are challenged by these differences, although recent developments in various fields are shedding some light on the subject. Genes do play a role in when puberty occurs, but it's a small one. Factors such as birth weight, body fat, nutrition, socioeconomic status and environmental exposures are likely more significant.

Adolescence is a time of significant hormonal changes, and puberty is a complex process that occurs on many different levels. Factors such as stress, brain maturation and even behavioral adjustments can institute a wide range of changes in gene expression. We now know that epigenetic changes influence the suppression and release of the hormone

Is a Calorie Just a Calorie?

Conventional wisdom suggests that a calorie is a calorie — that is to say, your body doesn't know the difference between the 50 calories you consume by eating a pear and the 50 calories you ingest from drinking some soda. Whether this is true is passionately debated. Certainly every calorie provides your body with a specific amount of energy, and in that regard they are identical.

One teaspoon (5 mL) of refined sugar provides 15.5 calories in the form of two very simple and unadorned carbohydrates in equal measure: glucose and fructose. But is consuming sugar any more harmful than consuming the newest kid on the block, sugar's more refined and sweeter cousin high-fructose corn syrup (HFCS)? The food industry often adds HFCS to processed foods because it rates higher than other sugars on the taste and likability scale. And as happens whenever a food additive becomes widely used, an active debate about its potential health risks is raging.

One question is, when your body processes sugar, does it treat glucose and fructose in the same way? Dr. Jonathan Purnell, an endocrinologist at Oregon Health & Science University, told me that glucose and fructose are processed differently by the body. "They both get broken down into energy, but they travel different metabolic paths. Also, they have differing energy efficiencies. The end result is that glucose yields more energy per molecule than fructose."

These differences have consequences for cells, organs and the body as a whole. When you consume too much fructose, your liver processes it in ways that are more likely to create fat that builds up in your liver and bloodstream (in the form of triglycerides) and insulin resistance. "Unfortunately, in our popular culture, 'carbs' are synonymous with sugar, which means most people are unaware of this difference," Dr. Purnell said. "However, foods that are rich in complex carbohydrates [such as vegetables and whole grains] — which are made up almost entirely of glucose strung together and which don't naturally contain increased concentrations of fructose — typically don't cause these unhealthy effects."

This is not to say that fructose is evil. When found naturally in fruit, where it's combined with other nutrients such as fiber, vitamins, minerals, phytonutrients and plain old water, it provides a healthy source of energy. It is virtually impossible to get too much fructose from eating whole fruit. The problem arises when fructose is selectively enriched in foods, especially processed foods; the fructose content of HFCS can be as high as 65 percent.

In the 1970s HFCS began to replace sucrose as the main sweetener of soft drinks, which, along with energy drinks and coffee beverages, are now probably the largest source of this carbohydrate in an average diet. About the same time, rates of obesity (along with those of metabolic syndrome and type 2 diabetes) began to rise rapidly. In 1970 about 15 percent of the US population qualified as obese. Today that figure is closer to one-third.

So how have scientists explained the link between sugar-added beverages and the rise of obesity in our population? Rodent studies have helped to connect the dots: obesity rates seem to depend on the amount of fructose consumed. For example, a 2005 study from Germany found that mice that drank concentrated fructose became obese, whereas those fed the equivalent amount of sucrose had an intermediate weight gain relative to consumption of plain water. Another study, published in *Scientific Reports* in 2015, found that ingesting fructose made mice sedentary, which would, of course, encourage weight gain.

It comes back to the fact that the body processes fructose and glucose differently. "Research shows that, as in the liver, the brain centers that control appetite and body weight [the hypothalamus] do not respond in the same way when exposed to fructose compared with glucose," Dr. Purnell told me. "When fructose was injected directly into this brain site of mice, it caused them to eat more. Their reaction to an injection of glucose was no different than for a control solution. But the fructose was less efficient at generating energy for the neuron, which means it stimulated their appetite. The mice needed to consume more fructose before they were satisfied."

Although it's difficult to establish causality, the same effects are thought to hold true for humans. A 2013 proof-of-concept study published in *JAMA* showed that volunteers who drank a beverage made up of glucose exhibited different brain activity patterns in the *hypothalamus* than when they drank a fructose beverage. They also reported a sense of fullness and satiety afterward that did not occur following the fructose drink. These findings align with Dr. Purnell's research. As he noted in an editorial accompanying the *JAMA* study, fructose promotes overconsumption of food by modifying the neurobiological pathways involved in regulating appetite. In our interview he explained, "The data tells us that because fructose is less satiating than glucose, you end up consuming more calories to achieve the same level of fullness."

Over the years, evidence has accumulated to suggest that high doses of fructose have a negative effect on cognitive function, particularly in males. It has also been linked with rising rates of nonalcoholic fatty liver disease and increased triglyceride levels, a risk factor for heart disease. Not surprisingly, research funded by the food industry is being actively generated to counteract these claims. However, we have a lot of proof that concentrated fructose is more harmful than other refined foods. The safest strategy is to assume that, at the very least, it will have a negative impact on food intake and body weight, and to avoid it in processed food products as much as possible, if not completely.

GnRH, which is instrumental in determining when puberty takes place. A 2016 Danish study of 51 healthy children, published in *Scientific Reports*, identified changes in patterns of DNA methylation at more than 450 sites that could predict the onset of puberty.

Menarche

Although time frames vary around the world as well as among individuals, the average age for menarche in North America is around 12.5 years old, with slight variations among racial groups. Data are scant, but over the past 50 years girls have gradually been getting their periods at a younger age. In the mid-19th century menarche occurred at about age 16, in 1900 it was at about 14 years old, and today it happens at about age 12. Different studies show different rates of change, but it is clear that the onset of menstruation has decreased over the past 150 years. Menstruation that starts at age 11 or younger is defined as early menarche, which is a risk factor for diseases including heart disease, stroke and breast cancer.

Because most breast cancers are fed by estrogen, experts recommend that a woman's supply of estrogen be kept as low as possible. In terms of her life cycle, when a girl begins to menstruate early, the time frame during which her body's cells are exposed to estrogen expands, theoretically increasing her breast cancer risk.

Early menarche has also been associated with depression in adolescence and with developmental issues in offspring. Girls who started menstruating before they turned 12 are more likely to give birth prematurely or to have a baby with a low birth weight, which contributes to the ongoing cycle of chronic disease.

A girl is more apt to experience early menarche if she was born prematurely, had a low birth weight or is obese. Some suspect the decline in the age of menarche in developed countries may be linked with the rising rates of obesity. The hormone leptin may link the two: girls with an above-average ratio of body fat and higher levels of leptin get their periods earlier than most of their peers. Leptin also affects the hypothalamus, the area of the brain associated with gonadotropin-releasing hormone (GnRH), which instructs the pituitary gland to begin releasing the hormones associated with sexual maturation. Studies have also associated early menstruation with exposure to environmental toxins, particularly endocrine-disrupting chemicals.

Adolescent Brains

Many of the major physiological upheavals that take place during adolescence relate to brain development. Puberty initiates a period of colossal reorganization and maturation in the brain. Take, for example, changes to the limbic system. This collection of brain structures is implicated in pleasure-seeking behavior and emotional responses, and it is closely connected to the *prefrontal cortex* — a term that parents of teenagers are likely to be familiar with after seeking answers to why their lovely child has suddenly turned into a terror.

The prefrontal cortex is responsible for executive functions such as decision-making, planning and organization. It also puts a check on impulsiveness. This part of the brain isn't fully developed until people reach their mid-twenties, which means that teens are predisposed to making hasty decisions based on emotional responses without fully assessing the consequences. Their rashness may result in the kind of risky behaviors typically associated with the teenage years, including smoking, drinking alcohol to excess and sexual promiscuity.

But an undeveloped prefrontal cortex isn't the only biological factor underlying adolescent difficulties. A study published in *Archives of General Psychiatry* in 2007 found that low birth weight could be linked with depression in female (but not male) adolescents. The researchers looked at 1,420 participants, 49 percent of whom were female. They found connections between low birth weight, adversity and the development of depression. Like girls with normal birth weight, those whose weight was less than ideal showed no signs of depression so long as they had not experienced any adversity. However, low birth weight made them more vulnerable to problems, with each additional adversity increasing their risk of developing depression. Adversities included socioeconomic factors like poverty and family violence, as well as physical problems like poor health and obesity. Thirty-eight percent of the low-birth-weight girls had at least one depressive episode between the ages of 13 and 16, compared to 8.4 percent of those with a normal birth weight. Only 4.9 percent of the boys in the study demonstrated any signs of depression.

Numerous studies have shown that biological changes in the brain make adolescents more vulnerable to stress. Stress is an environmental trigger that can spark changes in gene expression that may set the stage for mental illness. Stress can also trigger epigenetic changes that lead to physical pain — for instance, what experts describe as "heightened visceral hypersensitivity," a feature of painful gastrointestinal conditions such as irritable bowel syndrome (IBS).

Nutritional Needs in Adolescence

If adolescents seem to be hungrier than anyone else, it's because they are. The adolescent growth spurt, triggered by the pubescent boost in growth hormone, sparks appetite. The teenage body demands more calories than at any other time in life. Adolescent males need an average of 2,800 calories a day; females require an average of 2,200. That's 200 to 400 more calories a day than the average younger child or adult needs.

Although adolescents know a great deal about healthy eating, studies have shown that this knowledge is not likely to translate into nutritious food choices. Most teens tend to consume an abundance of calorie-rich and nutrient-poor processed foods and beverages. It's common for them to skip meals and eat a lot of junk food and fast food. They are also likely to avoid nutritious whole foods, which will have long-term consequences.

An absence of whole grains in the diet provides a case in point. For adolescent girls in particular, whole-grain consumption is linked with lower concentrations of homocysteine, a marker for stroke and cardiovascular risk. Whole grains also provide fiber. A 2016 study published in the journal *Pediatrics* found that breast cancer risk was reduced by as much as 16 percent in women who had high intakes of fiber. Some experts suggest that this positive effect may be because fiber helps to keep estrogen levels in check.

In adolescence, the combination of poor eating habits and higher nutritional needs can lead to nutrient deficiencies. These may show up in symptoms such as fatigue, moodiness, weakness and poor growth. A shortfall of nutrients can also increase the likelihood that a young person will develop obesity, cardiovascular disease, diabetes or osteoporosis as an adult, especially if there is a hereditary epigenetic predisposition.

Take folate, for instance. Studies show that adolescents are likely to be deficient in this B vitamin, which is a shame, as it is particularly beneficial during periods of rapid growth. Another consideration is that many women begin to take oral contraceptives as adolescents. These drugs are known to deplete folate and vitamins B_2, B_6, B_{12}, C and E. Once again, whole grains are helpful. Not only are they an easy way to increase levels of folate and other B vitamins, but these nutritious plant foods have many additional health benefits. One study of adolescents age 12 to 18 found that those with the highest consumption of whole grains had the lowest fasting insulin levels and the highest levels of folate.

Specific Nutrients Required by Adolescents

Although a balanced and varied diet of whole foods is the best overall eating strategy, the following nutrients are particularly beneficial in supporting development through the teenage years.

- **Calcium.** Adolescents have an increased need for calcium because up to half of their adult bone mass develops during this time. Calcium is most abundant in dairy foods, fish, dark leafy greens and legumes.

- **Iron.** A number of developmental processes that take place during adolescence depend on greater-than-usual supplies of iron. As tissues and muscles grow during the adolescent growth spurt, they must be properly oxygenated. That means they need a supply of hemoglobin (a protein in red blood cells) and myoglobin (a protein in muscles). The body requires iron to create both. In addition, in females the onset of menstruation and its associated blood loss depletes iron reserves, increasing the incidence of iron-deficiency anemia. While iron is abundant in many foods, not all sources are equally absorbable. Heme iron, which is found in animal foods such as meat, poultry and fish, is easily absorbed. Nonheme iron, found in plant foods such as dark leafy greens, legumes and whole grains, is not as easily utilized by the body. When obtaining iron from plant foods, it's important to simultaneously consume foods rich in vitamin C, such as citrus fruits, kiwis, bell peppers, Brussels sprouts and broccoli, as vitamin C enhances iron absorption.

- **Zinc.** Healthy growth and sexual maturation increase zinc requirements. This mineral is found in meat, poultry, shellfish, whole grains, beans, nuts and seeds.

- **Folate (vitamin B9).** Adequate intake of this vitamin helps to prevent anemia and support the rapid cell division that occurs during periods of growth. It works to create the building blocks of cells, to produce DNA and RNA, and to make red blood cells. Folate is found in dark leafy greens, vegetables, fruits, whole grains and legumes.

- **Vitamin B12.** This vitamin helps to make DNA and RNA, as well as red blood cells, and to prevent anemia. It has also been linked with healthy bones. Because it plays a role in creating and using the neurotransmitter serotonin, it may help to regulate mood. Vitamin B_{12} is found naturally only in animal foods: meat, poultry and fish. Adolescents who are vegetarian and vegan are at increased risk for B_{12} deficiency and should consider taking supplements.

- **Vitamin D.** This vitamin is needed for optimal bone health and immune system function. Inadequate intake during adolescence is particularly worrisome because a deficiency can affect peak bone mass and height. Vitamin D is primarily obtained through sun exposure, but even some teens who live in sunny climates have been shown to be deficient. Good amounts are found in fatty fish, specifically cod liver oil. Vitamin D_2, which the body must convert to active vitamin D_3, is found in mushrooms. Because it can be challenging to obtain adequate amounts of this nutrient through diet, and because dermatologists warn again sun exposure, vitamin D_3 supplements should be considered.

Some gene expression patterns linked with risk-taking behavior may be established in childhood, and possibly even earlier. A 2018 study published in the *Journal of Affective Disorders* found that 7-year-olds who at that age demonstrated hypermethylation in certain genes were more likely as 17-year-olds to engage in dangerous driving and substance abuse. But here's an interesting wrinkle: the effects are a two-way street. The study also noted that teens whose methylation was normal when they were children sparked changes to their DNA methylation if they were sedentary or engaged in risky sexual activity as adolescents. Interestingly, those who didn't exercise had higher methylation patterns, and those who were sexually active had lower methylation. Substance abuse moved the needle in both directions: changes in methylation increased substance abuse and increased substance abuse altered methylation.

While researchers can tell us that the expression of certain genes has changed in these adolescents, they still can't be sure of why that is happening. In the case of risk-taking behavior, for instance, their challenge is identifying the line between where behavior influences gene expression, and therefore brain development, and where brain development influences behavior. One problem with teens is that many have already started to "act out" by the time they are assessed. That leaves an unanswered question: How much has their behavior already influenced their brain development?

New research is attempting to resolve that uncertainty. In 2015 the Adolescent Brain Cognitive Development (ABCD) study, which will be the largest study of adolescent brain development in the United States, began to collect data on children who were nine years of age. The researchers imaged the children's brains and recorded their neural activity as they performed a variety of tasks, with a view to establishing a baseline before the turbulence of adolescence set in. Every two years for a period of 10 years, the subjects will return and be reassessed. With this set of data in place, researchers will be able to pinpoint the impact of specific behaviors on developing brains. They will also be able to identify how such behaviors are affected by brain development. In the future, this treasure trove of data will help to answer questions about the effects of behaviors on brain development. The behaviors being studied include playing video games and sports and using certain medications, as well as potentially riskier behaviors such as substance abuse and sexual activity. Eventually, the study will be able to link these effects to long-term health outcomes.

7

ADULTHOOD

If a plant in your yard seeks more moisture by growing deeper roots it will do so at the expense of its stem and leaves. In humans, increased allocation of energy to one trait, such as brain growth, necessarily reduces allocation to one or more other traits, such as tissue repair processes. The human fetus has a developmental hierarchy. At the top of this is the brain. Toward the lower end are organs such as the lung and kidney: these have reduced functions in utero and their development may be "traded off" to protect higher priority systems. The costs of trading off include, it seems, risk for disease in later life.

— DAVID BARKER AND KENT THORNBURG,
"THE OBSTETRIC ORIGINS OF HEALTH FOR A LIFETIME"

IN 1986, WHEN DAVID Barker first proposed that the nine months we spend in our mother's womb are likely the most impactful period of our lives, it went against the grain of public health dogma. In those days, it was pretty much assumed that chronic illnesses, such as heart disease and what was then called adult-onset diabetes, were the end result of poor diet and a sedentary lifestyle. Although there is no doubt that boosting your commitment to a variety of constructive habits (such as good nutrition and physical activity) benefits your health and well-being, Dr. Barker's work identified a fundamental flaw in this one-size-fits-all approach: the functional capacity of some of your organs and body systems is determined even before you are born. That means your fetal experience stalks you through life, influencing whether you will develop a chronic illness as an adult.

Today most authorities accept that Dr. Barker's ideas about the developmental origins of health and disease are at play in the larger canvas that is chronic disease. His original work focused on nutrition, but we now know that nutrition isn't the only prenatal factor that affects long-term health. The lifestyle patterns of previous generations on both the paternal and maternal sides spark changes in gene expression that may be heritable, contributing to the health of offspring for generations to come.

This chapter takes a look at the major chronic diseases of our time — obesity, diabetes, hypertension and cardiovascular disease, which are interconnected in numerous ways — including through the lens of fetal origins and *intergenerational inheritance*. Although cancer is also a serious disease that affects a significant number of people, for various reasons it is viewed as a disease of aging and is therefore discussed in chapter 8.

OBESITY

Over the past few decades, obesity has been increasing dramatically around the world. As of 2014, the worldwide incidence of the condition had more than doubled over the course of 30-odd years. Statistics from the World Health Organization (WHO) note that more than 600 million people qualified as obese in that year. Particularly concerning are data that indicate the condition is rising rapidly in children and adolescents. For instance, in 2017 *The Lancet* published a study based on WHO data that looked at 130 million people from all parts of the globe. Their conclusion: over the past 40 years, the number of obese children between the ages of 4 and 19 has increased by a factor of 10. Based on this and other information, it's not surprising that many experts are now using the term *epidemic* when discussing obesity.

The Wellspring of Many Problems

A major problem with obesity is that it is more problematic than simply being overweight. Obese people are not only likely to have a shorter life span, but are also at higher risk for many chronic diseases, particularly if they carry most of their weight around their middle. Obesity has been directly linked to:

- hypertension
- gallbladder disease

- osteoarthritis and related conditions such as gout
- some types of cancer
- several diseases of the pancreas, including pancreatitis and pancreatic cancer
- insulin resistance, which is a major risk factor for type 2 diabetes and cardiovascular disease
- heart disease (the Framingham Heart Study found that being obese doubled a person's lifetime risk of cardiovascular disease)

In fact, obesity has been called "a ticking time bomb" in terms of whether someone will become chronically ill. Moreover, a study published in the journal *Cell Systems* in 2018 found that you don't need to gain a lot of weight to put your health at risk. Even a small increase of 6 pounds (2.7 kg) is enough to activate markers associated with heart disease.

Participants in the study took only 30 days to gain their weight. Despite this short time frame, the researchers noted changes to their microbiome and immune system, as well as an increase in inflammation throughout the body. They could also identify the potential mechanisms triggering those effects: changes in the expression of 318 genes. Some genes became more active, while others were silenced.

A particularly surprising finding was that these epigenetic modifications increased the risk for cardiomyopathy, a condition in which the heart muscle becomes weakened. In an interview on the study published online, geneticist Michael Snyder, one of the lead researchers, commented that overeating for 30 days changes how the heart and all of its associated pathways function. In his opinion, the results aligned with how the human body works. "It's a whole system, not just a few isolated components, so there are system-wide changes when people gain weight," he said.

A Ticking Time Bomb for Chronic Disease

The potential effects of obesity start early: it has long been recognized as a complicating factor in pregnancy and childbirth. When pregnant women are obese, increased risks to the mother include gestational diabetes, various types of infection and preeclampsia (high blood pressure during pregnancy), and the fetus is at greater risk of being stillborn or having a birth defect. In addition, obese mothers are significantly more likely to be induced or to require a caesarean section, which has an impact on how the baby's microbiome develops.

The children of obese pregnant women are also more likely to develop chronic disease. For starters, they are at greater risk of having a high birth weight and/or of becoming

UNDERSTANDING YOUR BMI

Although it's not infallible as an indicator (one problem is that the standards fit Caucasian body types best), experts have traditionally used body mass index (BMI) to determine whether you are overweight or obese. Basically, BMI is a ratio of your weight to your height. Therefore, it is possible for a short person with very large muscle mass but little fat to be categorized as overweight or obese when, in fact, they are not. Generally, a BMI in the range of 18.5 to 24.9 is considered normal, between 25 to 30 is overweight, and greater than 30 is obese. Using these standards, very few people in developed countries qualify as underweight.

Another limitation of BMI is that it doesn't capture how fat and muscle are distributed on your body. From a health perspective, fat around your waistline is much more concerning than, say, fat in your thighs, because it is in such close proximity to vital organs such as your liver and pancreas. Some of that fat, known as *visceral fat*, may be hidden in the abdominal cavity. Visceral fat is very problematic. Current thinking is that it has a toxic effect (known as *lipotoxicity*) on your body because it releases substances that negatively affect your metabolism. Insulin resistance and systemic inflammation are among the potential results.

Most of the relevant research has used BMI as a measure, which is why it is mentioned often in this book. However, today most experts suggest using waist-to-hip ratio to estimate body fat. Divide your waist size by your hip size. If you are male, hope that it is at or below 0.95; if you are female, your risk starts to rise when it's over 0.85. Waist circumference measurement is even simpler. Males whose waist measurement is 37 inches (94 cm) or less and women whose waists are 31.5 inches (80 cm) or less are at low risk for weight-related health problems.

obese themselves. These factors increase their risk for a range of metabolic disorders, such as hypertension, insulin resistance and inflammation. Maternal obesity during pregnancy also increases the likelihood that her offspring will suffer from asthma and lung disease.

Fathers aren't off the hook: a 2017 study found that offspring were just as likely to inherit obesity from their father as from their mother.

What Causes Obesity?

Obesity is a complex disease that involves the interaction of many hereditary and environmental factors. We can trace some causation back to fetal experiences in the womb, and we know that obese fathers and mothers are likely to pass the condition on to their offspring. Although genes do not play a huge part in the actual risk for obesity, it does have a genetic component, in that certain genes that influence weight can interact with environmental factors, contributing to its development.

Long before we understood the impact of genes and epigenetics, experts had noted that obesity clustered within families, an observation supported by statistics. Heritability is estimated to be between 40 and 70 percent. The more obese you are, the greater the likelihood that obesity runs in your family. Identical twins are twice as likely to share the condition as fraternal twins. Some say obesity runs in families because of lifestyle and dietary habits. However, we know that adopted children are at greater risk of becoming obese if their biological parents — not their adoptive ones — are obese, which dispels the notion that unhealthy behaviors are the sole cause.

Thanks to the work of David Barker and scientists around the world who are studying the developmental origins of health and disease, we now know that certain people are programmed for obesity before birth. For instance, epidemiological studies show that men who were conceived during the Dutch Hunger Winter were more likely to become obese as adults than those who were conceived before or after the famine. As we learn more about epigenetics, we begin to understand why: If women are malnourished in the early stages of pregnancy, the nutrient deficiencies spark changes in gene expression in their offspring, disturbing systems that regulate energy balance throughout the body. Some of these epigenetic changes are heritable. We now know they can be passed on through at least two generations.

The Trail of Epigenetic Inheritance

Professor Mark Vickers of the University of Auckland, New Zealand, has a particular interest in the effects of maternal nutrition and the development of obesity and type 2 diabetes. He sees this trail of epigenetic inheritance as one of the root systems of the so-called obesity epidemic. As he noted in a 2014 paper, there is a cumulative effect. Obese parents produce offspring with a predisposition to obesity. One result is that, over successive generations, the population distribution shifts toward adults with increased body weight.

And yet not all of these at-risk children became obese — only a statistically significant number of them. Once again, your epigenome comes into play. Although your propensity for gaining weight is determined early in life, your genes are constantly adapting to their environment. That means your experience has a substantial impact on how your body reacts to its programming. If people's fate were written in stone, you would never find identical twins with significantly different weights, but it happens: one twin is obese and the other is lean.

When Finnish researchers looked at this phenomenon in 2013, they discovered some interesting things. First, the twins who were thin showed no signs of metabolic disease or inflammation even though their twin was obese. They also identified two categories of obese individuals who were twins: those who didn't accumulate liver fat and those who did. In other words, some obese individuals are, in metabolic terms, as healthy as lean people. Those whose obesity was classified as unhealthy suffered from metabolic syndrome and fatty liver, possibly due to inflammation and/or other unknown factors, while their twin siblings did not.

A more recent study from Germany's Max Planck Institute of Immunobiology and Epigenetics, published in the journal *Cell*, also looked at identical twins and concluded that differences in gene expression determine the predisposition to obesity. It linked these epigenetic changes with a specific protein known as TRIM28, which influences gene behavior. Mice with low levels of TRIM28 were obese, and those with adequate amounts of the protein were appropriately lean. When they looked at human identical twins where one of the pair was svelte and the other was obese, they found a similar pattern.

GENETIC GROUNDWORK

Scientists didn't begin to understand the genetic underpinnings of obesity until 1997, when they identified the first single gene variant linked with the condition. Today researchers are investigating more than 20 single genes related to obesity. For instance, studies have shown a strong relationship between fairly common single-nucleotide polymorphisms (SNPs) in the FTO gene, which is associated with fat mass and body mass index, and obesity in children. Adults with certain variants of this gene tend to be 8 to 10 pounds (3.5 to 4.5 kg) heavier than normal and are at increased risk for tipping over into obesity.

It should be noted that genes do not play a role in obesity unless they are expressed. How they are expressed is determined by a host of cellular processes, one of which is epigenetic mechanisms. In their quest to identify the causes of obesity, scientists are looking at epigenetic modifiers like, perhaps, the protein TRIM28, mentioned above. The environment is also on their radar. For example, some researchers have suggested that endocrine-disrupting chemicals (see "Endocrine Disruptors," page 90) collect in fat, where they have a negative impact on epigenetic mechanisms throughout the body. These changes disrupt the metabolism, promoting conditions such as insulin resistance, obesity and chronic inflammation.

While the genetic code you inherit from your parents is not by itself responsible for obesity, some genes are sensitive to environmental exposures, including to toxic chemicals. These genes are more likely to be adversely affected when the body adapts epigenetically, setting the stage for obesity.

The Obesogenic Environment

A major contributor to the development of obesity is what experts call our *obesogenic environment*, which encourages weight gain by, for instance, promoting high-calorie food that is deficient in nutrients. Unfortunately, the obesogenic environment is a prominent player in contemporary life. While it is already well known as a factor contributing to poor health in North America, the phenomenon has been spreading to low- and middle-income countries in tandem with growing prosperity in those regions.

In Africa obesity rates have been rising at an alarming rate, partly, say experts, because of the increasing availability of junk food and an increase in sedentary behavior as more people move from the countryside to urban centers. Moreover, many adults in Africa have been malnourished at various stages of their lives, including when they were in utero, predisposing them to obesity of developmental origin. Some medical professionals have equated the African "obesity crisis" with the HIV epidemic of the 1990s.

Obesogenic environments are fundamentally unhealthy. Worse still, other social and economic forces interact with this sickly state, cranking up its consequences. People are encouraged, often through expensive advertising campaigns, to overconsume nutrient-deficient foods that in some (perhaps many) cases are all they can afford or have access to. Clever marketing strategies support this strategy. For instance, a 2018 article in the *New York Times* reported that, in Africa, Coca-Cola reduced the size of its bottles to make the drink more affordable for poor people. And let's not forget the influence of technology: people joined at the hip to their personal communication devices are much more likely to live a sedentary lifestyle.

SODA, OBESITY AND TELOMERES

How familiar are you with telomeres? These stretches of DNA protein (see "Telomeres," page 227) are attached to the ends of your chromosomes, the structures that contain the DNA codes for your genes. Telomeres protect the chromosomes as cells divide. They have been linked with life span and the risk of certain chronic diseases (see "Telomere Length," page 228). And now, it seems, their health can be connected to the amount of soda you consume.

Here's how it works. In general, the longer your telomeres, the better. However, the older you get, the shorter they become. This is a natural process, but factors other than aging can also affect telomere length. In 2014 researchers looked at a group of people who regularly consumed 20 ounces (600 mL) or more of soda daily. The study, which was published in the *American Journal of Public Health*, reported that the soda-drinkers' telomeres shortened much more quickly than the norm — the equivalent of more than four and a half years in addition to the normal aging that would take place over the course of a year.

The researchers had included only healthy adults with no history of diabetes or cardiovascular disease in their study. The potential connections with metabolic disease are fascinating. Consider, for instance, that obesity is also associated with reduced telomere length — even for children. The authors of the study recommended that additional research be done to examine the pathways from "soda to cell." Understanding them might improve risk factors for cardiometabolic disease.

A Spiraling Effect

While obesity lays the groundwork for a raft of physical diseases, its "softer" effects shouldn't be ignored. In many countries a slender, elegant appearance is highly valued, and no more so than in France. In her memoir *You're Not Born Fat*, Gabrielle Deydier documented how being obese affected every aspect of her life. She had aced the interview for a job as a teaching assistant for children with special needs at a school in Paris, but after being hired for the job, she was warned by the headmaster that the teacher she'd be working with might be "difficult." Unfortunately, he didn't clarify what "difficult" meant. Like many people in France, the teacher was fat-phobic (*grossophobique* in French) and, quite simply, refused to work with Gabrielle, who weighed more than 300 pounds (135 kg).

What Is Leptin and Why Should You Care about It?

Leptin is a hormone that plays such a significant role in weight management it's been called the "obesity," the "starvation" and the "satiety" hormone.

With regard to satiety, leptin does two things: it stimulates the brain to make hormones that make you feel less hungry, and it simultaneously suppresses hormones that cause feelings of hunger. Ideally, it accurately reports to the brain when you have had enough to eat. Faulty signaling in this pathway has been linked with weight-management problems in many people.

Here's how it works. Leptin communicates directly with the hypothalamus, the part of the brain that regulates appetite, satiety and metabolism. Because most of the body's leptin is produced in fat cells, overweight and obese people — who have excessive numbers of fat cells — tend to have higher leptin levels than people of average weight. Leptin should ordinarily signal their brain to stop eating, but in effect there is a breakdown in communication in people with excess fat. This condition is known as leptin resistance.

Leptin resistance often leads to insatiable feelings of hunger and a desire to overeat. It has been compared to insulin resistance in type 2 diabetes, where the pancreas produces large amounts of insulin that the body is unable to use.

Another problem with leptin resistance is that it slows down metabolism, interfering with your muscles' ability to use glucose and fat as energy. This is the start of a vicious cycle. As fat builds up in muscle tissue, it promotes insulin resistance. Leptin pathways affect many different body systems, including endocrine functions, bone formation and immune and inflammatory responses. For instance, leptin miscommunication can be a trigger for chronic inflammation.

Researchers now believe that leptin resistance may be programmed in the womb. Studies using sheep and pigs have linked circulating leptin in utero with physiological roles related to energy balance. In simple terms, it seems that too much or too little nutrition in utero can increase the amount of circulating leptin later in life.

Leptin is regulated in part by epigenetic mechanisms. However, it may be worth noting that some people are born with mutations in the leptin receptor (LEPR) gene. These people are at significantly greater risk for morbid obesity and type 2 diabetes. And although it is a rare disease, these individuals are thus born with a leptin deficiency; when this occurs, it causes early-onset obesity and constant feelings of profound hunger. For these individuals, leptin replacement therapy has been effective at reducing hunger, and it does seem to promote weight loss.

Managing Leptin Resistance

Researchers are gradually identifying factors that might help people manage leptin resistance. Studies have demonstrated, for example, that diets rich in fructose (not from whole fruit, but from too much fruit juice and sweetened beverages) and fat (primarily saturated) can worsen leptin resistance. When leptin resistance exists, fructose and saturated fat further alter leptin's ability to communicate effectively once inside the brain. Their consumption can also raise blood triglyceride levels, which worsens leptin resistance.

In animal studies, imbalances in the gut microbiome have been associated with leptin resistance. Based on their species, there are four major categories of gut bacteria, two of which are linked with both obesity and leptin resistance. Specifically, obese people and those who are leptin-resistant share the same imbalance: an increased ratio of Firmicutes species relative to those belonging to the Bacteroidetes group. The question remains whether an altered gut microbiome creates leptin resistance or whether leptin resistance alters the microbiome.

Leptin resistance is also a risk factor for nonalcoholic fatty liver disease (NAFLD). Research suggests that nutritional supplementation and lifestyle changes may improve leptin levels in people with NAFLD. Human studies have shown that supplementing with 3,000 mg of turmeric daily for 12 weeks decreases serum levels of leptin compared with a placebo group. Similarly, for patients with NAFLD, supplementation with probiotics (friendly bacteria) and prebiotics (food for the friendly bacteria), along with a recommended weight-loss diet and increased physical activity, had a more favorable impact on leptin levels than the lifestyle interventions alone. For more information on NAFLD, see page 176, and for more on prebiotics and probiotics, see pages 282 and 284.

Arachidonic acid (AA) is an omega-6 fatty acid that in animal studies has been associated with impaired leptin signaling inside the brain. Diets rich in AA have been shown to increase the risk of leptin resistance and, perhaps not surprisingly, diabetes and obesity in humans. AA has also has been linked with chronic inflammation. Certain foods — specifically vegetable oils (such as sunflower, safflower, cottonseed and soybean oil) and animal foods (such as eggs, poultry and beef) — can raise AA levels in the body. In contrast, the omega-3 fatty acids EPA and DHA, found in foods such as oily fish, walnuts, flax seeds and chia seeds, have been shown to be protective against obesity in some people and may actually support weight loss in certain groups of obese people. It seems likely that increasing omega-3 fatty acids and improving the ratio between omega-6s and omega-3s in the diet may be helpful for maintaining a healthier weight and reducing leptin resistance. This can be easily accomplished by reducing consumption of vegetable oils rich in omega-6s while increasing those that are high in omega-3s.

It might be nice to dismiss this attitude as a peculiarly French proclivity, but it's not. Weight discrimination is equally alive and well in other parts of the world. This includes North America, where experts describe it as "stigmatizing." Overweight people are more likely to experience discrimination in every aspect of their lives, and, as research consistently shows, the constant stress of navigating a climate of fat-shaming takes a toll on physical and mental health.

Sadly, the indignities start at an early age. Being overweight is the most common cause of bullying at school. Fatter people are bullied more. The trauma of being bullied affects both the body and mental health. It can initiate hormonal changes that have been associated with immune system problems and even later-onset heart disease. Stress-related diseases, such as hypertension, may be another result. Bullying has also been shown to affect gene expression (see "Bullying," page 82).

Numerous studies have linked weight discrimination with unhealthy behaviors, like avoiding social interaction, and psychological distress. As Dr. Angelina Sutin wrote in her 2015 study *Weight Discrimination and Risk of Mortality*, the "cumulative effect of these hostile social interactions may be lower life expectancy." Once again, researchers could not pinpoint the exact mechanisms underlying this outcome. However, they identified a clear connection between weight discrimination and increased mortality — one that was comparable to other risk factors, such as a history of smoking.

Obesity, the Gut and the Immune System

Obese people have different ratios of bacteria in their gut compared to those who aren't overweight. In general, they have less diversity of bacterial species. Moreover, the bacteria they do have are associated with less-than-ideal metabolic processes related to energy storage and use. In fact, recent research suggests that the types of bacteria present in the gut, and how they interact, may be a driver of obesity. Other studies indicate that adjusting gut microbes might be an effective tool for weight loss.

When the bacteria in your gut get out of whack, the effects are systemic. These consequences include how your immune system responds to the environment. Dr. Susan Prescott, an expert on the immune system, believes that obesity has a chronic effect on the immune system. She points out that obesity, the metabolism and the immune system are closely linked. In her opinion, environmental toxins and lifestyles that limit exposure to a wide range of healthy bacteria are "prime suspects" in both the rising rates of obesity and the rapid increase in autoimmune disease and allergies around the world.

YOU ARE WHAT YOUR GRANDPARENTS ATE

Metabolic Syndrome

As for many other chronic conditions, the incidence of metabolic syndrome is on the rise around the world. The rising rates have been linked with numerous factors, including aging populations, chronic stress, sedentary lifestyles and nutrient-deficient diets. One problem is that, with the exception of abdominal fat, the symptoms of metabolic syndrome aren't obvious. As a result, it's been called a silent killer.

Metabolic syndrome is not a disease in itself. Rather, it is a cluster of conditions: people can be diagnosed with metabolic syndrome if they have three or more of the risk factors, which include hypertension, obesity, abdominal fat, elevated levels of triglycerides and insulin resistance. Each of these conditions is dangerous in its own right, but in combination they are synergistic, meaning that, when experienced together, the end result is worse than the cumulative effects of each taken individually. This constellation of disorders foreshadows the development of even more serious diseases, including cardiovascular disease, stroke and type 2 diabetes.

Researchers are urging people with a large waist circumference, even if their BMI falls within the normal range, to be screened for insulin resistance. Visceral fat, which collects around organs such as the pancreas, is linked with insulin resistance.

Given its connection with abdominal fat, it's not surprising that metabolic syndrome is closely linked with obesity, which has often been described as both a symptom and a cause.

A Harbinger of Things to Come

It's probably not surprising — as a 2018 study in the online journal *Diabetes, Obesity and Metabolism* found — that there is a clear link between three of the risk factors associated with metabolic syndrome and the likelihood that someone will develop type 2 diabetes. People with a BMI greater than 30 (which means they are defined as obese), triglycerides that exceed 80 mg/dL (4.5 mmol/L) and a fasting glucose level of 100 to 124 mg/dL (5.6 to 6.9 mmol/L) are more than 60 percent more likely to develop diabetes later in life.

If the triglyceride and fasting glucose levels don't seem alarming, that's because they aren't — they fall within the "normal" range. But for people in their forties, these slight elevations in metabolic markers serve as an advance warning system. Doctors can use these biomarkers to predict their likelihood of developing diabetes in the next 20 years or so and put them on a personalized program that mitigates the risk with strategies such as losing weight, getting more exercise and consuming a more nutritious diet.

Root Causes

Although they can pinpoint certain risk factors, the experts are at a loss to identify the exact mechanisms underlying the development of metabolic syndrome. As with virtually every chronic disease, a genetic/epigenetic component is involved. A 2015 paper published in the Czech journal *Physiological Research* concluded that metabolic syndrome, like all complex chronic diseases, results from gene–gene and gene–environment interactions that involve multiple genes and environmental factors. Like its close relative obesity, metabolic syndrome seems to be linked to glitches in the body's systems for regulating energy balance, and its roots can be traced back to the womb.

Numerous studies suggest that poor nutrition during critical periods of development (in utero and during early childhood in particular) influences metabolic processes such as how your body converts food to energy. Clare Reynolds is the lead writer of a 2015 paper on energy balance disorders published in the journal *Nutrients*. She reflected that the early nutritional environment plays a lifelong role in programming "many aspects of physiology and behavior, including metabolism, body weight set point and energy balance regulation." The good news is that good nutrition in the early stages of development can help to get any errors in metabolic programming back on track.

Exposure to toxins may also play a role in metabolic syndrome. In a 2017 paper, researchers from McMaster University in Hamilton, Ontario, linked early-life exposure to heavy metals and common chemicals, including pesticides and household products, with metabolic disorders such as elevated BMI, increased blood pressure in childhood and insulin resistance. They noted that the timing of the exposure is important: the more critical the developmental stage, the greater the effect it will have over the long term.

There is no smoking gun, but scientists are seeing strong indications that the risk of developing metabolic syndrome can be epigenetically transmitted to offspring over several generations. A 2016 mouse study published in *Cell Reports* showed that maternal metabolic syndrome produced metabolic abnormalities in three generations of offspring. The original changes in gene expression can likely be linked to some of the usual suspects: a diet high in sugar and unhealthy fats and low in quality protein.

Nonalcoholic Fatty Liver Disease

According to the US Centers for Disease Control and Prevention, as many as 20 percent of Americans suffer from nonalcoholic fatty liver disease (NAFLD). While it is normal for your liver to contain some fat, NAFLD is the result of excessive fat (in the form of triglycerides) building up in the liver's cells. A fatty liver is one in which fat accounts for at least 5 percent of the liver's weight. This condition accounts for over 75 percent of liver disease in the United States. It is also a growing health problem around the world; globally, the number of people with NAFLD has doubled in the past two decades, and it is estimated that 25 percent of adults suffer from some degree of fatty liver disease. The rising number of children is of particular concern. Ten percent of children are on the NAFLD continuum, a situation that has been described as a public health crisis.

Why is NAFLD becoming so widespread among children and adolescents? Some experts have linked its prevalence with the dramatic increase in obesity. But many young people who are not obese are being diagnosed with the condition. The obesogenic environment, which is characterized by sedentary behavior and excessive consumption of processed foods, has also been associated with development of the disease. Although it is a subject of heated debate (most of which is likely generated by sugar industry lobbyists), studies suggest there is a link between consumption of high-fructose corn syrup (HFCS), which is used to sweeten many soft drinks, and the rising rates of NAFLD in young people.

Multiple Risk Factors

While a number of genes have been associated with NAFLD, it's a complex condition and experts are entertaining the idea that a genetic predisposition may be just one of multiple risk factors. Studies have linked exposure to both air pollution and endocrine-disrupting chemicals with the disease. In these situations, researchers believe that early-life exposures may trigger epigenetic modifications that increase the risk of developing NAFLD.

A Stealth Operator

In the early stages of NAFLD it is rare to have symptoms. People often aren't aware they are developing the condition. However, during annual medical examinations, which usually include blood testing of cholesterol (a lipid panel) and a comprehensive metabolic panel (CMP), elevated levels of triglycerides and liver enzymes (AST, ALT) may show up. These results may be indicative of a fatty liver. It's a good idea to watch for a pattern of gradually increasing triglycerides and liver enzymes over time. If you wait until they are higher than normal to address them, it may be too late. Fatty liver is preventable, and the consequences of the disease are high.

Diet and Lifestyle Strategies for Managing NAFLD

While there is no agreed-upon conventional pharmaceutical treatment for NAFLD, diet and lifestyle interventions go a long way toward controlling and managing the condition. Because of their shared risk factors of poor diet, lack of physical activity and a sedentary lifestyle, many of the strategies to prevent and treat NAFLD are, not surprisingly, similar to those that improve insulin resistance, diabetes and metabolic syndrome.

Protective Foods and Nutrients

Foods and nutrients that can provide protection against fatty liver disease include:

- **Omega-3 fatty acids.** Studies show that a daily supplement of around 3 grams of omega-3s reduces blood levels of triglycerides and improves fatty liver (a decreased amount of fat is seen with ultrasound).

- **Vitamin E.** A deficiency in vitamin E, a potent antioxidant, is common in people with NAFLD. Foods high in vitamin E include almonds, spinach, sweet potatoes, avocados, chard, sunflower seeds and wheat germ. Research on vitamin E supplements for fatty liver has had mixed results but indicate that they may benefit people with nondiabetic and non-cirrhotic fatty liver disease.

- **Choline.** Choline, a water-soluble nutrient related to B vitamins, is involved in multiple pathways of liver function. Choline deficiency in humans is associated with NAFLD. The foods highest in choline are animal foods, especially egg yolks and also beef liver, salmon, shrimp and chicken. However, there are some good plant-based sources, including peanuts, Brussels sprouts, broccoli and cauliflower.

- **Coffee.** Although coffee has its pros and cons in general, drinking coffee regularly can be beneficial for people with liver disease. In some studies, daily coffee consumption reduced the progression of fatty liver to fibrosis and cirrhosis, and the more coffee, the better in those cases. Although the specific beneficial properties of coffee are not well understood, they seem to go beyond its antioxidant and caffeine content.

Foods and Substances to Avoid

- **Refined sugars.** Avoiding added sugars is crucial to preventing fatty liver disease. Table sugar, for example, is made up of two simple sugars, glucose and fructose, both of which play a role in the disease. Excessive glucose in the diet can lead to insulin resistance and type 2 diabetes. Fructose doesn't affect blood sugar levels, leading some people to believe it is better for you. However, fructose is metabolized in the liver, and high intake will boost fatty acid production, causing or worsening fatty liver. Fructose is found naturally in fruits and vegetables, and from those sources it isn't a cause for concern. But processed foods contain high amounts of fructose that can be detrimental to your health. High-fructose corn syrup (HFCS), a highly processed sweetener that contains more fructose than glucose, is particularly problematic. Its negative effects on the liver are more pronounced than those of other sugars. HFCS is found in conventional sodas, juices, energy drinks, candy and processed pastries and desserts. It is a cheap sweetener, so it is prevalent in many processed foods, including breads, ketchup, canned soups and salad dressings. Because it is often invisible and its use is so widespread, most people are likely consuming more HFCS than they realize.

- **Refined carbohydrates.** Avoid carbohydrates from refined grains, such as white bread, pasta, crackers and white rice. Excessive intake of refined carbohydrates increases triglyceride production in the liver and the risk of NAFLD. In general, avoiding refined carbohydrates will go a long way toward preventing or improving fatty liver disease. Healthy carbohydrates from whole foods such as vegetables, fruits, whole grains and beans should be consumed in balance with protein and fats.

- **Alcohol and acetaminophen.** These substances are liver stressors. Alcohol is metabolized by the liver and in excess can cause alcoholic liver disease. Even in the case of nonalcoholic fatty liver disease, alcohol places stress on the liver that can worsen the condition. Acetaminophen (Tylenol), a common over-the-counter pain reducer, is metabolized in the liver. Overdosing, either by taking too much at once or by taking smaller amounts over a long period of time, can cause liver toxicity and result in liver damage, especially when it is combined with alcohol.

Additional Strategies

- **Maintain a healthy weight.** Weight loss is a very effective strategy in the treatment of fatty liver disease. Studies show that an average loss of 7 to 10 percent of body weight improves fatty liver, cholesterol levels and insulin resistance and reduces liver enzymes. A loss of over 10 percent of body weight has been shown to completely reverse non-alcoholic steatohepatitis (see "A Dangerous Progression," page 180).

- **Increase physical activity.** Exercise of any type (aerobic or resistance) is very effective at reducing the degree of fatty liver, even in the absence of weight loss. On average, most studies showed positive effects with three to five days a week of exercise for 45 to 60 minutes.

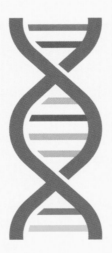

The Effects Are Systemic

Fatty liver disease is serious because its negative effects are not limited to the liver. NAFLD has a systemic effect throughout the body: chronic kidney disease, osteoporosis and colorectal cancer are among the conditions that may develop. It has become one of the most common causes underlying the need for a liver transplant.

The rising rates of NAFLD are also deeply intertwined with the increase in other chronic conditions. In animal studies, a fatty liver has been linked with insulin resistance, and when they coexist, the two conditions appear to rev each other up. One of insulin's jobs is to help glucose access muscle cells, and when the body's cells have a reduced ability to respond to insulin, blood glucose levels remain elevated. This triggers the liver to make more fatty acids and triglycerides. Up to 74 percent of people with type 2 diabetes have NAFLD, while up to 100 percent of obese people with diabetes have NAFLD. While each condition is harmful in its own right, together they work synergistically, increasing the risk and severity by more than a simple additive effect. In combination, they greatly increase the risk of developing other conditions, such as heart disease.

A Dangerous Progression

As fatty liver disease worsens, it may lead to nonalcoholic steatohepatitis (NASH). NASH develops when the liver swells and more fat accumulates, producing inflammation and fibrosis. The progression is slow and there are no obvious symptoms; the advancement of NASH has been compared to that of diabetes and hypertension. Eventually it can lead to irreversible scarring of the liver (cirrhosis), liver failure and, finally, the need for a liver transplant. Some experts are calling the rising rates of NASH a silent epidemic.

Other studies suggest that NASH may be linked to a methyl-deficient diet — one that is short in nutrients such as folate and vitamins B_6 and B_{12}. Studies have shown that when rats were fed a high-fat sucrose diet, low in methyl donors, they were more likely to develop NASH; however, when supplements providing methyl donors were included in their diet, the high levels of triglycerides that had accumulated in their liver thanks to the unhealthy diet were reversed. Numerous studies have linked imbalances in gut bacteria with both NAFLD and NASH, suggesting that targeted interventions to support the growth of beneficial bacteria might be useful.

Not all people with NAFLD progress to the more serious conditions. That raises a question: Are certain people more disposed to moving along the continuum toward cirrhosis? The answer is yes. There is evidence that individuals with certain SNPs in the PNPLA3 gene may have an increased risk of progressing to NASH, fibrosis and cirrhosis.

DIABETES

Although diabetes has been recognized as a condition since antiquity, early physicians understood little about how the disease actually worked. They knew that frequent urination was a symptom and that the urine of diabetics was unnaturally sweet. But it took until the turn of the 20th century for researchers to understand that the disease originated in the pancreas.

In 1893 the French pathologist Gustave-Édouard Laguesse recognized that tiny clusters of cells — now known as pancreatic islets — might play a role in diabetes. A subset of these cells produce the hormone insulin (among other substances), and Dr. Laguesse and his colleagues suspected that these secretions influence how the body processes carbohydrates. Experiments revealed that when the pancreas was removed, laboratory animals developed diabetes. This was a big step forward. However, scientists still didn't know which pancreatic substances were responsible for the disease. Perhaps not surprisingly, some dubious treatments, such as feeding raw pig pancreas to diabetics, were prescribed.

By the 1920s the location for a medical breakthrough in diabetes had shifted to Canada. In 1921 Toronto researchers Frederick Banting and Charles Best identified insulin, the key substance involved in causing the disease. Dr. Banting was awarded a Nobel Prize for the discovery, which become a landmark in terms of treatment. Diabetes was no longer invariably fatal; rather, it was now a chronic condition that could be controlled.

Understanding Diabetes

Fundamentally, diabetes is a disease in which the body cannot properly transform sugar (glucose) into energy within its cells. The pancreas produces insulin, which plays a significant role in regulating blood sugar (glucose) levels, by stimulating cells to absorb glucose and burn it for energy. One of insulin's jobs is helping your blood deliver glucose to your cells — glucose being the primary source of energy for most cells in the body. Although your body needs glucose for energy, high blood glucose levels, a symptom of diabetes, are problematic. When the pancreas doesn't create an adequate amount of insulin, or when insulin becomes less efficient at regulating glucose uptake, diabetes is the result. Diabetes is a serious condition in itself, but it is also a precursor to other diseases such as heart disease and kidney failure.

There are two basic types of diabetes: type 1, often called juvenile diabetes, and type 2, which is often identified as adult-onset. A third type, gestational diabetes, is a complication of pregnancy. As Susan Prescott notes in *Origins*, gestational diabetes is triggered by the significant metabolic and physiological shifts the mother must make to accommodate the needs of the fetus.

Gestational Diabetes

Six to 8 percent of pregnant women experience gestational diabetes. Women who are overweight or obese are more likely to develop the condition, as are those with a family history of type 2 diabetes. Women who smoke and those who come from certain racial groups — African Americans, Hispanics and various Indigenous peoples — are also at greater risk. Recent studies suggest that nutrition may play a role in its development. For instance, India's Mumbai Maternal Nutrition Project, which evaluated the effects of a daily nutrient-dense snack, found that the intervention reduced the rates of gestational diabetes by half, compared to a control group who received a snack low in micronutrients.

Gestational diabetes is most likely to occur after the 20th week of pregnancy and is usually temporary. However, although blood sugar levels typically return to normal after delivery, the condition leaves several problems in its wake. Women who experience gestational diabetes are 20 times more likely to develop type 2 diabetes later in life. The risk is highest during the first five years after giving birth. According to a recent study published in *PLOS Medicine*, they are also 2.8 times more likely to develop heart disease and almost twice as likely to end up with hypertension.

Babies born to mothers with gestational diabetes are more likely to be unusually large. They will be prone to respiratory problems, as well as to developing hypoglycemia (low blood sugar) as newborns. They are also at greater risk of developing type 2 diabetes as adults, likely as a result of epigenetic changes that took place while they were in utero.

Type 1 Diabetes

Type 1 diabetes, often called juvenile diabetes, is an autoimmune disease caused by a lack of insulin. Basically, the pancreatic islet cells that produce insulin are attacked by the body's immune system. This malfunction forces the pancreas to work harder at producing insulin in an effort to keep blood sugar levels under control.

Although genes definitely play a role in the development of type 1 diabetes, they don't tell the whole story. Certain genes predispose individuals to the disease, but researchers have observed that the highest growth rates are among children with low-risk or even protective versions of those genotypes. Familial patterns support the idea that genes are not the determining factor. According to the American Diabetes Association, the odds that fathers who have type 1 diabetes will pass on the disease to their children are 1 in 17. For women, they're 1 in 25 if your child was born before you turned 25, and only 1 in 100 if you gave birth after that. We also know there is a high discordance rate between identical twins, which suggests that epigenetic modifications are in play. If one twin has the illness, the other will develop it, at most, 50 percent of the time. This difference is especially compelling when diagnosis is made after the age of 15.

Researchers are beginning to explore the impact of epigenetic changes on development of the disease. For instance, they have identified associations between type 1 diabetes and altered gene expression resulting from modifications to DNA methylation and histone acetylation.

Where Are Its Roots?

So the question is, what precipitates type 1 diabetes? In a fascinating paper, Edwin Gale, a British expert on diabetes, points out that the disease was relatively rare when Banting and Best made their groundbreaking discovery in 1921. However, rates rose steadily around the world throughout the 20th century. Around 1955 they began to leap forward, and since roughly 1990 the rate of increase has accelerated. The steepest rise shows up in the number of preschool children developing the condition.

A look at the larger picture reveals that type 1 diabetes isn't the only autoimmune disease that is on the rise. Since the 1950s, the incidence of many others — including rheumatoid arthritis, lupus and thyroid conditions, such as Graves' disease — has also been increasing. Not surprisingly, experts now agree that nongenetic factors play a significant role in this scenario. Susan Prescott, who is an expert in early immune development, sees clear connections between environmental factors and the rising incidence of autoimmune diseases. She points out that the immune system is particularly sensitive to the lifestyle changes associated with contemporary life. These include energy-rich, nutrient-deficient diets, a sedentary lifestyle, exposure to environmental pollutants and toxins, increased hygiene that results in reduced microbial diversity, certain drugs and cigarette smoking.

The Highest Rate in the World

Finland has the highest rate of type 1 diabetes in the world. No one knows exactly why, but in 2016 researchers reported on some interesting findings after following about 200 newborns who were genetically at risk of developing the condition. Participants were divided equally among the Finnish province of Karelia, its Russian counterpart just across the border and nearby Estonia. After three years, 16 children in Finland, 14 in Estonia and only 4 in Russia had developed antibodies predictive of the disease. When the researchers compared the children's gut bacteria, they found dramatic differences in microbial composition between the children from Finland and Estonia and those from Russia, where the standard of living is much lower.

In a 2012 paper titled "Environmental Triggers of Type 1 Diabetes," researchers also cited geographic differences in the incidence of the condition. They noted studies of migrants that found increases in disease rates among population groups that moved from areas of low incidence to those that were high, and saw connections between less diversity in gut bacteria and higher incidence of the disease. These and other examples suggest links between the so-called hygiene hypothesis (see page 272) and type 1 diabetes.

Low vitamin D intake and childhood obesity have also been identified as potential factors. One Finnish study, published in 2000, used data on more than 1,000 children collected from well-baby clinics and school health-care units in that country. The research linked the incidence of type 1 diabetes with childhood obesity and rapid growth, particularly during the first three years of life.

Genes and Environmental Triggers

In 2002, when Edwin Gale published his paper, he speculated that type 1 diabetes might be the result of complex interactions between a genetic predisposition and environmental triggers. Subsequent studies have documented just that, and in hard-science terms. However, research along these lines is still in the early stages, and in many ways, trying to pinpoint the effects of environmental factors on the epigenome is like looking for a needle in a haystack. Identifying specific genes associated with a disease is just the first step. Sorting out how genes network with their world is far more complex. The interactions are varied: they include gene with gene, genes with the environment, and numerous external environmental effects, all of which may work together synergistically. These are extremely dynamic processes, and endless outcomes are possible.

Type 2 Diabetes

Type 2 diabetes is by far the most common form of the disease, accounting for about 90 percent of all cases. The International Diabetes Federation estimated that in 2017 425 million people suffered from type 2 diabetes globally and that more than half of those had been diagnosed with the condition since 2000. The word *epidemic* is often used to describe the rapid growth of the disease throughout the world. However, it can be tricky to separate the diabetes epidemic from the so-called obesity epidemic since the two are so closely linked. In fact, Paul Z. Zimmet, an epidemiologist and diabetes researcher in Australia, calls the combination "diabesity," which he feels is likely to become "the biggest epidemic in human history."

Diabetes takes a toll on the health of individuals, but the effects can be devastating to society as a whole. It is an expensive disease to treat. Moreover, by some estimates, the cost of medications to treat complications resulting from the disease is as much as four times the cost of those that treat diabetes itself. Complications associated with the condition include cardiovascular disease, damage to the nervous system and kidneys, poor blood flow to the extremities (which can develop into a need for amputation) and dementia, including Alzheimer's disease. Like other chronic illnesses, diabetes also incurs numerous social costs, ranging from missed workdays to early retirement.

Genetic Links

A number of large genome-wide association studies have identified genetic variants directly linked with type 2 diabetes. However, researchers have determined that each makes only a small contribution to development of the disease. We know that diabetes runs in families: research shows that if one sibling has the disease, their siblings from the same parents are three times more likely to develop the condition than a member of the general population. But while your genes may predispose you to developing diabetes, recent research indicates that they can also protect you from it. A group of Amish people in Indiana have a gene associated with low levels of a substance that protects them from metabolic diseases, including diabetes. They also have lower levels of insulin, and telomeres (see page 227) that are about 10 percent longer than those of their peers. Interestingly, they live about 10 years longer than their peers, on average to the ripe old age of 85.

Developmental Links

The current thinking is that type 2 diabetes is a multifactorial disease that occurs when a genetic predisposition is triggered by environmental factors. We've long understood that nutrition and a sedentary lifestyle play a role in whether the condition develops, and both have been shown to influence gene expression. This aligns with recent research, which suggests that you are more likely to develop type 2 diabetes as a result of epigenetic factors than because of your genes. Most compelling are studies of identical twins, who have exactly the same genome. When one twin has diabetes and the other doesn't, researchers have linked these outcomes to different epigenetic patterns associated with glucose tolerance.

Evidently, the propensity for type 2 diabetes originates in early life and develops (or doesn't) in response to environmental cues. Some experts now believe that about 25 percent of metabolic disease (obesity and diabetes) risk can be predicted by the prenatal environment. Both parents have an impact. Data from the Chinese famine linked high blood sugar in offspring with famine-exposed fathers as well as mothers. With fathers, the connection is epigenetic variations in sperm. With mothers, the risk is based primarily on what happens in utero.

We've long known that low-birth-weight children of mothers who were pregnant during the Dutch famine were more likely to develop diabetes later in life. If they were obese as adults, their risk increased even more. Low birth weight followed by rapid "catch-up" weight gain in early life leads to adiposity, and adiposity is a risk factor for diabetes because adipose tissue influences how glucose and insulin are metabolized. Disruptions in organ systems that affect metabolism may also be involved. For instance, both muscle and the liver play a role in how glucose is metabolized by insulin, and they can be impaired by poor nutrition in utero. So, too, can pancreatic function, which relates to insulin production.

If a mother has diabetes or develops gestational diabetes when pregnant, she is more likely to deliver a baby with a high birth weight. This, too, is a risk factor. Experts describe the relationship between birth weight and type 2 diabetes as U-shaped, with high risk at both extremes.

THE EPIGENOME

Evidence now suggests that disruptions to fetal development play out in the epigenome over the course of a lifetime. Follow-up studies on 442 subjects from the Dutch Hunger Winter have shown that a mother's nutritional status while pregnant can induce changes

DIABETES AND ETHNICITY

While those of us who reside in countries like Canada, Britain and the United States worry about the Western lifestyle and rising rates of "diseases of affluence," one of those diseases, diabetes, has been spreading like wildfire in Asian countries. As epidemiologist Caroline Fall points out, by 2025 it's expected that three-quarters of the world's 300 million adults with diabetes will reside in nonindustrialized countries, almost a third of those in India and China alone. Dr. Fall has been actively studying diabetes in India for 25 years, and in that country a major contributor to the problem is the transition from traditional rural lifestyles to increasingly urban ones. Along with that come behavioral changes, including a shift from manual labor to a more sedentary lifestyle and easy access to the kind of high-calorie, nutritionally deficient foods we tend to associate with the standard American diet.

But in capturing a national "diabesity" landscape, increased urbanization and socioeconomic growth are just part of the picture. History also comes into play. "A mother's nutritional status before she became pregnant makes a big difference in how her body responds to malnutrition when she is pregnant," Dr. Fall told me in an interview. "In Holland, the famine was short-term and women were well nourished before it happened, so there has not been an epidemic of diabetes in the country. But in India, generations of people have been poorly nourished. That's why Indian [and Chinese] people who move from rural to urban areas are much harder hit by exposure to an obesogenic environment. We think it's because of their history."

For many years Dr. Fall has worked closely with Dr. Chittaranjan Yajnik, who is also a specialist in diabetes research and maternal nutrition. Dr. Yajnik came up with the concept of the "thin-fat Indian." Compared with Caucasians, East Indians have a lower average BMI and strikingly low muscle mass, which makes them conventionally thin. However, they also have similar or higher levels of abdominal fat, which makes them disproportionately adipose, or "fat." This body type is present at birth, especially among the lightest and most undernourished newborns, and it persists through childhood. It also predisposes them to developing diabetes.

While the rising rates of diabetes in Asia are certainly a concern, vulnerability to diabetes related to ethnicity has also been noted in other parts of the world. For instance, statistics from the Centers for Disease Control and Prevention in the United States indicate that African Americans are almost twice as likely to develop diabetes as Caucasians. Moreover, the prevalence of the condition in this group has quadrupled over the past 30 years. African Americans are also more likely to experience greater disability from diabetes-related complications such as amputations, blindness, kidney failure and an increased risk of heart disease and stroke.

Native Americans, particularly the Pima Indians, and people of Hispanic origin also have a significantly higher risk of developing diabetes. In northern Canada, the rate of type 2 diabetes in the Inuit, once rare, is now comparable to that of the general population. In some Pacific Island nations, such as Fiji and Micronesia, about 30 percent of the population is affected.

While no one knows for sure exactly why the people in these various groups are more susceptible to developing diabetes, we can make some educated guesses. As Caroline Fall comments, "We think it's the clash between intergenerational undernutrition, which impairs fetal development, and the postnatal experience of plentiful food and low physical activity, which characterizes so much of contemporary life." In other words, it's a mismatch between historical experience and the obesogenic environment.

in methylation that continue into her child's adulthood. And other studies indicate that the risk resulting from epigenetic changes can be passed on through the generations. A 2009 study of mice, published in the journal *Diabetes*, showed that if a grandmother is undernourished, her grandchildren are more likely to be born with a low birth weight and to suffer from impaired glucose tolerance, even when her daughter was well nourished during pregnancy.

No Longer for Adults Only

In the past, type 2 diabetes was also known as adult-onset diabetes because it wasn't often found in children. However, over the past 25 years the incidence of the disease has increased dramatically in young people and children. This increase is especially prevalent in certain ethnic groups (see "Diabetes and Ethnicity," page 187) and in young people who reside in what might be described as disadvantaged neighborhoods.

While this is an alarming trend in itself, it's even more concerning because the disease progresses more rapidly in this age group than it does in older people. It is also less responsive to treatment. A 2012 study published in the *New England Journal of Medicine* found that within a few years of developing diabetes, almost half of the young people studied required daily injections of insulin to manage the condition. In addition, a standard drug used to control blood sugar levels failed to work in more than 50 percent of the subjects. Although we don't understand why this is the case, Susan Prescott speculates that the rapid growth and hormonal changes related to puberty may play a role in resistance to treatment among this age group.

The Obesity Connection

It is challenging to discuss diabetes without mentioning its connection to obesity. Most experts agree that obesity is the single greatest risk factor associated with type 2 diabetes. Not all people who develop type 2 diabetes are obese, but a higher percentage of obese people develop diabetes. Based on the evidence that the disease is almost twice as common in African Americans as it is in white people, one study published in *JAMA* in 2017 looked for racial factors in its development. However, when all other factors were adjusted for, the researchers concluded that obesity was the key cause of the disease. These results are supported by another study, the Diabetes Remission Clinical Trial (DiRECT), which was published in *The Lancet* in 2017. Those researchers found a clear link between weight loss and remission of type 2 diabetes. Eighty-six percent of patients who lost 33 pounds (15 kg) or more achieved remission, compared to only 7 percent of those who lost 11 pounds (5 kg) or less.

Almost 90 percent of people with type 2 diabetes are overweight or obese. Being overweight puts pressure on the body's ability to utilize insulin. Obese people are more likely to have what researchers describe as a cluster of pathologies, such as upsets in their metabolic and immune systems, less diversity in their gut bacteria and increased inflammation. While none of these factors is singularly responsible for the disease, they are all interconnected and likely work together, possibly synergistically, to create insulin resistance.

As noted elsewhere, obese people may be primed for type 2 diabetes thanks to growth-related events, including malnutrition during pregnancy and catch-up growth in early childhood. You are also more likely to develop excess abdominal fat and type 2 diabetes as an adult if your mother consumed too many calories while pregnant or if you were exposed to an obesogenic environment in early life. One study that looked at subjects over a period of 10 years found that higher rates of type 2 diabetes were associated with residing in a neighborhood that limited physical activity and, to a lesser extent, access to nutritious foods.

UNDERSTANDING INSULIN

Insulin, a hormone produced in the pancreas, plays a significant role in diabetes. It regulates blood sugar levels by stimulating the transport of glucose into your cells, where it is converted to energy. Type 2 diabetes results when there are problems with this process. Usually, a condition known as insulin resistance develops. More and more insulin is required to keep blood sugar levels in check, eventually wearing out the pancreas.

Over time, the combination of elevated blood sugar plus elevated insulin has negative effects on health. If blood sugar stays elevated for too long, chronic inflammation in the blood vessels is one result. This ultimately leads to diseases of the eyes, nerves, kidney, brain and heart. Nearly 70 percent of people with diabetes acquire heart disease, and most die of it.

In addition, if insulin levels stay elevated for too long, your fat cells are stimulated to grow, especially around the midsection, causing weight gain. When insulin resistance is long-standing, over time your pancreas "wears out." It can no longer produce sufficient insulin, a situation that often leads to the need for insulin replacement therapy.

Insulin Resistance and Obesity

What are the known causes of insulin resistance? Most experts agree that the strongest predictor is obesity. Fat cells are much more than energy-storage receptacles for the body; they are actually complex hormonal and chemical factories. Belly fat is particularly problematic because it creates hormones and inflammatory chemicals that worsen insulin resistance. Even if you have a normal BMI, a waist circumference of 40 inches (101 cm) or more if you are a man, or 35 inches (89 cm) or more if you are a woman, increases your risk of developing insulin resistance and type 2 diabetes.

Increased belly fat may also indicate that essential organs that regulate blood sugar, such as the liver and pancreas, are not functioning properly. Imaging studies of obese people show that they are storing too much fat in those organs, which can lead to nonalcoholic fatty liver disease (see page 176). This disease negatively affects the ability of the pancreas both to produce insulin and to respond to the body's needs for the hormone. A fatty liver becomes resistant to the clues insulin provides and loses its ability to appropriately perform certain tasks. These include storing excess sugar and releasing it into the bloodstream when blood sugar is low. Instead, a fatty liver continues to dump stored sugar into the bloodstream when it is not needed. For people with diabetes, this worsens their condition. Clearly, one strategy for managing diabetes is to identify strategies to reduce the amount of fat in the liver.

Additional Causes of Insulin Resistance

A sedentary lifestyle has a major impact on insulin resistance. Muscles use more glucose than any other tissue in the body, and they are incredibly effective at keeping blood sugar balanced and reducing insulin resistance following exercise. Numerous studies have documented the relationship between sitting for long periods of time and an increased risk for a variety of health problems, including cardiovascular disease and cancer. One review study, published in 2015 in *Annals of Internal Medicine*, concluded that the most significant risk associated with prolonged sitting (from 8 to 12 hours or more a day) was a 90 percent higher risk of developing type 2 diabetes. The researchers suggest that long periods of sitting generate changes in muscles that may have negative effects on how sugars and fats are metabolized, linking sedentary behavior to insulin resistance.

Certain medications also contribute to insulin resistance. These include corticosteroids, thiazide diuretics, beta-blockers and statins. Chronic insomnia and sleep apnea have also been linked with the condition, as has cigarette smoking.

Preventing or Controlling Type 2 Diabetes

Major medical organizations around the world, including the American Diabetes Association, the World Health Organization, the Canadian Diabetes Association and the National Health System in Britain, agree that lifestyle modifications can improve insulin resistance. Making appropriate lifestyle changes also helps with managing the symptoms of type 2 diabetes and may even be able to reverse the disease.

First and foremost among the recommended strategies are losing weight and increasing physical activity. If you are overweight, studies show that even if you have been identified as high risk for type 2 diabetes, losing just a small amount of weight (5 to 10 percent) can thwart its development. Research also shows that combining this amount of weight loss with increased physical activity (again, moderate — as little as walking for 150 minutes a week) reduces the risk by as much as 60 percent. If you are already taking diabetes medication, losing that small amount of weight may allow you to decrease the dose, which is beneficial over the long term. It almost goes without saying that if you smoke, quit. Also, if necessary, improve your eating habits: consume a nutrient-dense, whole-foods-only diet. Experts believe that if these interventions were widely adopted, over a 20-year period the incidence of diabetes might be reduced by a whopping 43 percent.

Weight Loss for Diabetes Management

Weight loss continues to be the single most effective strategy to treat or reverse diabetes. We know that losing 5 to 7 percent or more of your body mass can improve and sometimes reverse diabetes by improving insulin resistance. Increased physical activity — even a moderate amount such as 30 minutes of walking a day (ideally, more is better) — is also essential, not only for supporting weight loss, but also because it has a positive impact on insulin resistance.

Dietary Approaches to Losing Weight

As we learn more about the epigenome, it becomes increasingly clear that the single-variable approach, a traditional characteristic of nutrition research, has not adequately captured the many different effects that nutrition has on the human body. Nutrients engage in complex interactions with our genes, their variants and myriad epigenetic processes in ways we are only beginning to understand.

That being said, some dietary patterns have been well researched and may help manage type 2 diabetes by encouraging weight loss. However, it should be noted that medical concerns have been raised about the long-term effects of low-cal, low-carb and ketogenic diets. Also, because these diets limit the consumption of specific nutrients, they are not suitable for pregnant women.

A LOW-CALORIE DIET

Recently, research has emerged showing that it is possible to drive diabetes into remission by significant weight loss. One study compared 300 people who had been diagnosed with diabetes within the previous six and a half years. Half were assigned to a very-low-calorie diet (about 800 calories per day) for three to five months and stopped taking all their diabetes medications; the other half continued to follow standard diabetes protocols, taking their medications and participating in nutritional counseling. The group that restricted their consumption of calories lost on average about 30 pounds (13.6 kg) and almost half experienced remission of their diabetes. Only 4 percent of the standard-care group

METABOLIC AND BARIATRIC SURGERY

Metabolic and bariatric surgery aim to reduce stomach size or reroute the small intestine, with the goal of reducing the quantity of food consumed or the number of calories the body absorbs. These procedures are fairly dramatic and post-surgery they require strict caloric restriction. The associated weight loss has been shown to be very effective at reversing diabetes. Bariatric surgery in particular has been linked with significant metabolic improvements, which at least one study has associated with epigenetic changes that positively affect methylation levels.

achieved a similar result. It is important to note that diets this low in calories must be undertaken with medical supervision.

A LOW-CARB DIET

Studies show that when pregnant women follow a low-carb diet, they increase their risk of delivering a baby with a serious birth defect by as much as 30 percent. And a recent study linked adherence to a low-carb diet with an 18 percent increase in the development of atrial fibrillation (see "Heart Arrythmias," page 217.) However, a growing number of human studies indicate that a low-carbohydrate diet can improve some markers of diabetes. By facilitating weight and fat loss, it also reduces risk markers for heart disease. A moderately-low-carb diet consists of less than 60 to 100 grams of carbohydrate a day. In terms of macronutrient ratio, that works out to approximately 15 percent of daily calories from carbohydrates, 60 percent from fat and 25 percent from protein. (To put this into perspective, this is significantly less than the American Diabetes Association recommends, which is up to 180 grams of carbohydrate a day.)

A KETOGENIC DIET

A ketogenic diet is a very-low-carb diet that consists of less than 50 grams of carbs a day. These diets, which should be undertaken only under strict medical supervision, have been shown to reduce waist circumference and achieve weight loss in people with type 2 diabetes. Ketogenic diets are very effective at lowering blood sugar levels, so people with diabetes should expect that their medication will need to be adjusted accordingly.

A ketogenic diet maintains the body in a state of *ketosis*. That means the body switches its fuel source from carbs to fat. It should be noted as well that some scientists believe chronic ketosis is harmful and that ketogenic diets can increase LDL (low-density lipoprotein, or "bad") cholesterol in a small subset of people.

INTERMITTENT FASTING

Intermittent fasting (IF) is another recognized strategy for promoting weight loss that may also have particular benefits, such as lower fasting glucose, for people with type 2 diabetes. Animal studies indicate that it may be helpful in reducing insulin resistance. Additional benefits of IF include reduced waist circumference and decreased inflammation. Options for IF include:

1. Fasting for at least 12 hours (ideally 14 hours) between dinner and breakfast and limiting yourself to three meals a day;
2. Strictly reducing caloric intake by 500 to 600 calories for two days a week and eating normally the other days; or
3. Eating less than 800 calories for one day a week but maintaining a normal caloric intake the rest of the week.

A VEGAN OR VEGETARIAN DIET

Vegetarian and vegan diets are worth strongly considering for people with diabetes. In addition to promoting weight loss, they help to balance blood sugar and improve cholesterol levels. These diets are well established as preventive measures for diabetes, likely in part because of their high fiber content and above-average concentration of protective plant compounds, which among other benefits help to reduce inflammation. Increased intake of soy, which is a common source of protein in vegan and vegetarian diets, has been specifically associated with reducing the incidence of diabetes in women and Asian populations. Although human studies are scarce, in numerous animal studies genistein, a bioactive component of soy, has been shown to have an antidiabetic effect through its actions on pancreatic beta cells.

A NUTRIENT-DENSE DIET

We now know enough about nutrition and health to understand that the benefits of a healthy diet are derived from the combination of many different foods and nutrients and their cumulative and often synergistic effects on the human body. For people with diabetes, major medical organizations continue to promote diets based on mostly whole foods and that limit or entirely avoid highly processed foods, especially refined carbohydrates.

Within this category, the Mediterranean diet has been studied most with regard to preventing diabetes. It involves eating a moderate amount of protein along with primarily plant-based foods such as whole grains, fruits, vegetables, legumes and nuts, plus healthy fats obtained mainly from olive oil. The consumption of red wine, which has the benefit of slowing gastric emptying and thereby the rate as which blood sugar levels rise following a meal, is also recommended. In addition, red wine provides resveratrol, a plant compound also found in dark-colored berries and cocoa. Resveratrol has been shown to be a strong antioxidant, helping to protect the insulin-producing cells in the pancreas. However, be aware that cancer scientists now suggest that any regular intake of alcohol increases a person's risk for cancer.

New Tools for Diabetes Management

Recent research has shown that a few "superfoods" and "super supplements" have the ability to improve the genetic expression of certain proteins that can actually restore insulin function. The most studied of these proteins is called PPAR-gamma, and scientists are actively searching for ways to influence this powerful gene. In randomized controlled trials in humans, the following interventions had significantly beneficial effects on PPAR-gamma expression, and therefore insulin management, in particular groups of people:

- 1,000 mg of flaxseed oil supplementation, taken daily for 12 weeks by diabetic patients with heart disease;
- 1,000 mg of fish oil containing 180 mg EPA and 120 mg DHA, taken twice a day for 6 weeks by women with gestational diabetes;
- 250 mg of magnesium oxide, taken once a day for 6 weeks by women with gestational diabetes;
- 100 mg of CoQ10, a potent antioxidant, taken daily for 12 weeks by women with polycystic ovarian syndrome (PCOS), which is characterized by insulin resistance.

Additional "super nutrients" appear to be particularly beneficial in reducing type 2 diabetic risk factors. These include probiotics and prebiotics, fiber-rich foods that support friendly bacteria in the gut (see pages 282–288) and vitamin D, which helps with

Managing Diabetes with Diet

Unfortunately, experts can't seem to reach a consensus on the appropriate ratios of macronutrients for people with diabetes. Scientific recommendations continue to vary on the percentages of protein, fat and carbohydrates they should consume. As we learn more about genes and the epigenome, it seems likely that these differences in opinion reflect the possibility that there is no one-size-fits-all solution for managing diabetes through diet.

However, in general terms, all major diabetes organizations agree on the following:

- **Eat more vegetables.** Vegetables are rich in beneficial micronutrients, such as vitamins, minerals and protective plant compounds.

- **Consume enough fiber.** Twenty-five to 50 grams of fiber on a daily basis helps to keep blood sugar on an even keel. In addition, fiber nourishes the healthy bacteria in your gut. Obese people have an abnormal balance in their gut bacteria, which likely contributes to increased difficulty with managing insulin and keeping their weight under control.

- **Include healthy plant-based fats in your diet.** These include sources such as flax seeds, pumpkin seeds and extra virgin olive oil.

Carbohydrates

To date there is no scientific consensus about the amount of carbohydrate a person with diabetes should consume. However, all carbs are not created equal in terms of sending your blood sugar soaring. The glycemic index (GI) and glycemic load (GL) help to predict the impact that carb-containing foods will have on your blood sugar. Numerous studies have confirmed that diets with a large component of high-GI and high-GL foods increase the risk of diabetes.

Consider, for instance, that the foods that are key components of the standard American diet — refined sugar, white bread and white potatoes — all have very high GIs and GLs, while foods we designate as healthy, such as leafy greens, whole fruits, whole grains and legumes, have low GIs and GLs. Fats like olive oil and meats do not have a GI or GL because they contain no carbs and do not by themselves exert a noticeable effect on blood sugar.

When insulin therapy is required, all experts agree that it is essential to practice some form of carb-counting or monitoring, because the impact of carbohydrates on blood sugar will directly influence how much medication is required.

Fat

Experts generally agree that lower-fat diets are appropriate for people with diabetes, likely because fat is calorie-dense and caloric restriction is widely recognized as a strategy for losing weight. Diabetes organizations universally recommend reducing saturated fat intake to below 10 percent of daily caloric intake. Large epidemiological studies have associated consumption of saturated fat from animal foods (meat, dairy and eggs) with type 2 diabetes. Replacing saturated fats with monounsaturated fats — from nuts, seeds and olive oil — has been found to be protective against diabetes and to improve insulin resistance. Avoiding all highly processed trans fats (partially hydrogenated oils) has also been shown to significantly improve insulin resistance.

maintaining normal release of insulin from the pancreas. It's worth having your vitamin D level checked, because low levels are associated with insulin resistance. Vitamin D supplementation reduces low-grade inflammation in diabetics.

While these single nutrients show promising trends in research studies, the tried-and-true strategies for preventing, treating and reversing diabetes continue to be maintaining a healthy weight (or losing weight if overweight or obese), maintaining a physically active lifestyle, avoiding smoking, steering clear of energy-dense processed foods and consuming a whole-foods diet, primarily plant-based, that is rich in fiber, phytochemicals and healthy fats. These dietary and lifestyle choices, rather than fad diets, hold the keys to treating the diabetes epidemic.

HYPERTENSION

Hypertension, also known as high blood pressure, is one of the most prevalent chronic conditions everywhere in the world, affecting more than one billion adults. In 2017 the World Health Organization reported that around 40 percent of adults age 25 and over had hypertension. The rates are highest in Africa (46 percent) and lowest in the Americas (35 percent), where more men suffer from the condition (39 percent) than women (32 percent). In the United States, hypertension afflicts one in every three adults. New US guidelines, which have been widely criticized, were adopted at the end of 2017. The new standards mean that many people whose blood pressure used to be deemed normal are now classified as hypertensive; as a result, the number of people said to be suffering from the condition in America has jumped to 46 percent.

Hypertension is one of the constellation of disorders that comprise metabolic syndrome (see page 175). It is a serious problem because it increases your risk of much more severe disorders such as heart attack, heart failure, stroke and kidney disease. It is called a silent killer because there are often no noticeable symptoms.

So what is hypertension? When blood circulates throughout your body, it puts pressure on the walls of your blood vessels. Hypertension occurs when the pressure against those walls is consistently high. Not only does this gradually damage your blood vessels, but it makes your heart work much harder than necessary. Once your blood pressure is *consistently* high, your risk of developing a chronic illness increases over time.

"Consistently" means having a reading of more than 130/80 over a number of weeks. An occasional high reading is likely not cause for concern. For instance, you shouldn't be unduly alarmed if you register above normal when you visit your doctor; people's blood pressure often rises in response to physician visits, a phenomenon known as "white coat syndrome."

Hypertension, Ethnicity and Environment

In the United States hypertension is significantly more prevalent in African Americans than in other racial or ethnic groups. African Americans are likely to develop hypertension earlier, and the condition is more likely to result in complications such as heart disease and stroke. Some suggest this reflects the experience of being a person of color in America, and research backs this theory up. A number of studies that examined the living

LIFESTYLE AND BLOOD PRESSURE

Not surprisingly, lifestyle changes can benefit blood pressure. For instance, people who are overweight or obese have an increased risk of hypertension. For them, losing weight is a highly effective strategy. According to the Mayo Clinic, losing as little as 5 pounds (2.3 kg) can have a positive effect. In addition, being moderately active can make a big difference in managing hypertension. Studies show that moderate activity for just 30 minutes a day, most days of the week, can help to keep blood pressure under control. When your heart is stronger, it pumps blood more efficiently. The Mayo Clinic advises that increasing activity can lower systolic blood pressure (the top number) as effectively as some medications.

On the other hand, it is well known that smoking tobacco raises blood pressure (in addition to having numerous other negative health effects). So, too, does drinking too much alcohol. To maintain healthy blood pressure, moderate alcohol intake or less is recommended (a maximum of one drink a day for women and two for men).

Stress and anxiety also affect blood pressure. Ensuring that you get enough sleep, as well as incorporating deep breathing, meditation and other calming activities into your routine, can help to mitigate the negative effects of stress.

conditions of African Americans found connections between residing in a poor neighborhood, such as Detroit's inner city, and elevated blood pressure, suggesting that epigenetic changes linked with poverty and stress may be involved.

In the population as a whole, environmental factors such as stress and a sedentary lifestyle have been linked with hypertension, just as they have with obesity and diabetes. Although there seems to be a genetic connection, most experts think genes have only a small impact on the condition — there are too many different genes involved in its development, each playing a tiny role. Dr. Susan Prescott suggests that the immune system might also play a role, along with inflammation and oxidative stress. She believes hypertension may result when several physiological mechanisms work together synergistically.

The Developmental Origins of Hypertension

A woman's nutritional status during pregnancy is a significant factor in whether her offspring are prone to developing hypertension. In a paper linking maternal nutrition, a low nephron count and adult hypertension, Dr. Susan Bagby wrote that, as of the year 2000, more than 80 publications had linked low birth weight with a higher incidence of hypertension later in life. When fetal growth is restricted because the mother is undernourished, the development of abdominal organs such as the kidneys, liver and pancreas is likely to be affected.

Take the kidneys, for instance. If there aren't enough nutrients to sustain robust development, a fetus will develop an inadequate number of filtering units, called nephrons. Fewer nephrons and smaller kidneys are not in themselves problematic, because babies with low birth weights are small, so the organ size and capacity are fundamentally balanced. The problem lies in what happens after the baby is born. Poor nutrition in utero alters the baby's metabolism. Enhanced appetite and, consequently, accelerated early growth are likely results of this nutritional programming. So not only is the child's kidney function less than ideal, but they are likely to have a larger body mass, which puts further pressure on the kidneys.

Even so, as Dr. Bagby noted, being overweight is not a necessary prerequisite for developing hypertension. It is, however, an additional risk factor. A much more significant factor in whether someone will end up with hypertension as an adult is how they grow early in life. Children whose BMI increased rapidly between the ages of three and 15 were most vulnerable. Interestingly, even if this acceleration leveled off by the time they turned seven and they subsequently achieved a normal BMI, their risk of developing hypertension remained high. If they continued to gain more weight than usual until age 15, they were at increased risk for both hypertension and diabetes.

In 2002 David Barker and Johan Eriksson were among the authors of a longitudinal study based on the health data of more than 8,000 Finnish people born between 1934 and 1944 — the Helsinki Birth Cohort Study (see page 24). The researchers looked at specific aspects of the subjects' childhood and whether they had developed hypertension as adults. Of the group sampled, just over 1,400 suffered from hypertension (determined by medication prescribed to treat the condition). All had low birth weights and were either short or thin at birth but soon grew rapidly to compensate. From the age of eight and onwards their BMIs were above average.

Twenty-five percent of the subjects whose BMIs were high at age 12 subsequently developed hypertension, compared to 9 percent of people whose birth weight was high but who had a low BMI. Because the data allowed researchers insight into the socioeconomic status of their subjects, they were able to note that the growth dynamics had the greatest impact on subjects whose socioeconomic status was low when they were children. These findings resonate with some of the research on African Americans. In the Helsinki study, living conditions in adult life did not affect the risk of developing hypertension.

Hypertension and Salt

Unless you've been living off the grid for several decades, you probably think salt is to blame when blood pressure soars. From a plumbing perspective, this makes sense. When sodium is consumed in excess, blood levels of this essential mineral are likely to rise. To balance the excess, more water enters the bloodstream. This increases the overall volume in the blood vessels, which can lead to an increase in blood pressure. So it's not surprising that over the years studies have shown that reducing sodium can lower blood pressure.

Not Everyone Is Salt-Sensitive

Conventional wisdom has long held that a high intake of sodium contributes to hypertension. However, that's definitely not the whole story. While a low-sodium diet may help to improve blood pressure for some people over the short term, a number of recent studies have thrown conventional wisdom about dietary sodium into question.

Dr. Lynn L. Moore was the lead author of a 16-year study published in 2017 that looked at the role sodium plays in hypertension. While her team found "no evidence that a diet lower in sodium had any long-term beneficial effects on blood pressure," they did conclude that an intake of certain dietary minerals helped to keep blood pressure levels in check. Their findings indicated that when sodium is consumed with high levels of potassium, magnesium and calcium, lower blood pressure levels are the likely result.

Another study (derived from the second National Health and Nutrition Examination Survey study in the United States), which followed 7,000 adults for 13 years, showed that a low-sodium diet (less than 2,300 mg per day) actually *increased* the risk of death from heart disease. And research published in *The Lancet* in 2016 demonstrated that the link between sodium and blood pressure represents more of a bell curve: sodium intake either below 3 grams a day or over 7 grams a day can increase the risk of hypertension.

It may seem counterintuitive to link too little sodium with hypertension, but salt is an essential electrolyte. Electrolytes support proper levels of fluid in your body and provide electrical balance to keep your cells working together. If they become imbalanced (for instance, with too much calcium or potassium and not enough sodium), you may experience a wide range of symptoms, such as muscle spasms, an irregular heartbeat or even convulsions. Changes in blood pressure may also show up.

We now know that some people can consume high amounts of salt and have no trouble excreting it. Other people do not excrete excess sodium as easily, and when their kidneys can't keep up with the demand, hypertension is the result. In other words, the current dietary guidelines on sodium intake may not be relevant for some people.

Salt Sensitivity May Originate in the Womb

Birth size may play a role in how you process sodium. In a 2011 study published in the *American Journal of Clinical Nutrition*, which used data from the Helsinki Birth Cohort Study, researchers identified a link between salt intake, low birth weight at full term, and hypertension. The elderly men and women studied were more likely to be salt-sensitive (resulting in hypertension) if their birth weight was less than 6.7 pounds (3,050 g). Within this group, the researchers identified a clear link between higher daily intake of salt and elevation of the subjects' systolic blood pressure. They speculated that this association might be linked with fetal undernutrition that affected kidney development in utero. These findings suggest that individuals who are born at full term but with a low birth weight might benefit from reducing their dietary intake of sodium.

Researchers have also been exploring the role that genes play in the development of hypertension. We now know that numerous genes and gene variants are associated with whether individuals are sensitive to salt, and that when hypertension is caused by salt sensitivity, epigenetic modifications are implicated in development of the disease.

Dietary Strategies for Managing Hypertension

Even if you have been "programmed" for hypertension by your fetal and childhood development, diet can go a long way toward preventing and even treating it, if necessary.

Avoid Processed Foods

Although hypertension is a complex condition, there's little doubt that the rising rates are linked to the high levels of salt in processed foods. The current American Heart Association guidelines recommend no more than 2,300 mg of sodium intake per day — about 1 teaspoon (5 mL) of table salt — but most Americans consume 3,400 mg or more. The foods that contain the highest amounts of added sodium are processed foods and fast foods, so for many people, the easiest way to limit sodium is to avoid these. A side benefit will be reduced intake of added sugars, poor-quality fats and refined grains, all of which adversely affect health.

Increase Intake of Certain Nutrients

Avoiding processed foods also increases the nutrients you obtain. Not only do whole foods contain more vitamins, minerals and phytonutrients, but these nutrients work together synergistically. Studies have shown, for instance, that combining certain foods can dramatically increase their disease-fighting properties. Nutrients that help you maintain a healthy blood pressure include the following:

- **Potassium**, which is abundant in fruits and vegetables, is particularly crucial for managing blood pressure. Unfortunately, it is often lacking in the standard American diet. Potassium helps to balance sodium in the blood. It also helps to relax blood vessel walls, which can further reduce blood pressure. The recommended intake of potassium is 4,700 mg a day, but most people don't achieve that goal. Strategies to increase your consumption of potassium include snacking on high-potassium fruits (bananas, kiwis, mangos, melons and pears), switching out bread and pasta for sweet potatoes, and adding a green salad to every meal. If you find it difficult to eat enough fruits and vegetables on a daily basis, consider adding a freshly pressed juice or smoothie to your diet from time to time.

- **Magnesium** is very important for heart health because it helps to relax blood vessels. Many people are magnesium-deficient, not just because of low dietary intake, but also because magnesium in the body is easily depleted. Magnesium deficiency can be caused by chronic stress, alcohol consumption and certain drugs, including proton pump inhibitors (used to lower stomach acid production), diuretics (ironically, used to treat hypertension) and even some antibiotics. Magnesium is found in unprocessed foods such as whole grains, beans, nuts and dark green leafy vegetables. People who have hypertension should make a special effort to ensure that they obtain adequate amounts of magnesium from their diet. They may also need to supplement with additional magnesium.

- **Calcium** also helps your blood vessels relax. Consumed along with potassium and magnesium as part of a healthy diet, it helps to keep blood pressure in check. The best approach is to focus on obtaining it through a diet based on whole foods, including dairy foods, dark green leafy vegetables (such as collard greens and kale), almonds, broccoli, bok choy, beans and fish such as sardines and salmon.

- **Vitamin D** deficiency seems to increase the risk of hypertension. Studies have been inconclusive about why this might be. The best approach is to have your doctor test your blood levels of vitamin D. If necessary, supplement with vitamin D_3 to ensure optimal levels.

Specific Dietary Approaches

Since hypertension is a major risk factor for heart attack and stroke, numerous dietary approaches to managing the condition are being studied. Here are a few examples:

THE DASH DIET

The Diet to Stop Hypertension (DASH diet) is a well-researched dietary plan that has been shown to lower blood pressure within two weeks. While the initial goals of the diet focused on improving and reversing hypertension, additional studies have shown that if it is followed over the long term, it can have multiple benefits. It promotes weight loss and reduces the risk of stroke, heart failure, osteoporosis, kidney stones and some types of cancer. The DASH diet is recommended by the American Heart Association and the National Heart, Lung, and Blood Institute and is included in the US guidelines for treating hypertension.

The DASH diet is based on consumption of whole foods. It is rich in fruit, vegetables, whole grains, low-fat dairy products, beans, nuts, seeds and lean meats. It focuses on foods that are rich in nutrients associated with lower blood pressure, specifically potassium, calcium and magnesium. It also limits sweets and sugar-sweetened beverages.

THE PORTFOLIO DIET

Originally developed for reducing cholesterol levels (see "Diet and Cholesterol," page 208), this vegetarian diet was found to lower blood pressure as well. The portfolio diet includes the usual suspects in heart-healthy dietary approaches: fruits, vegetables and whole grains. It also emphasizes foods containing soluble fiber (such as whole-grain oats and barley, legumes, okra and eggplant), nuts, soy protein and plant sterols (found in whole grains, legumes and sesame, pumpkin and sunflower seeds). Research suggests that the portfolio diet is more effective than the DASH diet for reducing blood pressure; in fact, it was found to be as effective as a standard starting dose of blood pressure medication. However, compliance may be challenging.

THE MEDITERRANEAN DIET

Recent research has linked the Mediterranean diet, discussed on page 195, with lower blood pressure in study participants. It is rich in fruits, vegetables, whole grains, nuts, seeds and healthy fats, especially extra virgin olive oil. This diet is recommended by many cardiologists and the American Heart Association, among others.

HEART DISEASE

Heart disease is a serious health problem not only in and of itself, but also because it is the most expensive disease to treat. Cardiovascular disease (CVD), which used to be viewed as a disease of affluence, has migrated from Western countries to those that are less developed. It is now the number-one cause of death around the world. According to the World Health Organization, in 2015 almost 18 million people died from cardiovascular disease, including 7.4 million from coronary heart disease and 6.7 million from stroke. In the United States alone, the Centers for Disease Control and Prevention report that over 600,000 people die from heart disease every year, accounting for one in every four deaths.

It Begins in the Womb

In 1997 Johan Eriksson and David Barker published the first of the more than 120 papers they collaborated on, based on information obtained from the Helsinki Birth Cohort Study. Published in the *British Medical Journal*, the paper reported their finding that babies whose growth was restricted in utero by poor maternal nutrition had an increased risk of heart disease as adults. Subsequent studies examined growth and adiposity in childhood, concluding that the highest rates of heart disease occurred in males who were thin at birth but gained weight rapidly as children; by the time they were seven years old, the at-risk males had an average or above-average BMI. Drs. Barker and Eriksson identified a slightly different pattern of catch-up growth in females. For the women they studied, thinness at birth wasn't the issue; rather, coronary heart disease was more strongly associated with short body length at birth.

Perhaps not surprisingly, Drs. Eriksson and Barker also found strong similarities in the childhood growth patterns of people who developed heart disease and those who ended up with diabetes. People with diabetes had, as children, experienced a rapid weight gain that continued past the average. The adults who suffered from a stroke were short at birth and had grown more slowly as infants than other children. As the doctors reported in a study published in the *International Journal of Epidemiology* in 2008, low birth weight and slow growth during infancy are linked with an increased risk of coronary heart disease and stroke later in life, likely because this growth pattern inhibits liver growth and influences liver metabolism, which may alter how the body metabolizes cholesterol.

Eighteen percent of the study participants whose development conformed to this model took lipid-lowering drugs.

These findings align with other research into developmental origins for CVD. Data from the Dutch Hunger Winter showed that people whose mothers were pregnant during the famine were twice as likely to develop heart disease as adults. And David Barker's original findings linked low birth weight with chronic disease later in life. He found that people who weighed 5 pounds (2,300 g) at birth were three to five times more likely to develop CVD than those who weighed 9 pounds (4,090 g). We now know that epigenetics participates in these outcomes. Basically, factors that influence fetal development impact the expression of several genes involved in growth and metabolism. Metabolic syndrome, diabetes and hypertension are all linked to metabolism, and all of these conditions are major risk factors for CVD.

NOT A DISEASE OF AFFLUENCE

Although various theories on the social determinants of health have been around since the 1800s, epidemiologists such as David Barker and Anders Forsdahl (see "Hunches about Links," page 19) were among the first to use statistics to identify links between low socioeconomic status and illness. Their work showed that the origins of CVD are more likely to be located in poor living conditions than in comfort and prosperity. Over the course of decades, a substantial amount of research has emerged to support this point of view.

Chronic Stress and Heart Disease

Stress has long been associated with heart disease. In fact, many believe it qualifies as a unique risk factor for the illness. One of the advantages of our developing knowledge of epigenetics is its promise to identify some of the mechanisms underlying how environmental impacts, such as stress, lead to the development of disease. Adverse childhood experiences have a significant impact on long-term health, so it shouldn't be surprising that numerous studies are now linking heart disease and related conditions with negative experiences early in life.

For instance, studies have specifically linked poverty with heart disease. A paper published in the *American Journal of Epidemiology* in 2009 concluded that people who grew up in economically deprived circumstances are 82 percent more likely to develop heart disease than those from more prosperous backgrounds. A 2006 study, based on data from the Johns Hopkins Precursors Study, looked at white male physicians, all of whom had gone on to successful and productive lives. Those from low socioeconomic backgrounds had a significantly higher BMI at all the life stages documented by the study, and they were twice as likely to develop CVD before reaching the age of 50.

This is yet another example of early-life experiences significantly altering gene expression. Marcus Pembrey was one of the authors of a 2011 study (limited to men) published in *Epigenetic Epidemiology* that examined more than 20,000 DNA sites across the genome. By connecting the dots, the researchers could identify epigenetic changes resulting from childhood experiences that were affecting the men's DNA as adults. Half of the subjects came from affluent homes — the top 20 percent in terms of socioeconomic status — whereas the remainder grew up in households that fell in the bottom 20 percent. When the researchers measured methylation levels, they discovered major differences between the two groups. In the disadvantaged group, methylation levels were affected at 1,252 sites. The men from privileged backgrounds were affected at only 545 sites. The methylation changes tended to occur in clusters, suggesting that entire networks of genes had been epigenetically modified by the men's childhood experiences.

Like other studies, Pembrey's research paints a picture that captures the long-term health effects of early social disadvantage. As he speculated in an interview with *New Scientist*, the genes of the disadvantaged subjects may have changed their behavior as a protective response, to help them survive a challenging childhood. However, over the long term, the differential methylation patterns may have increased their risk of developing serious health conditions such as heart disease and diabetes.

Heart Disease and Genes

Looking at the genome in general, approximately 60 SNPs are commonly linked with the risk for CVD. Many of these overlap with those connected to the risk for ischemic stroke, which is caused by decreased blood flow to the brain. A 2018 study published in the journal *Circulation: Cardiovascular Genetics* identified almost 200 widespread genetic variants in people of European ancestry that worked together to predict the risk for CVD. People with a high number of these variants are at increased risk of developing early-onset coronary artery disease ("early onset" is defined as prior to the age of 40 for males and 45 for females). The researchers noted that charting a significant number of these SNPs could serve as an early warning system, identifying people with a heightened likelihood of developing the disease.

However, the number of people with these variants who actually develop CVD varies widely. From a genetic standpoint, heart disease is multifactorial, which means it involves hundreds of different genes, each of which makes only a small contribution to its development. In addition, those genes have complex relationships not only with each other but also with their environment, which includes the impact of external influences ranging from nutrition and level of physical activity to exposure to toxins, access to green spaces, socioeconomic status and social networks. In other words, it's your genes in combination with your epigenome that determines whether you will develop CVD.

Heart Disease and Cholesterol

Conventional wisdom suggests that high cholesterol and heart disease go hand in hand. However, this assumption is far from proven. While high levels of LDL ("bad") cholesterol can cause plaque to form in the arteries, nearly half of heart attacks occur in people who appear to have normal cholesterol levels. At least 30 percent of people with heart disease have no known risk factors. For them, early-life changes may be underlying causes.

Your Body Needs Cholesterol

Cholesterol is not bad. In fact, this steroid compound is crucial for several important jobs. For starters, your body needs it to create cells and keep them functioning. It supports the walls of all your cells but is particularly important for your brain. About a quarter of the cholesterol in your body resides in your brain, and it plays a key role in the construction of the cells in your central nervous system. Cholesterol is a component of the membrane surrounding every cell. It connects nerve cells and the myelin sheath, helping to transmit nerve impulses and keep your nervous system humming. Moreover, your body needs cholesterol to make steroid hormones and vitamin D, and to produce bile, which is necessary for digesting dietary fats.

More Than Diet

Most people produce about 75 percent of their cholesterol in their liver, while the remaining 25 percent is absorbed from their diet. Your body can adjust for the amount of

DIET AND CHOLESTEROL

The idea that foods high in dietary cholesterol, such as eggs and shellfish, and those high in saturated fat, such as red meat, raise cholesterol and therefore cause heart attacks is an oversimplification. For most people, dietary cholesterol has little or no impact on blood cholesterol levels. However, a 2019 study of almost 30,000 people, now being actively debated, did identify a link between excess dietary cholesterol and an increased risk of CVD. The evidence linking saturated fat consumption with high LDL levels is also under debate. Intake of saturated fat raises both "good" (HDL) and "bad" (LDL) cholesterol. It may also modify LDL cholesterol, making it less harmful.

Recent research suggests that another dietary factor may be playing a more significant role in the development of heart disease. A 2015 study published in *JAMA* linked added sugars in the diet with an increase in mortality from CVD. Added sugars are found primarily in processed foods. In addition to the usual suspects (sodas and energy drinks), various forms of sugar are added to a wide range of foods, including breakfast cereals and even "healthy" options such as yogurt. Given what we now know about the potential health risks, if you are consuming any kind of prepared food, it's wise to check the ingredient list for added sugars.

In terms of blood cholesterol, here's the basic problem: a high intake of added sugar is linked with lower HDL cholesterol levels. It has also been shown to produce higher levels of small-dense LDL, a subtype of LDL cholesterol that is more likely to cause plaques in blood vessel walls. In addition, excessive sugar (as well as alcohol and refined grains and flours) can increase triglyceride levels, which are an independent risk factor for both heart disease and nonalcoholic fatty liver disease (see page 176). Moreover, a diet high in sugar and refined carbohydrates is often lower in fiber, a nutrient that plays a key role in keeping cholesterol levels balanced. So, all in all, added sugar is a basketful of bad news.

A diet of fiber-rich whole foods high in healthy omega-3 fatty acids will help to keep cholesterol under control. Dr. David Jenkins, an endocrinologist and research scientist at the Li Ka Shing Knowledge Institute of St. Michael's Hospital in Toronto, led the research team that developed the glycemic index. He subsequently developed a plant-based diet that has been shown to reduce LDL cholesterol in people whose cholesterol levels are not genetic in origin. The portfolio diet is a modified vegetarian diet that helps to not only reduce total and LDL cholesterol levels but also lower blood pressure (see page 203). Studies have shown that the portfolio diet can reduce LDL cholesterol by as much as 30 percent.

cholesterol you consume by increasing or decreasing the quantity your liver produces. Genetics, early-life development, diet and lifestyle all play a role in cholesterol levels. As noted earlier, several genes linked with metabolism are affected by prenatal experiences, which also may influence how the body metabolizes cholesterol.

For most people, genes play only a small part in determining blood cholesterol levels. But for a small percentage, their impact can be quite significant. For example, familial hypercholesterolemia is a gene defect that causes people to lose the ability to eliminate the LDL particles their liver produces. This deficiency can lead to extremely high levels of LDL, increasing the risk that heart disease will develop early in life.

Another genetic factor is the APOE (apolipoprotein E) gene. People with certain variants of this gene tend to absorb more dietary cholesterol and have higher LDL levels. If you are one of these people, reducing your consumption of cholesterol-rich foods can be an effective way to keep your cholesterol levels in check. However, recent research shows that for the general population, broad recommendations to avoid cholesterol-rich foods won't lower levels of "bad" cholesterol.

Women and Heart Disease

Although we know that there are sex-related differences in the risk of developing heart disease, the area does not appear to be well researched. As noted, Johan Eriksson and David Barker found that males who developed heart disease later in life were more likely to be thin at birth, whereas females were more likely to have a short body length. While it has long been thought that hormonal changes related to menopause increase the risk of CVD in older women, experts are now taking a serious second look at that assumption.

In the summer of 2018, a study published in the journal *Heart* concluded that various reproductive factors may increase women's risk for heart disease and stroke. Researchers followed more than 250,000 women for an average of seven years. They found that girls who began to menstruate before they turned 12 were 5 percent more likely to develop coronary heart disease, 10 percent more likely to suffer from cardiovascular disease, and 17 percent more likely to have a stroke.

A propensity to miscarry is another risk factor. Women who have had three or more miscarriages are more than twice as likely to develop heart disease as those who never miscarry. And women who have obstetric complications, including preeclampsia and gestational diabetes, are more likely to suffer cardiovascular disease as they age. Early menopause (before the age of 47), whether artificially or naturally induced, also increases heart disease risk. Researchers suggest that improved screening for women with identifiable risk factors such as these could help to prevent heart disease from developing.

The good news is that breastfeeding has a preventive effect in warding off CVD. Epidemiologist Dr. Sanne Peters has studied breastfeeding from the maternal perspective. In one 2017 study of Chinese women, she found that breastfeeding reduced the risk of CVD in mothers by about 10 percent. Her data showed that the longer the mothers breastfed, the greater the reduction in risk.

Atherosclerosis

What can an ancient Egyptian mummy teach us about clogged arteries? Known as atherosclerosis in medical terminology, this dangerous condition results when arteries become blocked by a buildup of plaque. Atherosclerosis is far and away the primary cause of heart attacks. It can also cause stroke, peripheral arterial disease and aneurysms.

Atherosclerosis has replaced infectious diseases as a leading cause of death in the developed world, and although pinpointing the causes has proved challenging, conventional wisdom suggests it is a "lifestyle disease" of the modern era. It has been linked with a high dietary intake of meat, certain kinds of fat and, perhaps, refined carbohydrates. Other factors associated with the condition include sedentary behavior, cigarette smoking and that inevitable fact of life, simply getting older.

Current lifestyles notwithstanding, evidence suggests that the disease was stalking humans long before fast-food chains set up shop and the couch-potato way of life became something approaching the norm. Research indicates, for instance, that our preindustrial ancestors were (statistically speaking) about as likely to suffer from atherosclerosis as contemporary humans. And, just like us, the longer they lived, the more blocked their arteries became.

Long ago, some citizens of ancient societies enjoyed the luxury of having their bodies wrapped up and preserved after they died, in hopes of improving their journey into the afterlife. Fortunately for us, some of those mummies, along with others preserved by natural forces, are still intact. And they have a few things to teach us about heart disease.

When a group of scientists used modern technology to scan the bodies of 137 mummies, they found calcified plaque in more than 30 percent of the preserved remains. These individuals dwelled in locations as diverse as ancient Egypt, Peru, southwest America and the Aleutian Islands. Surprisingly, the findings were relatively consistent across all the geographical locations, even though the diets of the embalmed specimens were quite diverse. Indigenous plants varied among the locations, as did protein sources, which ranged from mainly seafood to the meat of domesticated animals.

The study, which was published in *The Lancet* in 2013, found just two commonalities among the populations: the use of fire for cooking as well as for warmth, and the likelihood, given the times in which they lived, that humans suffered from reasonably high levels of chronic infection. As the researchers noted, in hunter-forager horticultural societies that didn't have access to antibiotics, about 75 percent of mortality could be attributed to infectious disease. The disparate diets and high levels of physical activity of these ancient citizens led the researchers to conclude that current knowledge, which tends to identify atherosclerosis as a lifestyle disease, is at best incomplete.

Inflammation: A Common Thread

As scientists move forward on understanding atherosclerosis, exposure to smoke (today often in the form of tobacco smoke) seems to be linked with development of the disease. Basically, smoke provokes inflammation. Recent scientific thinking is shifting toward chronic inflammation as the underlying cause of heart disease, and away from the traditional wisdom that identifies high cholesterol as the main perpetrator in the development of plaque.

Consider, for instance, that cholesterol levels are normal in about half the people who have a heart attack. Significantly as well, most of the data linking fat and CVD come from prosperous European and North American societies. Although total fat consumption is only part of the equation, the Prospective Urban and Rural Epidemiological (PURE) Study — a large cohort study published in *The Lancet* in 2017 — which looked at more than 135,000 individuals from 18 countries, found no connection between fat intake and CVD or heart attack.

Without dwelling on the details, atherosclerosis results from a gradual buildup of harmful substances. Among these are fatty streaks in the arteries. The fatty streaks can be linked to the risky lipid profile associated with babies who were small at birth and grew slowly during the first two years of their lives. As Barker and Eriksson found, by the time these babies were adults approaching 60, their HDL cholesterol was lower and their triglycerides were likely to be higher than usual. Children whose mothers smoke or have high cholesterol themselves are also more likely to have fatty streaks. And it may be worth noting that many risk factors for CVD, such as high triglycerides, increased blood pressure and various measures of adiposity, begin to show up in children. When they occur in clusters, the risk rises.

Most experts agree that the fatty streaks in the arteries progress to atherosclerotic plaques in adulthood by propelling inflammation. Atherosclerosis develops slowly over a long period of time. By the time plaque shows up, the disease process is well underway.

What do the mummies with surprising rates of atherosclerosis tell us about inflammation? Exposure to smoke was one of only two commonalities among the mummy populations. Today the connection between cigarette smoke and inflammation is well established. Even from an early age, smokers have higher levels of inflammation, which promotes development of plaque (smoking is also one of the major risk factors for heart disease). So it's reasonable to assume that our ancestors had high levels of inflammation along with plaque.

C-REACTIVE PROTEIN

C-reactive protein (CRP) is a substance produced by the liver that rises in response to inflammation. These days physicians can identify inflammation by measuring CRP levels. Consistently high levels have been linked with numerous conditions, including immune-mediated skin diseases, periodontitis (gum disease), kidney disease, obesity and type 2 diabetes, as well as atherosclerosis.

CRP is integrally connected to the immune system: its levels increase as part of the body's natural reaction to infections, trauma and allergens. When your body is fighting an infection, your CRP rises to battle potentially harmful pathogens as part of the body's defense system. Once the job is done, CRP should return to normal levels. When that doesn't happen, inflammation becomes problematic.

PLAQUE AND THE IMMUNE SYSTEM

Scientists now believe that inflammation is implicated in the formation of artery-clogging plaque, thanks to a malfunction in the immune system. In fact, atherosclerosis has been described as a chronic inflammatory and immune disease. When the body's innate immune-system response misfires, it generates inflammatory substances that create plaque.

Dr. Susan Prescott is a world expert on immune system development, and her research supports the conclusion that the immune system plays a starring role in the development of plaque. As she noted in her book *Origins*, for more than a century experts have been speculating that infections, a common cause of elevated CRP, may promote, if not actually cause, atherosclerosis. However, so far that theory hasn't held up. Although bacterial DNA has been detected in plaques, the evidence isn't strong enough to identify infection as a primary cause of plaque development; for example, antibiotics do not prevent CVD.

However, gut bacteria do play a prominent role in our immune system (see below and chapter 9). And although the research is still in its early stages, researchers are actively studying links between gut microbiota and numerous inflammatory diseases. We know, for instance, that specific probiotics, such as *Lactobacillus reuteri*, reduce inflammation, and that patients with certain inflammatory conditions, such as Crohn's disease, are deficient in particular groups of intestinal bacteria. Emerging evidence suggests that a diet high in fiber that promotes the development of friendly gut bacteria and the production of short-chain fatty acids may protect against CVD by lowering inflammation.

THE ROLE OF MICROBES

The hygiene hypothesis (see page 272) provides another connection between inflammation and infection. Its basic premise is that modern environments have become too clean. Many children are dirt-deprived. By not allowing them to play in the mud or limiting their exposure to animals, their parents may be increasing their risk of developing chronic diseases later in life. When children's exposure to infectious agents like bacteria is inadequate, their immune systems don't develop robustly. This likely creates a predisposition to inflammation.

Thomas McDade, a biological anthropologist with a particular interest in how inflammation develops and contributes to the diseases of aging, found that CRP levels were much lower in people who lived in less developed countries than in residents of the United States. For example, Filipino children who grew up in rural areas with high levels of microbial diversity had much lower levels of CRP as adults. The underlying dynamic, suggests Susan Prescott, is part of a natural process. In the course of frequently battling infections, inflammation rises and falls, creating more effective regulatory pathways that can switch inflammation on or off as required. If there aren't enough infections to fight, the pathways aren't as robust, which likely sets the stage for chronic inflammation later in life.

Biologically, the basic premise of the hygiene hypothesis resembles the "thrifty phenotype" idea — the theory that malnourishment in the womb creates a predisposition to fat storage that may be maladaptive in times of plenty. As Dr. McDade commented in a 2012 paper, it seems likely that our bodies "could not anticipate the highly sanitized, low-infectious disease environments currently inhabited by humans in affluent industrialized settings." Because the human immune system is still quite plastic in early life,

Remedying Chronic Inflammation

As we learn more about the connections between inflammation and various disease states, we are also gaining insight into why inflammation develops and learning techniques for managing it. An interesting side note is that researchers now suspect that statins — one of the most frequently prescribed medications in the world — may be beneficial in treating heart disease not so much for their cholesterol-lowering abilities, but rather because they reduce inflammation, as measured by CRP levels. Some evidence indicates that their anti-inflammatory benefits result from their influence on epigenetic mechanisms, specifically histone modifications.

Food and Inflammation

There are numerous connections between elevated CRP and diet. We know, for instance, that certain foods promote inflammation. These include refined carbohydrates, such as grains from which the bran and germ have been removed (refined wheat, rice and corn are the major offenders), processed sugars (including high-fructose corn syrup) and processed deli meats. Excessive alcohol intake is also known to promote inflammation, as is smoking cigarettes. Susan Prescott also suggests that a high-fat, low-fiber diet may encourage inflammation by negatively influencing the composition of gut microbiota.

Various diets, including the Mediterranean diet and the Pritikin diet, can reduce inflammation. In general terms, these diets tend to be high in vegetables, fruits, whole grains, nuts, seeds and healthy fats. The Pritikin diet, in conjunction with regular exercise, has been specifically shown to reduce levels of CRP in the blood.

As popular diets come and go, however, it is becoming increasingly clear that one size does not fit all. Genetic research suggests that some people may be more prone to inflammation than others, and that the same dietary changes may not work for everyone. For example, although studies on the benefits of polyunsaturated fatty acid (PUFA) supplementation in general have been contradictory, it may benefit people with certain genotypes. Among this group, consumption of omega-3 fatty acids has been shown to reduce inflammation by altering epigenetic markers such as DNA methylation.

Inflammation has also been linked with the ratio of omega-3 to omega-6 fats in the diet. The standard American diet leans toward lower intakes of omega-3s and higher intakes of omega-6s, a ratio that is thought to drive systemic inflammation and contribute to the development of atherosclerosis.

And let's not forget your gut. Consuming a high percentage of plant-based foods supports positive ratios of beneficial bacteria in your gut. Some of these microbial companions produce short-chain fatty acids (SCFAs), which help to lower inflammation. SCFAs have also been shown to influence gene expression in ways that reduce the production of inflammatory cytokines, a protein usually produced by the immune system.

Stress and Inflammation

Chronic psychological stress also plays a role in systemic inflammation. Cortisol, one of the body's stress hormones, influences inflammation. Some evidence indicates that when cortisol levels remain elevated because of chronic stress, immune cell receptors become less sensitive to the hormone, reducing its ability to control inflammation. In addition, we know from animal studies that chronic exposure to stress changes gene expression in immune cells, making them more pro-inflammatory. Interestingly, these patterns of pro-inflammatory gene expression have also been found in young adults exposed to the chronic stress associated with low socioeconomic status.

Stress-reduction techniques can be effective for moderating the effect of stress on inflammation. A systematic review showed that mind–body interventions (MBIs) such as yoga, tai chi and meditation decrease the expression of pro-inflammatory genes. A regular dose of physical activity is also a great inflammation fighter: numerous studies have demonstrated the anti-inflammatory benefits of exercise. A 2017 study published in the journal *Brain, Behavior, and Immunity* concluded that just 20 minutes of moderate exercise, including walking on a treadmill, resulted in a reduction of TNF (tumor necrosis factor), a pro-inflammatory cytokine.

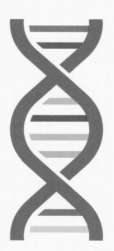

he suggested that "a poorly educated immune system may be the result" of our overly pristine environments. He believes that, just as we expose infants and children to cognitive and social stimuli to promote brain development, we also need to open them up to a broader range of diverse microbes to encourage development of their immune systems. In so doing, we may reduce their chances of developing chronic inflammation and, perhaps, atherosclerosis as well.

CONNECTING THE DOTS

While we don't have all the answers, it seems likely that chronic inflammation is a response to a variety of environmental factors. These include poor nutrition and toxic exposures, including to cigarette smoke, as well as a lifestyle that is deficient in microbes. As noted above, evidence suggests that a propensity for chronic inflammation may begin in the womb. We know, for instance, that babies with a low birth weight (and possibly those at the high end of the birth weight spectrum too) are born in a pro-inflammatory condition.

In 2017 Thomas McDade used data from the Philippine birth cohort mentioned above to connect the dots between epigenetic changes in childhood and chronic inflammation as an adult. His research found that quality of nutrition, the robustness of microbial exposure and socioeconomic status in childhood could predict DNA methylation in nine genes involved in regulating inflammation. It's one more step along the circuitous path linking the various biological mechanisms at work in early life that predispose individuals to developing heart disease as adults.

HEART DISEASE, INFLAMMATION AND SOCIAL DISADVANTAGE

The more we learn, the stronger the connections grow between heart disease, chronic inflammation and social disadvantage. Poverty is associated with poor nutrition for various reasons, not the least of which is overconsumption of processed foods, which tend to exacerbate inflammation. Inflammation has also been linked with childhood mistreatment. One 2017 study found that more than 10 percent of people with high levels of CRP had experienced some form of abuse in the first decade of their life, and their levels of CRP were commensurate with the severity of the abuse. We know that CRP is elevated with stress or hormonal surges. The jury is still out on whether CRP is just a marker of inflammation or a pathological agent.

Notably, overweight and obese people have significantly higher levels of CRP. Susan Prescott speculates that chronic inflammation may be one of the links between CVD and obesity, because adipose fat tissues release substances that promote inflammation.

Heart Arrhythmias

Have you ever heard the term "holiday heart syndrome" and wondered what it meant? It was coined in 1978, and it refers to the association between drinking too much alcohol and the onset of disturbances in heart rhythm, most commonly atrial fibrillation. The expression came about when physicians noticed that patients who didn't have underlying heart disease were more likely to experience heart arrhythmias after weekends and holiday periods when they drank more alcohol.

Heart arrhythmias occur when the electrical impulses that coordinate your heartbeat don't work properly. Heart arrhythmias also include bradycardia (a slower-than-normal heartbeat) and tachycardia (when your heart beats too fast). Atrial fibrillation (AFib), which is characterized by an erratic heartbeat, is the most common form of arrhythmia. According to a 2019 study published in the journal *Heart Rhythm*, about 25 percent of adults over 40 in the United States are at risk for AFib. AFib afflicts about 35 million people worldwide. The number of people with the condition is growing rapidly, and death rates linked to AFib, as either the primary or contributing cause of death, have been rising for more than 20 years.

The main danger associated with atrial fibrillation is ischemic stroke, which occurs when blood clots form in the heart and travel to the brain; the risk increases fivefold in people with AFib. Because the heart beats so erratically, blood is not properly pumped out of it, so it pools and is likely to clot before traveling to the brain. AFib is estimated to be the root cause of about 20 percent of ischemic strokes.

The risk for atrial fibrillation increases with age. In addition to alcohol consumption, risk factors include hypertension, diabetes, obesity, hyperthyroidism and chronic kidney disease. Other potential perpetrators include electrolyte imbalances, stress and prescription medications. Based on a survey of 1,300 patients with AFib, the 2019 study identified common triggers. These included drinking coffee (28 percent) and lack of sleep (21 percent). The consensus was that when two or more triggers were combined, the likelihood of experiencing an episode increased. It should be noted that other studies have specified that moderate tea and coffee consumption is problematic for people with AFib.

In addition, AFib has been linked with participation in football and endurance sports, such as marathon running.

A Developmental Component

Heart arrhythmias have a hereditary component: certain genes are associated with increased risk. They may also be traced back to fetal development. A 2017 study published in the *Journal of the American Heart Association*, which used data from the Helsinki Birth Cohort Study, found a U-shaped association between birth weight and incidence of AFib: babies born with either a low or high birth weight were at increased risk. The authors also discovered that, independent of birth weight, the offspring of obese mothers were approximately 35 percent more likely to develop AFib than those born to mothers whose BMI was in the normal range. They suggested that prepregnancy lifestyle interventions to reduce maternal obesity might have a positive effect on AFib risk in future generations. In addition, the study identified tall stature as a risk factor, which may account for the higher incidence of AFib among males.

While recognizing that the mechanisms are not fully understood, the authors of the study speculated that epigenetic changes in utero might contribute to development of the condition. Both obesity and AFib are linked with inflammation, and AFib is also highly reactive to environmental triggers like air pollution. A 2015 study published in *Heart Rhythm* linked early-life exposure to secondhand smoke, either in utero or in childhood, with an increased risk of developing the condition. Recently, scientists have begun seeing connections with the immune system. Immune cells secrete certain substances that have been linked with arrhythmias. In 2017 scientists reported that macrophages, a type of white blood cell known for fighting off infections, help your heart to beat in a regular fashion.

Common Triggers

Triggers for AFib include alcohol consumption, stress, food sensitivities, electrolyte imbalances and exposure to toxins.

ALCOHOL CONSUMPTION

Epidemiological research shows that alcohol consumption plays a definite role in triggering AFib, even in people with no previous signs of heart disease. Binge drinking in particular is known to interfere with the heart's conduction system, triggering irregular beats. In people with a history of AFib, alcohol consumption may also increase the release of certain neurotransmitters associated with heart rhythm. (However, at least one study found it had no effect on people without a history of AFib.)

STRESS

Numerous studies have linked various types of stress, including perceived rather than actual stress, with increased risk for AFib. A 2018 study based on data from the Swedish Longitudinal Occupational Survey of Health showed that people experiencing job stress were 50 percent more likely to develop AFib. Another study published that year in the *American Journal of Cardiology* connected traumatic life events with the development of AFib in women over 45. And a 2015 study published in the *Annals of Internal Medicine*, based on the Reasons for Geographic and Racial Differences in Stroke (REGARDS) research, identified high levels of perceived stress associated with low income as a risk factor for AFib.

Although the immediate concern with AFib is that it will lead to stroke, the anxiety associated with having an out-of-control heartbeat is in itself problematic, and concerns have been raised about the long-term effects of the disease on mental health and quality of life.

FOOD SENSITIVITIES

Although the evidence is largely anecdotal, food sensitivities have also been associated with AFib. Many people report reacting to tyramine, a compound that occurs naturally in aged and fermented foods (it has also has been linked with migraine headaches). Major offenders include aged cheeses, such as Cheddar, or those that contain streaks of mold, such as various types of blue cheese, as well as fermented foods like sauerkraut and soy sauce.

Monosodium glutamate (MSG), an ingredient used as a flavor enhancer in many processed foods, and aspartame, an artificial sweetener, are potentially problematic for people with AFib. Although there have been no peer-reviewed studies, many people with AFib report that consuming either MSG or aspartame can trigger an episode. In the digestive process MSG produces free glutamate and aspartame releases aspartate. Both substances are neurotransmitters and are known to be excitotoxins, which means they overstimulate the brain and possibly the heart via their influence on the vagus nerve. These substances are used extensively in processed foods because they encourage "addiction" to certain flavors.

Recent research, including a study under the auspices of the Mayo Clinic, is looking at the links between AFib and autoimmune conditions. Other studies have investigated connections with dysbiotic gut bacteria. An out-of-whack microbiome could play a role in triggering AFib by activating the autonomic nervous system, which is actively linked to the gut via the vagus nerve. Another gut connection is through the immune system, which some research, including studies of histamine intolerance, has linked with AFib. Histamine intolerance can produce a very broad range of symptoms. In general, reactions result from deficiencies related to the functioning of the DAO or HNMT gene, which hamper the body's ability to process histamine. In addition to heart arrhythmias, these deficiencies have been linked to a wide variety of autoimmune conditions, including gluten sensitivity and inflammatory bowel disease. High amounts of histamine are found in certain foods, such as those belonging to the nightshade family, which includes tomatoes, potatoes, peppers and eggplant. Many prescription drugs can also trigger a histamine reaction, as can consuming spicy food or food that causes bloating.

ELECTROLYTE IMBALANCES

Electrolytes are chemicals that conduct electricity in your body. They include charged forms of sodium, calcium, potassium and magnesium. Your heart muscle uses these minerals to carry electrical impulses, and when they become unbalanced, an irregular heartbeat may result. A common electrolyte imbalance occurs with too much sodium and too little potassium. These elements are intricately linked and, unfortunately, are likely to be unbalanced in the standard American diet. The main culprit is overconsumption of processed foods, which are notoriously high in sodium. According to the *Harvard Heart Letter*, every day the average American consumes between 2,500 and 7,500 mg of sodium. The RDA for potassium is 4,700 mg, of which a typical North American is likely to get only 2,500 mg a day. Potassium is also depleted by certain medications, such as corticosteroids and diuretics, which may be a factor in explaining the rapidly rising rates of AFib in older people.

While potassium is important on its own, consuming more of it also helps your body excrete excess sodium. Evidence suggests that improving the balance between these two minerals benefits heart and vascular health (see "Hypertension and Salt," page 200). The best way to increase your intake of potassium while lowering your intake of sodium is to eat more whole foods, especially fresh fruits, vegetables and legumes.

When it comes to keeping your heart rhythm regular, magnesium is a particularly significant electrolyte because it supports efficient functioning of your heart's electrical system. Not only is it sadly lacking in the standard American diet, but lifestyle factors such as stress and certain prescription medications deplete the body's magnesium stores. For more on dietary sources of magnesium, see "Dietary Strategies for Managing Hypertension," page 202.

EXPOSURE TO TOXINS

Heart arrhythmias have also been linked with numerous environmental toxins, including pesticides, traffic-related air pollution and exposures to propane or chlorine gas, paint thinners and heavy metals. While studies have identified some of these triggers, they have not provided much insight into the mechanisms that lead from the trigger to an AFib attack. However, they are worth mentioning because AFib rates are rising so rapidly and the causes are so diverse.

RADIATION THERAPY

In recent years, radiation therapy (RT) has emerged as a serious concern in relation to CVD. While RT is an important part of therapy in many types of cancer, as survival rates for cancer improve, its potentially negative side effects have come into focus. Many medical professionals, cardiologists in particular, believe RT is being used in situations where the benefits do not outweigh the risks. As a result, radiation-induced heart disease (RIHD) is a growing concern. The risk is highest among women who get radiation to the left breast, over the heart. Patients should ask their cardiologists about the issue before having treatment.

According to a 2013 study published in the *New England Journal of Medicine*, the effects of RT begin to show up as soon as five years after treatment. The larger the dose of radiation, the greater the risk of a subsequent heart attack. RT has also been linked with heart arrhythmias. RT generates *reactive oxygen species*, which are highly toxic substances. It can also alter the electrical patterns of the heart, and it has a significant impact on the expression of numerous genes.

Studies have identified links between RT, heart arrhythmias and changes in gene expression related to histone modifications, RNA-based mechanisms and DNA methylation. These epigenetic modifications may result from a panoply of factors that include inflammation and vascular disease as well. However, experts agree, these changes to gene expression endure long after the radiation treatment is over.

PHYSICAL ACTIVITY AND CHRONIC DISEASE

Unless the world has been passing you by, you know by now that exercise, even in moderate amounts, is very, very good for you. Not only does it help you maintain a healthy weight, strengthen your muscles and stay mobile, but it also reduces your risk for a wide variety of illnesses, ranging from type 2 diabetes and cardiovascular disease to some types of cancer. And, oh yes, it also helps to perk up your mood, improving your mental health.

In recent years researchers have been toiling away, exploring the mechanisms that might make all of these benefits possible. Is there something going on at the cellular level that might help to explain why exercise can affect your risk for chronic disease? Not surprisingly, some of the answers are rooted in your epigenome. In a comprehensive review paper published in *Acta Physiologica* in 2017, exercise physiologist Joshua Denham highlighted the growing body of research linking exercise with epigenetic changes that may reduce your risk for a wide variety of illnesses. Improvements can occur quite quickly in certain genes. In one mouse study, offspring that inherited a propensity for obesity and metabolic syndrome turned their regrettable legacy around in just eight weeks, thanks to an intervention that combined diet and exercise. Interestingly, human studies that track visible physical improvements also indicate that eight weeks is an appropriate time frame within which to expect results.

In 2014 scientists at Sweden's Karolinska Institute published a study that followed 23 men and women for a period of three months. The subjects cycled for 45 minutes three times a week, using only one leg; muscle biopsies of their legs were taken both before and after exercising. As expected, the exercised leg showed physical improvements. But the biopsies also revealed new methylation patterns in some 7,000 genes: those associated with insulin response, inflammation and how the body processes energy.

Numerous studies have also noted connections between exercise and beneficial changes to DNA methylation. For instance, exercise has been shown to modify DNA methylation to increase expression in genes associated with tumor suppression and decrease the activity of genes that encourage the growth of cancer cells.

In another study, researchers from the Mayo Clinic explored the benefits of 12 weeks of high-intensity interval training (HIT) for both younger and older people. They found a surprising result: the older you are, the more likely your genes will respond to the effort. More than 400 genes in muscle cells were expressed differently in the subjects who were older than 64. In the younger group, only 275 were affected. However, it's important to note that people over 50 should be very cautious about introducing anything other than moderate exercise into their lives. Extreme exercise is particularly risky for older adults, who may have undetected cardiovascular disease. And even physically fit people should be wary of engaging in endurance sports such as marathon running. Many cardiologists feel that exercising beyond a certain point may damage your heart, in addition to straining joints and ligaments.

Still, evidence indicates that exercise can help you stay biologically young by keeping your telomeres long (see page 227 for more about telomeres). A German study of both sedentary and active people from different age groups found that a group of committed runners with an average age of 51 had exceptionally youthful telomeres — just slightly shorter than the telomeres of runners in their twenties.

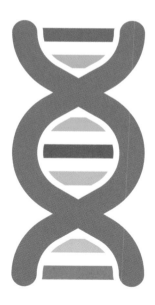

8

AGING

> The essence of chronic disease is not a single, overwhelming disruption of the body occurring either at conception or in middle age. There are pathways to disease. ... Health through a lifetime is launched by the mother and a strong launch in the womb goes a long way to ensuring a good score.
>
> — DAVID BARKER, *NUTRITION IN THE WOMB*

IF YOU'RE LOOKING FOR the fountain of youth, a good start might be to ask Robert Marchand for directions. For most of his working life the ebullient Frenchman was a kind of jack-of-all-trades: firefighter, sugarcane planter and lumberjack are just three of his many occupations. He also spent time as a prisoner of war during the Second World War. When he was 35, Marchand showed an aptitude for cycling, finishing seventh in the Grand Prix des Nations, an annual event in France where both professional and amateur cyclists compete. The problem was, earning a living didn't leave him much time for training, so he didn't return to cycling until he was almost 70. At that point he was able to stick with the sport, and by the time he turned 100, he was setting world records.

Robert Marchand is a textbook case of aging well. He shows us that growing older is not only about staying alive; it also involves maintaining your physical and mental health. When it comes to aging, the word *resilience* often crops up, usually in the context of traits such as the ability to recuperate or to overcome challenges. Monsieur Marchand obviously possesses resilience. In 2014, when he was 102, he broke his own centenarian record, pedaling 16.7 miles (26.9 km) in one hour. In 2017 he earned another spot in the history books when he cycled more than 14 miles (22.5 km) around a track in exactly an hour.

His secret is a general approach to life that conforms to most healthy-living guidelines. He says he eats lots of vegetables and fruits and, until recently, a little bit of meat (now he doesn't eat any). He also drinks a small amount of coffee. And, says his coach, he likes to set goals for himself.

So we can guess that an apparently healthy diet, plenty of exercise and a "can do" attitude have helped to keep Robert Marchand young at 107. One thing we know for sure is that, unlike many older people, he has strong muscles — an attribute that on its own supports good health and works to keep chronic inflammation at bay.

WHAT IS AGING?

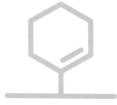

Senescence:

The point at which cells exhaust themselves and stop dividing but do not die.

Aging is a complex process. Why do some people age well and others seem to grow old before their time? Many different elements contribute to how successfully we weather the advancing years, including things that took place while we were still in the womb. Aging, in essence, results from the accumulated effects of countless tiny changes, many of them epigenetic, that occur over the years.

In biological terms, aging takes place in your cells. All parts of your body contain cells. For various reasons, scientists can't say for sure how many, but it's about 37 trillion, according to a 2013 estimate published in *Annals of Human Biology*. It's remarkable: we start life as a single cell and, through the process of replication, end up with this huge quantity of busy cells, all doing different jobs to keep our bodies running.

Your body is constantly creating new cells through a process known as division. These cells age and replicate at different rates depending on where they are located; for example, cells in the heart turn over slowly and those in the intestines are on the speedy side. Sadly, this process begins to slow down around the age of 35. Our cells gradually become "old." They reach a point, known as *senescence*, where they can no longer replicate themselves.

And since, in very simple terms, your life span is determined by your cells' capacity to divide, as they exhaust that ability, you begin to age.

Telomeres

When she was growing up in the Australian state of Tasmania, Elizabeth Blackburn was interested in the natural world, which isn't surprising because she comes from a family of scientists and physicians. Like many children, she enjoyed home-based scientific experiments, such as collecting tadpoles in jars, but unlike most kids, her innate curiosity inspired a unique journey. In 2009 she shared the Nobel Prize in Physiology or Medicine with two collaborators.

Professor Blackburn has devoted much of her professional life to studying *Tetrahymena*, a type of single-celled animal that is widespread in freshwater ponds. Because it lives near the surface of ponds in algae, she calls it "pond scum." As a scientist she became interested in chromosomes, particularly in their end sections, which are known as *telomeres*. Since pond scum has an abundance of telomeres, it became the focus of her work.

Which brings us back to cell division. Telomeres come into play when cells divide. They have been likened to the plastic tips at the ends of shoelaces that prevent them from fraying. Some cells divide thousands of times, and all of the DNA within them needs to be copied. Telomeres live at the ends of chromosomes and protect them, helping to keep them stable during the process of replication. However, every time a cell divides, the telomeres tend to shorten a bit. The length of telomeres and the rate at which they shorten have been linked with aging.

So here's another curious thing about pond scum: it has an abundance of telomeres and, unlike in most other

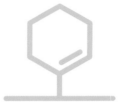

Telomeres:
Bits of DNA at the end of a chromosome that protect it during cell replication.

Telomerase:
An enzyme, often referred to as "anti-aging," that maintains telomeres, helping to keep them long.

organisms, they don't shorten when its cells divide. As Blackburn and her team discovered, *Tetrahymena* have the ability to produce an enzyme that prevents the telomere ends from shortening. They named this enzyme *telomerase*. Basically, telomerase synthesizes and adds a new segment of DNA with each division, to make up for the telomere segment that was lost and prevent the chromosome from aging.

Telomere Length

We know that genes play a role in both telomeres and aging, because scientists have identified rare genetic diseases known as telomere syndromes that are associated with premature aging. In addition, by studying centenarians and their offspring, we've been able to connect long lives with a greater incidence of certain genetic variants. Thanks to genome-wide association studies, scientists were able to pinpoint a number of single-nucleotide polymorphisms (SNPs) associated with telomere length (TL). However, when it comes to genes, aging and TL, while TL seems to have a genetic component, the genetic variants identified so far account for only a small portion of the differences in TL and its relationship to longevity.

So what's the connection, if any, among telomere length, the rate at which telomeres shorten and getting old? Shortened telomeres are associated with old age, but in scientific terms, age is not necessarily chronological. Aging is a cellular process, defined by shortened telomeres and, indirectly, your body's ability to produce telomerase. Scientists now believe that abnormalities in TL can serve as an early warning of disease and mortality independent of chronological age. As a result, much current research is directed toward gaining a better understanding of TL and its impact on health and illness at various stages in life. While shorter telomeres have been associated with many metabolic and inflammatory conditions (including dementia and cardiovascular disease), it remains to be resolved whether accelerated telomere shortening is a cause or a consequence of aging and disease.

FETAL DEVELOPMENT AND TELOMERE LENGTH

Although the science is still developing, many researchers believe there is a strong link between early-life TL and later susceptibility or resistance to disease. Some suggest these relationships may originate in utero. For instance, a 2007 study published in the *American Journal of Clinical Nutrition* found that children with a low birth weight were more likely to have shorter telomeres, along with altered immune function. In a 2013 paper published in the journal *Psychoneuroendocrinology*, researchers identified a number of factors that affect telomere length throughout the life span. These include maternal stress during pregnancy, childhood adversity, depression and an unhealthy lifestyle.

If TL is affected by experience, it seems logical that the longer your telomeres are at birth, the better your health is likely to be throughout life. Although there are no human studies to support this notion, a 2012 study of zebra finches found that TL in early life was a strong predictor of life span in a group of these birds. The authors of the paper made a case for the involvement of "telomere biology" in the interactions between genes and the environment that take place in the womb. They suggested that TL and telomerase are plastic in utero and that TL may be influenced by what happens in the womb. As we know, stressful experiences during pregnancy may initiate long-term epigenetic effects. These authors argued that the epigenetic changes produced by stress may influence the "telomere biology system."

Other research, although sparse, supports this point of view. One 2011 study in which Elizabeth Blackburn was involved found that young adults whose mothers were highly stressed while pregnant were much more likely to have shorter telomeres than a comparable control group whose mothers were not stressed. As the researchers pointed out, shortened telomeres, as well as reduced telomerase activity, have been consistently linked with susceptibility to disease. They also noted that telomerase activity can be improved by behavioral interventions that reduce stress, such as counseling and stress management.

LIFESTYLE CAN SLOW DOWN THE CLOCK

Telomere length seems to depend on two things: the length of your telomeres at birth and the degree of erosion that occurs throughout life. While preliminary research suggests that it may not be possible to turn back the clock, you may be able to take steps to slow its pace. For instance, a 2008 pilot study published in *Lancet Oncology* found that just three months of intensive lifestyle changes in a group of 30 men with low-risk prostate cancer increased telomerase activity in certain immune-system cells, thereby contributing to telomere maintenance. However, in that study no changes in TL were noted.

In a follow-up study, 10 of the men who were initially studied were enrolled in a program involving comprehensive lifestyle changes, including diet, activity, stress management and social support, for a period of five years. A control group whose lifestyle modifications were described as minor was also actively monitored over the same time period. The researchers found that TL increased significantly in the group following the lifestyle program but decreased in the control group. In other words, the more participants adhered to rigorous lifestyle changes, the longer their telomeres became. It should be noted the sample was small and there were limitations to the study group: the participants were all older men afflicted with low-risk prostate cancer. Testing those findings with larger trials based on broader segments of the population would be helpful.

WHAT DOES IT ALL MEAN?

Since then a number of studies have looked at the effects of lifestyle changes on TL, but the results are inconsistent. Based on what we know about the health benefits of exercise and its positive impact on certain diseases, such as cardiovascular disease and some types of cancer, it seems reasonable to assume that it might induce favorable changes at the cellular level. However, studies have shown that *extreme* exercise (whether endurance or resistance) actually shortens telomeres. Although more research is clearly needed, at the moment it seems that middling amounts of moderately intense exercise are probably the safest strategy for preserving telomere length.

The question is, are long telomeres associated with any health risks? The answer is maybe. Although research is still in the early stages, both longer and shorter telomeres have been linked with increased risks for certain types of cancer. Unlike other cells, which replicate themselves into nonexistence, cancer cells have an endless ability to divide. That means one of their challenges is to keep their telomeres from shrinking, which they address by increasing their production of telomerase. Does the ability of telomerase to slow down the aging process outweigh its potential to promote cancer? Again, this has not been determined. Preliminary mouse studies indicate there is no risk, but this is currently a topic of active debate. However, there's little doubt that the relationships among telomeres, telomerase, cancer and aging have opened the doors to exciting new research on many different fronts.

Nourishing Your Telomeres

A variety of food components may be capable of either decreasing or increasing TL. The trouble is that dietary studies are far from definitive. For instance, the Mediterranean diet, which is highly regarded in terms of its overall health benefits, produced mixed results when it came to TL. A study published in the journal *Clinical Nutrition* in 2016 looked at a group of more than 500 subjects with high cardiovascular risk. In the group that followed the Mediterranean diet for five years, longer telomeres were noted only in the women, not in the men.

There is also evidence to suggest that specific nutrients may have an impact on TL. For instance, a 2016 study published in the *Journal of Nutrition* reports that various nutrients could positively influence expression of the TERT gene, which has been linked with telomerase activity. These include genistein (found in soy, sunflower seeds, broccoli and other foods); epigallocatechin gallate (EGCG), a polyphenol known to be a potent cancer fighter (found in green and black tea, pecans and raw cranberries); and sulforaphane (found in brassica vegetables such as cauliflower, kale and collard greens).

The study also noted a number of specific nutrients associated with telomere length, including folate, vitamin B_{12}, niacinamide (a form of vitamin B_3), vitamins A, C, D and E, and the minerals magnesium, zinc and iron. Data from the Nurses' Health Study linked dietary fiber, specifically from cereals, with longer telomeres in middle-aged and older women. However, as the researchers have noted, nutrients likely interact with one another, and because so little research has been done at this point, recommending specific nutrients with a view to promoting longer telomeres is probably premature.

CANCER

There is little doubt that worldwide cancer rates are rising. One reason is that cancer is associated with growing older, and populations around the world are aging. Also, obesity is one of the major risk factors for cancer, and it has been described more than once as a global epidemic. So it's probably not surprising that globally cancer is a leading cause of death and that almost 40 percent of men and women will receive a cancer diagnosis during their lifetime.

The four most common cancers worldwide are breast cancer (in women), lung cancer (both men and women), prostate cancer (in men) and colon and rectal cancer (both men and women). The good news is that in some jurisdictions, such as the United States, the death rates from cancer have been steadily declining. According to the American Cancer Society, over the past two decades the US cancer mortality rate has fallen by more than 25 percent, thanks to fewer smokers, early detection and advances in treatment.

However, occurrence rates, mortality risk and which types of cancer are most prevalent differ geographically from a global perspective, and racially and ethnically within the United States. For instance, in developing countries, lung cancer is the most common type in men, whereas prostate cancer prevails in developed countries. In the United States, race has an impact on the development of prostate cancer: African-American men

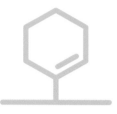

Reactive oxygen species (ROS):

A type of unstable molecule containing oxygen, often called a "free radical." Traditional wisdom is that when ROS build up, they cause cellular damage, a process often compared to rust collecting on a car. However, recent research suggests that in some contexts ROS may be beneficial.

Oncogenes:

Genes that have been altered from the norm, either by mutation or by increased expression, providing them with the potential to initiate the growth of cancer cells.

Tumor-suppressive genes:

Genes that work in a variety of ways to prevent the development and growth of cancer cells.

are about 70 percent more likely to develop prostate cancer than their Caucasian or Hispanic counterparts. In 2015 African Americans were 14 percent more likely to die from cancer than white people.

A Disease of Aging

As scientists learn more and more about cancer, it is becoming increasingly clear that it is primarily a disease of aging. The incidence of cancer increases with age, and some of the molecular changes associated with growing older overlap with cancer-related processes. Like aging, cancer is usually the cumulative result of many forms of stress that take place over a long period of time. Among other factors, both cancer and aging are fueled by increased production of reactive oxygen species and may include certain epigenetic changes, particularly those associated with DNA methylation.

What Is Cancer?

Cancer is, fundamentally, a disease in which your body's cells grow and divide uncontrollably. Two different classes of genetic activity precede its development: increased expression of *oncogenes*, which promote cell growth, in combination with decreased expression of *tumor-suppressor genes*, which have the opposite effect, inhibiting cell growth. Cancer depends on the mutually supportive activity of both types of genes.

Essentially, cancer develops when the systems that control how cells divide and multiply become imbalanced. Pinpointing causality is challenging because the loss of equilibrium may be the result of many different interactions, some of which may have synergistic impacts. These include damage to DNA, oxidative stress, lifestyle factors and epigenetic changes, accumulated over time. As the

Canadian Cancer Society states, "Very few cancers have a single known cause. Most cancers seem to be caused by a complex mix of many risk factors." The disease may also develop in people who have no risk factors.

Contrary to popular belief, in many cases cancer is not a death sentence. These days it tends to be treated as a unique type of chronic disease. Over the past few decades, advances in cancer treatment have allowed many survivors to live longer. However, ongoing care is often required for disabilities associated with the treatment, including chronic pain, chronic fatigue or outcomes that may damage certain bodily functions, such as radiation- or chemotherapy-induced heart disease. After treatment, survivors should follow the diet and lifestyle recommendations for preventing cancer recurrence.

THE OBESITY-INFLAMMATION-CANCER CONNECTION

Chronic inflammation (see "Inflammation: A Common Thread," page 211), which is strongly associated with being overweight or obese, can increase your risk of developing cancer. Excess belly fat produces hormones that raise levels of insulin, estrogen and leptin, all of which have been linked to cancer development.

Are Your Genes Involved?

In recent years, the idea that certain people are at high risk for developing cancer because they have specific genes has gained considerable traction. The media have highlighted two variations in the BRCA gene in particular. These so-called cancer genes, which appear to run in families, are powerful predictors of the risk for developing breast and/or ovarian cancer. However, according to the US National Cancer Institute, only about 5 to 10 percent of cancer risk is heritable in the sense that the genes your parents passed on to you are the cause; most genetic changes that cause cancer are acquired during one's lifetime, "as the result of errors that occur as cells divide or from exposure to carcinogenic substances that damage DNA, such as certain chemicals in tobacco smoke."

The Epigenome Is a Key Player

In the 1980s scientists discovered links between lower-than-normal DNA methylation and colorectal cancer, thus identifying the first epigenetic changes associated with the disease. Today scientists agree that, in humans, alterations to the epigenome are a hallmark of all types of cancer. And changes to gene expression are one mechanism with the potential to affect both the development of cancer and its progression.

As a 2010 paper titled "Epigenetics in Cancer," published in the journal *Carcinogenesis*, stated, "epigenetic modifications may be the key initiating events in some forms of cancer." In summary, the researchers concluded that most of these changes are heritable, and that many are established when the embryo is modifying generic cells to differentiate them for their specialized functions by way of altering gene expression. Throughout a lifetime, this heritability can be modified — positively, in ways that inhibit various cancer-signaling pathways, or negatively, which may set the stage for development of the disease.

What Causes Cancer?

Most of the cellular changes leading to cancer occur in response to environmental influences from one or more of the following factors: smoking, drinking alcohol, obesity, chronic inflammation, carcinogens (chemicals that cause cancer), physical inactivity, viruses and radiation. For instance, smoking is linked with lung cancer; high-risk forms of the human papilloma virus can cause cervical cancer; the environmental toxin benzene, which is a component of gasoline and is widely used in products such as plastics and pesticides, has been linked with leukemia; and radiation exposure can trigger thyroid cancer.

The environmental influences on cancer development are compelling. Consider, for example, a 2018 study, published in the journal *Environmental Health*, that examined health data on more than 5,000 flight attendants, 80 percent of whom were women. Although it's long been known that flight attendants have an increased risk of melanoma and breast cancer, those studied also had increased rates of several other types of cancer, including uterine, cervical, thyroid and gastrointestinal cancers. The incidence of nonmelanoma skin cancer was more than four times greater than the norm, and they were twice as likely to develop breast cancer. The researchers suspected that exposure to potentially carcinogenic substances, such as pesticides and flame retardants, as well as higher levels of cosmic ionizing radiation come into play. They also noted the potential impact of disrupted sleep patterns, which have been identified as a cancer risk. These sorts of environmental factors can have an impact on the expression of both oncogenes and tumor-suppressor genes.

Cancer's Roots May Lie in Fetal Life

Today we know that the risk for developing certain cancers can be traced back to fetal experiences. For instance, some evidence suggests that newborns who are significantly larger than average are at increased risk for breast, ovarian, prostate, testicular and colon cancers. In addition, numerous epidemiological studies conducted by David Barker and his associates linked some types of cancer (among them breast, ovarian, lung, colorectal and prostate) with various physical characteristics. These include the relationship between birth weight and length, the growth of pelvic bones and the shape of the placental surface at birth. Likely these markers are affected by a range of environmental impacts in utero, including hormone levels, toxic exposures and nutrition. (Evidence does show that mothers with wide hips have higher estrogen levels, which affects *progenitor cells* of the breasts, ovaries and pancreas.) We know that this "programming" may alter the epigenome and that its effects are not immediately obvious. As Susan Prescott wrote in her book *Origins*, "some of the environmental risk in cancers may be inherited quite early and not manifest for many years."

MAMMARY GLAND DEVELOPMENT

Take breast cancer, for instance. As noted, it is the most common cancer worldwide, and although genetics can play a role in its development, more than 70 percent of breast cancers are not linked to heritability.

The mammary glands begin to develop in utero, likely around the fourth week of gestation, a highly sensitive period in fetal development. Breast cancer has been linked with both high and low birth weight. Moreover, numerous researchers have linked the increased incidence of breast cancer over the past 50 years with exposure to various environmental chemicals that mimic the effects of estrogen. The degree of the consequences depends on the dose and when the exposure took place during the developmental process. Moreover, laboratory studies have linked fetal exposure to endocrine-disrupting chemicals (see "Endocrine Disruptors," page 90) — found in certain herbicides and air pollution — with various developmental problems in the mammary glands that scientists suspect are linked with breast cancer.

The DES Story

In 1938 Dr. Charles Dodd made an exciting discovery when he and his team of scientists succeeded in creating the first synthesized version of a natural hormone. Diethylstilbestrol (DES), which imitates natural estrogen, was initially prescribed to ease the troublesome symptoms of menopause. The word then spread among physicians that this drug, which was more powerful than natural estrogen, could be used to improve pregnancy outcomes, a use that caught fire thanks to a 1948 article (based on imprecise research) published in the *American Journal of Obstetrics & Gynecology*. In 1953 the first controlled, randomized, double-blind study on the use of DES during pregnancy was published in the same journal, and it concluded that DES did not show any benefit with regard to preventing miscarriage. However, by that time the drug was well established, and it continued to be widely prescribed, likely because pharmaceutical companies actively disputed the study's conclusions.

A Popular Drug

With the enthusiastic support of its manufacturers, DES gained traction, as drugs do, and it soon became a popular remedy for a broad range of conditions, including pregnancy-related nausea. Physicians at the Royal Children's Hospital in Melbourne, Australia, even prescribed the hormone to overly tall prepubescent girls to stunt their growth. The American agroindustry bought into the program and began routinely feeding DES to cattle and chickens to achieve various cost-effective benefits. The practice was soon questioned when this "off-label" use was linked with undesirable side effects, such as breast development in male humans. By 1959 the FDA had prohibited the use of DES in chicken feed, but that ban didn't take effect for another seven years, and the eventual ban on its use in cattle feed wasn't enforced until 1980.

Making Sense of Unusual Connections

Unfortunately, pregnant women had to wait until 1971 before even a modicum of action was taken on their behalf. That year, alarming research was published in the *New England Journal of Medicine* that linked prenatal exposure to DES with development of a highly unusual type of vaginal cancer in female offspring. Under normal conditions, clear-cell adenocarcinoma (CCA) occurs rarely and only after women have passed menopause, but in the late 1960s clusters of young women suffering from the disease began to appear.

When the link between DES and CCA was finally established, the FDA recommended that doctors stop prescribing the drug. However, they did not ban it outright, and DES continued to be prescribed in the United States, where, estimates suggest, about 4 million fetuses were exposed to the drug. DES was also prescribed widely in other parts of the world, where similar side effects were reported. After various trials in the court of public opinion (and eventually in the legal system), in 2000 the FDA finally acted to withdraw approval for the use of DES in humans.

A Multitude of Consequences

We now know that use of the drug significantly increased the risk of a multitude of health problems, particularly in the group known as "DES daughters." The daughters of women who took DES while pregnant are considerably more prone to fertility problems. If they do manage to get pregnant, they are more likely to experience an ectopic pregnancy or to develop pre-eclampsia (also knowns as toxemia). They are also at higher risk of having a miscarriage or delivering a premature or stillborn baby. By the time they reach 40, DES daughters are twice as likely as unexposed women to develop breast cancer, and that rate increases as they age. Moreover, their mothers are 30 percent more likely to develop breast cancer than women who did not take DES.

DES sons may also experience negative health effects. Although the studies are inconclusive regarding some of these risks, it is possible that they will have an increased incidence of noncancerous growths on their testicles and other genital abnormalities, such as undescended testicles, that may be a risk factor for testicular cancer. Animal studies have linked DES exposure in males to an increased risk of prostate cancer. Since DES sons as a group are only now beginning to turn 50, when the rate of prostate cancer traditionally starts to increase, we don't yet have epidemiological evidence to verify this connection.

Regrettably, as the years pass, evidence is emerging that the negative effects of DES exposure are being passed on to a third generation. Research suggests that some DES granddaughters are having menstrual difficulties, such as late menarche and irregular periods. These markers may indicate greater susceptibility to malignant tumors, a theory supported at this point only by mouse studies. Unexposed grandchildren of "DES lineage" mice have a greater frequency of cancerous tumors in the reproductive tract. Again, as is the nature of cancer, these cancers showed up as the mice aged. It will clearly be some time before we know the full impact of the DES experiment.

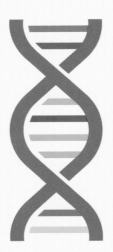

OTHER LINKS

Several other cancers can also be traced back to experiences in the womb, via exposures to toxins, such as cigarette smoke or alcohol, and environmental contaminants, such as heavy metals, air pollution and radiation. When a pregnant woman eats carcinogenic dietary compounds like nitrosamines (found in processed meats), it increases the risk that her offspring will develop brain tumors. In recent history, use of the estrogenic drug DES (see "The DES Story," page 236) provides one of the most vivid and alarming examples of the impact a pharmaceutical drug can have on fetal development. Sadly, we likely won't fully understand the effects of this biological time bomb for several generations to come.

Nutri-Epigenomics and Cancer

It's now generally accepted that diet can influence gene expression, which is the focus of the emerging science of nutri-epigenomics. Not surprisingly, these interactions are very complicated, but in general terms we know that certain nutrients and bioactive components of food affect various metabolic pathways. In the case of cancer, some of these nutritional powerhouses may be able to modify how carcinogens are metabolized. The phytochemical content of fruits and vegetables, in particular, may help to prevent cancer by influencing changes in gene expression that are protective against it.

Some of the most effective cancer-fighting foods and compounds include cruciferous vegetables, carotenoids, polyphenols and isoflavones.

Cruciferous Vegetables

Cruciferous vegetables, such as broccoli, Brussels sprouts, cabbage and cauliflower, provide sulforaphane and indole-3-carbinol, both of which have been shown to elicit direct epigenetic effects, which may help to protect against cancer. Regularly eating these vegetables reduces your risk of developing cancer, may slow down its development if the disease has taken hold, and may improve the efficacy of chemotherapy. It may be more beneficial to consume cruciferous vegetables raw. Chopping and chewing helps to activate their protective compounds, while overheating can inactivate them.

In 2012 researchers reported on the results of the Shanghai Breast Cancer Survival Study, which looked at 5,000 female survivors of breast cancer. For those who ate the most cruciferous vegetables within the first three years following their diagnosis, the risk of death associated with the disease decreased by 62 percent, and the risk that the cancer would recur decreased by 35 percent. The more cruciferous veggies consumed, the greater the protection against stomach, lung, colon and rectal cancers as well.

Carotenoids

Carotenoids are pigments found most abundantly in red, green, orange and yellow fruits and vegetables. Research has demonstrated that the more of these compounds you consume, the less likely you are to develop cancer. Beta-carotene is the most familiar carotenoid; others include lutein, lycopene, zeaxanthin and beta-cryptoxanthin. Some carotenoids suppress tumor growth by influencing gene expression. The effects of lycopene on prostate cancer have been well studied and although the results have been mixed, an extensive literature review published in 2015 linked higher intakes of lycopene (abundant in tomatoes) with a lower risk of developing the disease.

Polyphenols

Polyphenols are potent plant chemicals found in a wide variety of foods, including green tea, turmeric, red wine and soybeans. They appear to significantly alter the epigenome of cancer cells by inhibiting DNA methylation. Some of the best-known polyphenolic compounds are catechins, curcumin and resveratrol.

Catechins are found in a number of foods, the best known of which is green tea. In terms of cancer protection, the most effective catechin appears to be EGCG. This chemical is protective against a variety of cancers, likely through its ability to inhibit the activity of the gene DNMT, which codes for a protein that regulates DNA methylation and is linked to numerous diseases in addition to cancer.

Curcumin, the main component of the spice turmeric, also appears to inhibit DNMT activity. In addition, it may decrease the expression of certain oncogenes, among other cancer-protective benefits.

Resveratrol, found in red wine and fruits such as red grapes, blueberries and raspberries, is well known as an antioxidant. But it also has anticancer and anti-inflammatory effects in the body, thereby providing further protection from cancer (although some research indicates that it has a negative effect on the pancreas and muscle development in offspring). In laboratory studies, resveratrol has been shown to reduce the growth of several different types of cancer, including liver, skin, breast, prostate, lung and colon cancer cells.

Cancer, Diet and Lifestyle

Diet and lifestyle certainly have a bearing on cancer development, likely through their interactions with the epigenome. The World Cancer Research Fund International estimates that about 20 percent of all cancers diagnosed in the United States are related to being overweight or obese, physical inactivity, excessive alcohol consumption and/or poor nutrition. Most experts agree that regular cancer screenings to ensure early detection are important. Screening tests are commonly available for cervical, colon, breast, lung and prostate cancers. The screening test for colon cancer can actually prevent cancer from developing, because early cancer cells (polyps) are removed during the test.

Cancer Prevention Strategies

The following strategies come from the World Cancer Research Fund International, the World Health Organization (WHO), the American Institute for Cancer Research and the American Cancer Society.

DIETARY STRATEGIES

- **Consume a nutrient-dense whole-foods diet heavy in a wide variety of plant foods.** All major medical organizations agree that a plant-based diet, high in whole foods and low in red meat and highly processed foods, can lower the risk of developing cancer. Up to 45 percent of colon cancer cases could be avoided through diet and lifestyle changes alone. Plant-based diets are rich in phytochemicals, which may protect your body from precancerous changes and help to reduce inflammation.

- **Limit your consumption of energy-dense foods.** These include processed foods. Foods that are high in calories and low in nutrients encourage weight gain and increase your risk of developing insulin resistance and ultimately diabetes. Having type 2 diabetes increases the risk of cancer of the liver, pancreas, endometrium, colon, rectum, breast and bladder.

- **Limit your consumption of red meat.** Convincing evidence links red meat — which includes beef, pork and lamb — with the development of colorectal cancer. The International Agency for Research on Cancer (IARC) classifies red meat as a "probable carcinogen." Abstinence is not necessary: you can eat up to 18 ounces (510 g) a week without increasing your cancer risk. But it is important to avoid charring meat when cooking. The blackened areas of overcooked meat contain carcinogens called heterocyclic amines (HCAs), and frequent exposure to these compounds has been linked to an increased risk of pancreatic and colon cancer. Moreover, burning fat from meat being grilled creates polycyclic aromatic hydrocarbons (PAHs), another potential source of carcinogens that are linked to stomach cancer. When grilling meat, using a marinade can reduce both HCA and PAH levels.

- **Avoid highly processed meats.** Both the IARC and the WHO consider processed meats, such as lunch meats, hot dogs and bacon, to be carcinogens. Even low consumption on a daily basis (think four strips of bacon or one hot dog) can increase your risk for colon cancer. Curing (adding nitrites or nitrates) and smoking meat can lead to the formation of N-nitroso compounds (NOCs) and PAHs, both of which are considered carcinogenic. In addition, heating bacon and hot dogs produces more PAHs. Choosing "nitrate-free" processed meats is not a risk-free alternative; these meats are often preserved with celery juice, which is rich in nitrates. At this time, using nitrates from a "natural" source for meat preservation is not thought to alleviate the overall negative health effects.

- **Avoid artificial sweeteners and foods with added sugar.** Emerging evidence suggests that artificial sweeteners increase the risk of obesity, which has been associated with some types of cancer. Laboratory studies from the 1970s, which have been widely criticized, linked the artificial sweetener saccharin with bladder cancer. However, the FDA subsequently concluded that small quantities of artificial sweeteners do not increase cancer risk. The problem is, many people drink a lot of diet soda and, as the Harvard Medical School warns, we don't know what health impacts this level of consumption might have over many years. As for sugar, some scientists now see cancer as a metabolic disease, and a growing body of related research indicates that cancer cells are fueled by sugar.

- **Limit consumption of salty foods and foods processed with sodium.** Highly salted food can damage the stomach lining, increasing the risk of stomach cancer.

- **Avoid deep-fried foods.** Laboratory studies have found that exposure to acrylamide, a chemical that is produced when foods are deep-fried, increases the risk for several types of cancer. In humans, regular consumption of deep-fried foods has been linked with a significant increase in prostate cancer risk.

LIFESTYLE MODIFICATIONS

- **Be as lean as possible without becoming underweight.** Being overweight or obese is strongly linked with an increased risk for postmenopausal breast, colon and rectal, endometrial, esophagus, kidney and pancreatic cancers. It also raises the risk of developing non-Hodgkin lymphoma, multiple myeloma and gallbladder, liver, cervical, ovarian and aggressive prostate cancer.

- **Be active for at least 30 minutes every day and avoid excessive sitting.** Experts recommend standing and walking around for 5 minutes after sitting for 30 minutes. Increasing physical activity directly lowers the risk of several types of cancer, including breast, endometrial, prostate and colon cancer.

- **Do not smoke or chew tobacco.** Ninety percent of all lung cancer is due to smoking.

- **Limit alcohol intake.** Experts recommend a maximum of two drinks per day for men and one for women. They also agree that abstinence is best, as any amount of alcohol increases your risk for breast, mouth, throat, esophageal, liver, colon and rectal cancer. The more you drink, the greater the risk.

- **Do not combine alcohol with smoking.** Combining alcohol and smoking is dangerous. A 2006 study published in *Alcohol Research & Health* found that combining alcohol with tobacco use synergistically increased the risk of cancers of the oral cavity, throat and larynx. Other studies found even greater increases in risk associated with these combined exposures. Research published in 2004 demonstrated that people who drank heavily and smoked had a 300 times higher risk for these cancers than people who neither drank nor smoked.

Isoflavones

Several isoflavones (found primarily in soy and fava beans) have been investigated for their anticancer properties. Genistein is the most studied of these *bioactive compounds*. This *phytoestrogen* is protective against many forms of cancer, specifically breast cancer, although it seems to also inhibit cervical, prostate, colon and esophageal cancers. In particular circumstances genistein has been shown to improve expression of miRNA (a type of RNA molecule), histone acetylation and/or DNA methylation. It can even reactivate tumor-suppressor genes. A common misconception is that it is wise to avoid soy, but human studies show that soy consumption does not increase the risk of breast cancer and may actually lower it.

Common Carcinogens Associated with Food Production

Many pesticides used in food production contain known carcinogens. These include certain synthetics, such as organochlorines, creosote and sulfallate, some of which have been banned in certain jurisdictions. Others, such as DDT (which has been banned worldwide, although it is still in limited use in some areas) and lindane, are known to promote the growth of tumors. Occupational exposure to these chemicals has been linked with the development of various cancers, in particular lymphoma and leukemia.

However, when it comes to preventing cancer, controversy remains about whether it's preferable to eat an organic diet — consisting of food produced without the use of pesticides and herbicides — or a so-called conventional diet. A large prospective study that followed more than 600,000 women in the United Kingdom for over nine years showed little to no decrease in the incidence of cancer associated with consumption of organic food, except possibly for non-Hodgkin lymphoma. However, a French

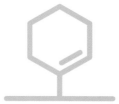

Bioactive compounds:
Chemicals in food that work with your metabolism to promote health.

Phytoestrogen:
A form of estrogen that occurs naturally in plants; it is commonly found in soy products.

study that followed 70,000 people for five years, published in *JAMA Internal Medicine* in 2018, concluded that frequently eating organically produced food could reduce the risk of cancer by as much as 25 percent.

PLANT FOODS LOWER CANCER RISK

There is strong evidence that a diet rich in whole plant foods reduces the risk of cancer. So if it's a challenge to purchase organic food, buy conventionally produced produce instead. Use the Environmental Working Group's Clean 15 and Dirty Dozen resource (www.ewg.org) to help you reduce your dietary exposure to pesticides and herbicides.

BPA EXPOSURE

BPA (bisphenol A) is a chemical commonly used in food packaging, such as plastic water bottles. It is currently banned in Canada and the European Union because it is a known endocrine disruptor that has been shown to stimulate certain cancer cells to grow in laboratory studies. Reducing your exposure to BPA may be protective against ovarian, breast and prostate cancer.

OSTEOPOROSIS

I love to walk. I live in a large city and walk everywhere, not only because I enjoy walking but also because I believe it is very good for my health. And so it is, as are my regular Pilates classes and my sessions at the gym, where I do about 40 minutes of weight-bearing exercise every visit. I do this partly because, as a woman who is on the downside of 50, I need to work harder to keep my bones strong. I know I'm particularly vulnerable to developing osteoporosis, which among other problems increases my risk for fractures. That concerns me. I know that breaking a bone could have catastrophic results, not only because I'm familiar with the research, but also because it's an experience that resonates within my family.

Cascading Effects

If you've ever broken a bone, you'll know that one result is reduced mobility. If you are an elderly person who breaks a hip, the experience is all too likely to initiate a cascade of events that may ultimately result in death. Fractures limit mobility, and the subsequent lack of activity accelerates bone density loss. A significant percentage of people who break a hip never fully recover, and as many as 50 percent will die within six months.

My late mother-in-law was one of those people. Although she had a number of health problems from the time she turned 80, she continued to live an independent and enjoyable life until she had a fall and broke her hip, not too long after her 90th birthday. Like many people, she never fully recovered, and her health began to deteriorate quickly. Statistics show that after breaking their hip, about 15 percent of people who have been living independently need to move to long-term nursing care. My mother-in-law was a case in point. Over a relatively short time span she moved from living in her own apartment to an assisted-living retirement home and finally to a nursing home, where she soon passed away.

Common and Costly

Declining bone mass and bone density are linked with growing older, which makes osteoporosis a particularly frightening disease. Your vulnerability dramatically increases as you age, and if you are female, you are at even greater risk. About 10 percent of women aged 60 have osteoporosis, and by the time they reach 90 years of age, 66 percent of women suffer from the disease. While men are not as susceptible, once they have their 60th birthday their risk gradually rises, ranging from 10 to 16 percent. After the age of 50, one in two women and one in five men will suffer a fracture due to osteoporosis.

Osteoporosis is one of the two most common musculoskeletal disorders of old age (the other is osteoarthritis). The toll it takes is not just personal, nor is it limited to the disease itself. Among other effects, serious fractures limit mobility, which can take the joy out of daily living, resulting in emotional disorders such as depression. And the global burden is increasing as populations age; according to statistics provided by the International Osteoporosis Foundation, disability resulting from osteoporosis has an economic impact even greater than that caused by cancers, excepting only lung cancer.

Links to Fetal Development

While numerous diet and lifestyle strategies can help to prevent or at least delay the onset of the disease (see "Preventing Bone Loss," page 246), more and more science is supporting David Barker's observations that babies with a low birth weight have lower bone mass and an increased risk of developing osteoporosis later in life. Since a fetus obviously has little use for its skeleton, bone mass is a likely sacrifice if it needs to prioritize its development.

As Dr. Barker pointed out in his 2008 book *Nutrition in the Womb*, "The strength of a bone depends on its size and the density of the calcium salts within it. ... Low birth-weight babies have a lower bone mass which persists throughout their lives. People who were small at birth or who did not thrive during infancy also have life-long alterations in two hormones, growth hormone and cortisol, which influences bone mass. These alterations lead to both lower peak bone mass and to more rapid loss of bone mass with age."

A 2009 study published in the journal *PLoS Medicine* used data from the Helsinki Study of "very low birth weight adults" — those whose weight was less than 3.3 pounds (1,500 g), compared to an average full-term birth weight of about 7.7 pounds (3,500 g) — to establish that by the time they reached young adulthood, babies who were born prematurely and with a low birth weight had significantly lower bone mass and density than their peers who were born at term. The researchers pointed out that premature birth deprives babies of a period of development in the third trimester that is significant in terms of bone mineralization. These babies are born with less than ideal bone mineralization and are likely compromised in developing bone mass during childhood.

In her book *Origins*, Susan Prescott observed that birth weight and how much an infant weighs can predict both growth hormone and cortisol levels later in life. Children who weigh less than normal during their first year and/or grow slowly throughout childhood have a much greater risk of breaking a hip later in life. The question is, what maternal factors are linked with these results?

The Importance of Maternal Nutrition

The fetus begins to develop a skeleton at about five weeks of gestation. As Dr. Prescott noted, the processes involved in skeletal development depend on certain hormones and the availability of various nutrients, such as vitamin D, calcium and phosphate. Anything that interferes with these processes can increase the baby's risk of developing

Preventing Bone Loss

Bone is the material from which your skeleton is built. In addition to providing support and protection for your organs, bone produces blood cells that help to protect you from infection. It also acts as a reservoir for minerals, particularly calcium and phosphorus, so your body can draw on them in times of need.

Your body is constantly breaking down old bone and making new bone, using cells called osteoclasts and osteoblasts. Starting in utero and throughout childhood and young adulthood, your body creates new bone faster than it breaks bone down. Around the time you turn 30, your bone mass peaks. It remains stable for a period of time, but then eventually starts to decline. This process may result in osteoporosis.

Factors Influencing Bone Loss

As an adult, your challenge is to slow down the process of bone loss. Throughout adulthood a poor diet, smoking, excessive alcohol consumption, some medications and certain diseases can speed up the pace at which your bones break down or the speed at which new bone forms. Other influences include inflammation, hormonal changes, a sedentary lifestyle and excess stress.

INFLAMMATION

Adults with decreased bone density have been found to have higher levels of C-reactive protein, a blood inflammatory marker. We know that people with certain inflammatory autoimmune conditions, including rheumatoid arthritis, SLE (systemic lupus erythematosus) and celiac disease, are more likely to develop osteoporosis for various reasons, in addition to the chronic inflammation associated with those conditions. For example, in rheumatoid arthritis the antibodies that attack an individual's own tissue also promote osteoclast (bone-breakdown) activity. In addition, the steroid medications often used to treat these conditions have been linked with slower bone regeneration and an increased risk of fracture.

HORMONAL CHANGES

Females over age 50 are the group at greatest risk for developing osteoporosis. During and after menopause, estrogen levels drop significantly, and that hormone plays a crucial role in supporting osteoblasts, which create new bone. When the Danish Osteoporosis Prevention Study followed more than 1,500 menopausal females to try to identify risk factors for osteoporosis, the researchers found that genes may play a role. A variation in the MTHFR gene (C677TT) was associated with significantly lower bone mineral density at the neck of the femur (thigh bone), the hip and the spine, and the incidence of fractures increased more than twofold when women had this SNP. A meta-analysis of MTHFR genotype studies confirmed these findings.

A SEDENTARY LIFESTYLE

Sitting for long periods increases your risk of osteoporosis. Lack of physical activity in adulthood contributes to an increase in bone resorption, which is linked with decreasing bone mass. On the other hand, people who are physically fit have been shown to have higher bone mineral density. Standing more often, in addition to engaging in weight-bearing exercises such as walking and jogging, will reduce your risk of bone loss. Resistance exercises and movement that includes high-impact weight-bearing will promote bone formation and reduce age-related bone loss.

EXCESS STRESS

Chronic physiological stress causes elevated levels of the hormone cortisol, which can reduce bone mass by influencing the rate of bone resorption and formation.

TOBACCO AND ALCOHOL

Although the causal connections aren't clear, both cigarette smoking and drinking too much alcohol have been associated with lower bone density.

Supporting Healthy Bones Through Diet

Generally speaking, the best dietary approach for promoting bone health is similar to those that support the prevention of other chronic diseases: plenty of whole foods, including whole grains, which, among other nutrients, tend to be high in bone-friendly minerals like calcium and magnesium. Omega-3 fatty acids have also been shown to promote bone health. Eliminating processed foods is also important. Among other concerns, they are high in salt, which promotes calcium loss. Sodas are also problematic, as they are high in phosphates, which interfere with your body's ability to absorb calcium. Here are some additional tips to keep your bones healthy:

- **Emphasize anti-inflammatory foods.** A diet low in inflammatory foods slows the rate of bone loss in postmenopausal females. Data from the Women's Health Initiative linked a diet high in inflammatory foods with an increased risk of hip fracture in white women younger than 63. Processed foods are known to provoke inflammation.

- **Choose foods with a high mineral content.** Minerals are important for bone health, in part because bone is made of about 35 percent type 1 collagen and 65 percent inorganic minerals. Calcium and phosphorus are the most abundant minerals in bone; magnesium is present in smaller amounts. Phosphorus is easily obtained through diet, but deficiencies of calcium and magnesium are common. Research shows that ensuring an adequate intake of these minerals at all stages of life is critical for maintaining healthy bone mass.

- **Increase your vitamin D intake.** Vitamin D controls the concentration of calcium and phosphorus in the blood, which affects the amount of these minerals that can be used and stored in the bones. Many people may need to take a supplement to ensure adequate levels of this vitamin.

- **Eat more prebiotics.** Prebiotics are found in foods that contain nondigestible dietary fiber, which becomes a fuel source for your gut bacteria (see "Prebiotics," page 282). In animal and some human studies, dietary calcium and magnesium absorption was increased with a higher intake of prebiotics. More research is needed to understand the full effect your gut flora has on osteoporosis risk, but in the meantime, a diet high in fiber makes sense.

- **Take a probiotic.** A Swedish study published in the *Journal of Internal Medicine* in 2018 found that taking a probiotic supplement containing the bacterium *Lactobacillus reuteri* reduced bone loss in a group of women 75 to 80 years old by almost 50 percent when compared to a control group that received a placebo. *L. reuteri* is known to have an anti-inflammatory effect, which may account for these positive results.

osteoporosis later in life. Disruptive factors include medical conditions such as maternal diabetes, preeclampsia and hypertension, as well as whether the mother smoked, her fat mass and her level of physical activity, particularly during late pregnancy.

Naturally, good maternal nutrition helps the baby develop strong and healthy bones. A longitudinal study published in 2009 in the *Journal of Bone and Mineral Research* specifically linked a mother's diet during pregnancy with greater bone size and higher bone mineral density in nine-year-old children. The researchers concluded that when mothers consume a "prudent" diet during pregnancy — one abundant in whole foods and low in processed food — their children will develop healthy bones.

While following a balanced diet based on whole foods is always a good idea, some specific nutrients, such as calcium and vitamin D, are particularly important for developing and maintaining bone mass. Numerous dietary and lifestyle modifications have been shown to be helpful in preserving bone, thereby helping to prevent fractures (see "Preventing Bone Loss," page 246).

Scientists are also exploring the role of leptin (see "What Is Leptin and Why Should You Care about It?" page 172), a hormone traditionally associated with appetite and weight management. Leptin affects the growth and development of osteoblasts, the cells that synthesize bone, and studies indicate that the amount of leptin a fetus receives depends on the quality of the mother's diet and her fat stores. Researchers have studied leptin concentrations in umbilical cord blood and have linked high levels of the hormone with positive bone mineral density.

SARCOPENIA

Unless you are in your twenties or younger, your muscles are probably not as strong as they were yesterday. The problem is, quite simply, you are getting older. While aging takes a toll on your body in general, it is particularly unkind to your muscles, which were in their prime around the time you turned 25. At that point they were poised for decline, and if you're preparing to celebrate your 80th birthday, you won't be happy to learn that almost half of your youthful muscle mass is gone.

The loss of muscle mass — and, perhaps more significantly, muscle strength — associated with aging is known as sarcopenia. Factors that contribute to it include neurological decline, hormonal changes, inflammation, a decrease in physical activity, poor nutrition and chronic inflammatory diseases such as rheumatoid arthritis. However, the seeds that develop into sarcopenia are sown very early: in the womb and during early infancy. As David Barker writes, "Slow growth in the womb and during the first few months after birth is accompanied by a reduction in the amount of muscle that is laid down. People with low birthweight tend to have low muscle mass throughout their lives."

Over the years, numerous studies, some of which were done by Dr. Barker's colleagues, have confirmed his findings: more muscle at birth means better glucose control as an adult and a longer life without frailty. The research includes epidemiological as well as more biologically focused studies. For instance, animal studies have shown that when a fetus doesn't receive adequate protein or calories, certain biological pathways associated with protein synthesis are affected. One result is that the baby is born with fewer skeletal muscle fibers, and those it has developed aren't of optimum quality.

Muscle Mass Matters to Health

Muscle mass accounts for as much as 60 percent of body mass. Maintaining muscle mass and strength throughout your lifetime is vital to health and well-being because muscles connect with many bodily functions. As anyone who has been confined to bed for even a relatively short time can tell you, muscle strength declines rapidly. It's a compelling reminder of the "use it or lose it" dictum.

Muscle is metabolically active tissue, and its loss can set the stage for more serious consequences. The reduced activity associated with illnesses such as arthritis and osteoporosis may set off a cascade of negative effects that increase the risk of other conditions such as diabetes and heart disease.

The Obesity Factor

While biological and metabolic changes are the driving forces behind sarcopenia, obesity can also make a significant contribution. Factors associated with obesity, such as excessive calorie intake, sedentary behavior and chronic inflammation, can lead to sarcopenic obesity. This condition is defined as the confluence of sarcopenia and obesity, and it's particularly problematic because both conditions work together to increase potential risk.

People who are not obese have an appropriate balance between muscle mass and weight. Obese people are likely to have muscle mass that is far too low in relation to their

Nutrition and Lifestyle Approaches for Preventing Sarcopenia

Interventions that focus on improved nutrition and increased physical activity are likely to show positive outcomes in both preventing and slowing the progression of sarcopenia.

Eat More Protein

Adults over 50 need more dietary protein than younger people. Older people don't metabolize protein as efficiently, so they need more of it to make the same amount of muscle. Bear in mind, however, that consuming too much protein can lead to kidney damage, especially among the elderly.

The current recommended protein intake for healthy younger adults is 0.8 grams per kilogram of body weight — that's 54 grams of protein a day for a 150-pound (68 kg) adult. But this amount isn't sufficient to prevent sarcopenia in older adults. Studies show that adults over 50 should consume at least 1 gram and up to 1.5 grams of protein per kilogram of body weight, or 68 to 102 grams of protein a day if you weigh 150 pounds. Unfortunately, studies have shown that as many as 35 to 40 percent of older adults don't meet that requirement.

The easiest way to increase your protein intake is to eat more food from animal sources, such as eggs, fish, poultry and meat, because these foods are a rich source of "complete" protein. Complete protein delivers all nine of the essential amino acids that your body needs and can't create itself. Some whole grains, such as amaranth, quinoa and buckwheat, also provide complete protein, although in small amounts relative to food from animal sources. Most other plant foods provide "incomplete" protein, which means they don't contain a full range of essential amino acids. However, eating a variety of plant foods throughout the day will provide the required amount of these nutrients. Beans and legumes (including soybeans), nuts, seeds and whole grains provide the best plant-based sources of protein.

Because plant-based foods aren't as protein-dense as animal foods, it can be a challenge to get enough protein if you are following a vegetarian or vegan diet. As a result, more and more people are including protein powders — based on sources such as peas, hemp, rice and whey (from dairy) — in their diets. Protein powders are a processed protein source (some contain added sugars and other additives), but they can be an effective strategy for boosting protein intake.

We now know that for older people, timing impacts how effectively the body uses protein. A 2017 study published in the *American Journal of Clinical Nutrition* looked at a sample group of Quebec residents age 67 to 84 and concluded that consuming protein at breakfast is beneficial. The researchers found that spreading out protein intake evenly over three meals a day — rather than consuming the majority at lunch and dinner, which is the norm — resulted in greater muscle mass and strength than when little or no protein was consumed in the morning.

Optimize Vitamin D Intake

Low levels of vitamin D are associated with low muscle strength in older adults. Supplementing with vitamin D not only increases muscle strength and function, but has also been shown to reduce the incidence of falls.

Exercise Regularly

When it comes to supporting your muscles, exercise is at least as valuable as good nutrition. Resistance exercise — movements that force your skeletal muscles to contract — has been shown to increase strength and decrease frailty in older adults. Aerobic exercise — movement that increases your pulse rate and respiration — can increase strength and can also improve gait and overall quality of life. Ideally, a minimum of 20 to 30 minutes, three times a week, of either type of exercise is recommended, although as little as 10 minutes a day has been shown to reduce frailty and lengthen life span.

Recent research originating at the Mayo Clinic suggests that exercise can, in effect, slow the aging process at the cellular level. Although aerobic exercise and strength training were both shown to be very beneficial, when it comes to building muscle mass, strength training had the greatest overall benefit for older people. The researchers were most surprised by the influence exercise had on gene activity. In participants older than 64, almost 400 genes were impacted. The relevant genes are believed to affect the mitochondria by producing energy to feed muscle cells. Apparently exercise acts at the cellular level by encouraging cells to make more proteins, which feed your body's energy needs. More importantly, exercise increases mitochondrial function and improves muscle metabolism.

It's important to remember that your workouts don't need to be heavy-duty to produce results. A study published in the journal *Experimental Gerontology* in 2017 found that, for people over 50, low-intensity workouts are just as beneficial as those that are more intense. It also noted that, for this group, there was no benefit in increasing the number of workouts from two to three per week. As one of the researchers suggested, it's possible that older people don't have the capacity to recover from the inflammation generated by exercise as quickly as those who are younger, and that their bodies need more time between workouts.

weight, which makes the physical demands of daily living more challenging. Lower muscle mass, obesity and physical inactivity are associated with higher levels of intermuscular adipose tissue (IMAT), which is fat that has infiltrated skeletal muscle tissue. Increased IMAT influences the composition of the muscles, leading to a lower proportion of lean muscle, and can decrease strength and mobility. Experts believe that when obese people suffer from muscle impairment, the two conditions act synergistically to increase the risk of negative health outcomes.

DEMENTIA AND ALZHEIMER'S DISEASE

Dementia is not an actual disease; rather, it is a collection of symptoms linked with loss of cognitive functions associated with aging, including memory. While it is not an inevitable part of growing older, dementia is a major health concern for people over 65, because at that point the risks of developing the condition begin to increase. In the United Kingdom, for instance, dementia afflicts about 2 percent of people between 65 and 69. Twenty years later the risks have risen dramatically: between the ages of 85 and 89 about 20 percent of people suffer from dementia. Over time, annoying symptoms such as occasional forgetfulness can evolve into more serious problems, such as disabling confusion that may eventually progress to incapacity. At its severest stage, dementia may result in complete dependence on others to manage the demands of daily life.

Alzheimer's disease (AD) is a subset of dementia and the most common form of the condition. Sixty to 80 percent of dementia cases qualify as AD, which is a progressive disorder of the brain that gradually destroys memory and cognitive skills. More than 50 million people worldwide have AD, and the rates are expected to double every 20 years, which is comparable to predictions about diabetes.

A Tangled and Twisted Web

Alzheimer's disease is named after a German neurologist, Dr. Alois Alzheimer. In the early 1900s Alzheimer decided to examine the brain of a deceased woman, 51 years of age, who had symptoms we would now associate with the disorder. The doctor's curiosity was piqued because his patient was extremely young to be so severely afflicted. With the help of new technologies he was able to identify major abnormalities in her brain tissue, particularly in the region associated with language and memory. The autopsy revealed clumps (now known as amyloid plaques) and twisted wads of fibers (now called tau tangles). Both are made from protein particles that already exist in a healthy brain. The problem is, in patients with AD they somehow become malformed.

Within the scientific community there is wide discussion and disagreement about what initiates the toxic cascade that eventually leads to dementia. It has been described as the battle of the proteins, or "plaque versus p-tau." Recent studies suggest that p-tau (the tangles) is more strongly linked with cognitive decline than plaque (the clumps). These are hotly debated theories that are well beyond the scope of this book. However, in some respects the focus on these abnormalities may have narrowed the peripheral vision of researchers, limiting opportunities to identify other contributors to the disease that may be more easily modified. For instance, there is now strong evidence for what experts call vascular dementia — abnormalities in blood vessels that lead to the disease — which links it with diabetes.

Genes and Alzheimer's

Current evidence suggests that, for most people, Alzheimer's disease — particularly the late-onset type — results from a combination of genes, lifestyle and environmental factors. Whether it strikes early or late, it may have a "familial" connection, which means a parent or grandparent also suffered from the condition. Early-onset Alzheimer's disease (EOAD) typically shows up between the ages of 30 and 65 and is much less common than late-onset Alzheimer's disease (LOAD). About 60 percent of people with EOAD have one of three specific gene variants that predispose them to developing the condition. However, scientists do not yet have a clear idea of why the remaining 40 percent or so do not end up with the disease.

Genetic links to LOAD, the form most people are at risk of developing, are far less compelling. However, scientists have been able to identify a variant of one gene, ApoE-4, that increases the risk. People with two copies of this variation have a 15 percent greater risk of developing LOAD, and an average age of onset that is lower by 10 years. The ApoE gene is strongly associated with the immune system, which recent research indicates may play a role in LOAD. Interestingly, another variant of the ApoE gene, ApoE-2, has been linked with a *reduced* risk of developing the condition. Studies now show that a number of genes associated with the immune system influence AD development, both increasing and reducing the risk.

Roots in the Fetal Environment

Even though AD usually doesn't manifest until quite late in life, scientists are beginning to suspect that its seeds are sown much earlier, possibly in the womb. For instance, researchers Bryan Maloney and Debomoy Lahiri, of the Indiana University School of Medicine, have proposed that AD and some other forms of dementia are linked with epigenetic changes that may originate in utero (possibly even via imprinted parental genes). Acknowledging David Barker's work as their inspiration, they developed a model — Latent Early-life Associated Regulation, or LEARn — that helps to identify specific epigenetic changes occurring during development that lead to Alzheimer's later in life. Triggers for these changes may include in utero exposure to toxins such as heavy metals or pesticides, dietary factors such as folate supply, or maternal medical conditions such as high cholesterol or inflammation.

If, for instance, a fetus is exposed to a toxin, any potential effects on its development likely won't be apparent at birth. In the case of AD, the impact would remain latent for about six decades before manifesting. Drs. Maloney and Lahiri use leaded gasoline as one example. Although it was banned in the United States in 1996, according to their LEARn model it will take about 50 years for levels of AD to decrease in response. That means the effects of the ban may not become noticeable until children born after 1996 reach the at-risk age for LOAD.

Those Pesky Bacteria

The impact of gut flora is another potential factor that researchers are currently exploring in relation to dementia. It is well known that the composition of your gut bacteria gradually changes over time and, generally, its diversity declines with age. Paul O'Toole, a microbiologist affiliated with Ireland's University College Cork, is particularly concerned about the lack of variety that typically characterizes the diet of older people. A diet that lacks diversity — often described by the cliché "tea and toast" — has a similar effect on bacterial composition, limiting microbial richness. Dr. O'Toole has linked age-related microbiota scarcity with a range of health effects, from cardiometabolic and inflammatory processes to cognitive decline. Among other concerns, the loss of diversity in core groups of beneficial bacteria affects the production of health-promoting compounds made by bacteria, such as short-chain fatty acids. This process may be linked with reduced cognitive function and Alzheimer's disease. (For more on the microbiota, see chapter 9.)

Good News on the Horizon

In the United States in recent years, the percentage of older adults with dementia, including AD, has declined dramatically, from 11.6 percent in 2000 to 6.8 percent in 2012. Researchers who drilled down into data from the Framingham Heart Study believe the decline may be linked with a trend toward higher education levels, which parallels a reduction in most vascular risk factors (except for obesity and diabetes). Although participants in the Framingham study tend to be more educated and affluent than most people, researchers agree this decrease suggests that the risk of developing AD can be modified by factors that may be controllable.

Risk Factors for Dementia and Alzheimer's Disease

Emerging evidence indicates that making healthy dietary and lifestyle choices and reducing exposure to environmental toxins before the warning signs become obvious could at least delay and possibly even prevent the development of dementia, including AD. Identifying risk factors and intervening early is the most promising strategy.

Obesity

While some of the evidence linking obesity with dementia is contradictory (it has been suggested that using body mass index to evaluate obesity may be responsible for certain discrepancies), several studies have linked excess abdominal fat, particularly in middle age, with an increased risk for dementia. As one 2010 study published in *Annals of Neurology* concluded, the more belly fat you have, the more your brain will shrink later in life. A number of common pathways suggest links between the two conditions. For instance, obese people are more likely to suffer from chronic inflammation, a risk factor for dementia. They are also more likely to have a sedentary lifestyle and to suffer from health conditions such as diabetes and high cholesterol, which also increase the risk of developing dementia.

Diabetes

Type 2 diabetes and AD are so closely linked that AD is sometimes called "type 3 diabetes." A 2008 literature review, published in the *Journal of Diabetes Science and Technology*, identifies impairments in how the brain utilizes glucose and metabolizes energy as biological markers signaling the onset of dementia. It concludes that AD is a form of diabetes that selectively afflicts the brain. Some researchers suspect that the APP (amyloid precursor protein) gene, which affects insulin pathways, is the common link. Among other functions, these pathways influence metabolism, which supports how the nervous system functions, providing a possible connection with the brain.

Cholesterol Levels

As noted, the ApoE gene has been linked with LOAD in a small percentage of people. This gene also plays a role in how we process and use cholesterol and other fats, so researchers are looking at how cholesterol is processed in the brain and whether that is connected with cholesterol levels in the blood. One recent study, published in *Neurology*, found that high blood cholesterol levels were significantly related to the brain plaques associated with AD. Chronically impaired blood flow to the brain results in vascular damage, reducing the body's ability to clear the clumps of plaque.

It's also worth noting that many of the risk factors for dementia and Alzheimer's disease overlap with those for heart disease. These include hypertension, high cholesterol, lack of exercise, obesity, tobacco smoking and a nutritionally deficient diet lacking in fruits and vegetables. People with high cholesterol often have hypertension and diabetes as well.

Inflammation

Some researchers, such as the authors of a 2015 paper published in *Lancet Neurology*, believe inflammation plays a significant role in the development of AD. In their opinion, it's much more than a "mere bystander" that is activated by the plaques and tangles, but is rather an active participant, contributing "as much or more to the pathogenesis as do the plaques and tangles themselves."

Researchers now believe that in many ways AD (and dementia in general) may be a degenerative inflammatory disease linked with long-term nutritional deficiencies and poor lifestyle choices, such as alcohol abuse and inadequate physical activity. They also believe chronic stress may be involved. We do know that conditions such as systemic inflammation and obesity may impede certain interactions between the immune system and the brain, accelerating progression of dementia.

High Homocysteine Level

Elderly people tend to have higher levels of homocysteine, an amino acid naturally produced by the body. This increase may result from reduced kidney function or because older people are less efficient at absorbing vitamin B_{12}. High levels of homocysteine have been linked with conditions including heart disease and stroke in addition to dementia. A 2002 study published in the *New England Journal of Medicine* concluded that "an increased plasma homocysteine level is a strong, independent risk factor for the development of dementia and Alzheimer's disease."

Keeping your homocysteine low may slow the progression of dementia. Lifestyle factors such as diet, smoking, obesity, sedentary behavior and stress can increase blood levels of homocysteine, as can numerous prescription and over-the-counter pharmaceuticals. Taking some widely prescribed medications, such as H2 antagonists or proton pump inhibitors (used mainly to treat excess stomach acid), reduces the body's ability to absorb vitamin B_{12}, which helps to keep homocysteine under control.

Supplementation with vitamins B_2, B_6, B_{12} and folic acid is a proven therapy for reducing blood levels of homocysteine. One 2012 study, the VITACOG trial, showed that supplementation with vitamins B_{12}, B_6 and folic acid reduced levels of homocysteine in people older than 70 who already suffered from mild cognitive impairment.

Nonalcoholic Fatty Liver Disease

Not only do the risk factors associated with NAFLD (such as type 2 diabetes, obesity and hypertension) contribute to cognitive impairment, but a 2016 study published in the journal *Neurology* identified NAFLD as an independent risk factor for age-related cognitive decline. Another study, using data from the Framingham Offspring Cohort, found that by the time they reached middle age, otherwise healthy adults with NAFLD already demonstrated the lower brain volume associated with memory loss.

Alcohol Abuse

A French study found that very heavy drinkers were three times more likely to develop dementia than people who consumed alcohol in moderate quantities.

Severe Head Injury

Although the whys and wherefores aren't totally understood, severe head trauma increases the risk of developing dementia, including AD. It has been suggested that inflammation may be the link, as head trauma is followed by inflammation in the brain.

Brain Food

Following a Mediterranean-style diet (see "A Nutrient-Dense Diet," page 194) can help to lower your risk of developing dementia. Among its benefits, the Mediterranean diet helps to keep inflammation under control by focusing on foods that are known to be anti-inflammatory. It also includes fish, which supply the omega-3 fatty acids EPA and DHA. These nutrients help older adults maintain brain function, and a deficiency has been linked with smaller brain volume, an indicator of age-related cognitive decline. While there is no research that supports their benefit for people who already have AD, several studies indicate that these fatty acids may improve brain function in people suffering from milder forms of cognitive impairment linked with aging.

Increase Your Intake of Antioxidant-Rich Foods

Oxidative stress, which is linked with the production of free radicals (think of a sliced apple turning brown when exposed to air), is known to be an underlying process in the development of dementia. Your body regularly produces reactive oxygen species (ROS), which are necessary for certain cellular processes. However, when too many of these substances are generated, they must be neutralized through various antioxidant defenses. In general terms, a high dietary intake of antioxidants — found in numerous whole foods, particularly plant foods, as well as coffee and chocolate — can help to reduce the impact of oxidative stress.

Some specific antioxidants have been studied with regard to their effect on dementia and AD. Research shows, for instance, that people with dementia have lower blood levels of vitamin C and beta-carotene, two potent antioxidants found in citrus fruits, kiwis, mangos, berries, carrots, sweet potatoes and dark leafy greens. A 2018 study, published in the *American Journal of Geriatric Psychiatry*, found that curcumin, a compound found in the spice turmeric, improved memory and mood in a group of adults between the ages of 50 and 90 who took curcumin supplements twice daily over a period of 18 months. When researchers examined brain scans, they found that those who were taking the supplements also had significantly fewer clumps of plaque and tangles of p-tau than a control group taking a placebo.

Other studies have shown that compounds in cinnamon inhibit tau tangling. Interestingly, cinnamon has also been shown to lower blood sugar levels in people with diabetes, which may be another link with AD. It's probably worth noting that many herbs and spices (including kitchen staples such as parsley) are particularly high in antioxidants, which in theory could help to counteract the oxidative stress associated with AD development.

A Sedentary Lifestyle

Researchers at UCLA found that the longer you spend sitting, the thinner your brain becomes. If you sit for more than three hours a day, every additional hour decreases the thickness of your medial temporal lobe — which is linked with memory function — by 2 percent. From the opposite perspective, other studies have linked regular physical exercise with improved cognitive function and a reduced risk of dementia.

Exposure to Toxins

Exposure to environmental toxins, including pesticides and aluminum, has also been associated with an increased risk of developing dementia.

Lifestyle for Brain Health

Diet isn't the only way to help keep your brain healthy. A study published in 2015 in *JAMA Neurology* showed that people with higher cognitive reserves (defined in this study as more than 16 years of education) had a lower risk of dementia. While that doesn't mean everyone should go back to school, it does help to explain why lifelong social and intellectual engagement is so important for all adults, and especially elderly people.

There is now strong evidence that staying active also helps to prevent cognitive decline. Aerobic exercise in particular shows promise for preventing dementia, not only for its cardiovascular benefits but also because it helps to increase blood flow to the brain.

Unfortunately, there is currently no known treatment that will cure, delay or stop the progression of dementia. The best approach is to consume a healthy diet and engage in a lifestyle that exercises both your mind and your body. These steps will also lower your risk of heart disease and diabetes and help to control inflammation, your blood pressure and cholesterol levels, all of which have an impact on the aging brain.

SLEEP AND HEALTH

While we've long understood that there are many benefits to a good night's sleep, scientists still don't have many answers that directly support the relationship between sleep, health and well-being. They do know that an adequate amount of restful sleep improves memory, mood and immune function, and that sleep supports the body's repair and recovery processes. People who regularly get about eight hours of restful sleep feel better and are less likely to develop certain diseases. On the other hand, those who sleep poorly or for less than six hours per night are more likely to end up with a number of conditions, including heart disease, diabetes, hypertension and obesity. Poor sleep can even decrease one's life span: several large-scale studies have shown that sleeping five hours or less per night increased mortality risk from all causes by about 15 percent.

The Circadian Clock

Humans evolved as diurnal creatures, which means we are active and alert during the day and sleep at night. The simple truth is that our biology has not evolved beyond that rhythm. When we try to buck the system, illness and inflammation may follow. Studies indicate, for instance, that night-shift workers, particularly women, have an increased risk of developing various types of cancer. Women who work night shifts over the long term are 32 percent more likely to develop breast cancer, a risk that rises to 58 percent for female nurses working the night shift. Night-shift workers are also at higher risk for lung and digestive cancers, diabetes and obesity. In fact, the International Agency for Research on Cancer has classified shift work as a "probable carcinogen" for humans.

The Role of Hormones

The circadian clock dictates the times we feel tired or awake, and one of the ways it does that is by releasing hormones such as melatonin. Melatonin has far-reaching effects within the human body. It impacts the ability to fight infections and the incidence of certain types of cancer, and it correlates with inflammation levels in the body. As you age, your body gradually produces less melatonin, a process that has been linked with increased insomnia and poor sleep in older people.

Both short- and long-term sleep deprivation have numerous health consequences, from undermining your immune system to increasing your risk of hypertension. Not getting enough sleep can create hormonal imbalances that impair glucose regulation, which over time can lead to diabetes. Insomnia and short-term sleep deprivation have also been associated with heightened levels of inflammatory chemicals in the body, including C-reactive protein (CRP), a well-known risk factor for heart disease and obesity. Even children experience negative effects from disturbed sleep, exhibiting higher levels of CRP and other indicators of inflammation.

MAGNESIUM

Magnesium deficiency has been associated with insomnia, as well as stress and anxiety, and adequate levels are known to promote more restful sleep. Among its many functions, the mineral interacts with neurotransmitters that promote sleep. In one small study of elderly people, those who were given 500 mg of magnesium daily over the course of eight weeks fell asleep faster and slept more deeply than the control group. Foods that provide magnesium include whole grains, dark leafy greens and nuts and seeds.

Gene Expression and the Circadian Clock

We now know that circadian rhythms are influenced by gene expression, and that some of the negative effects of sleep disturbances can be connected to epigenetic changes. For instance, animal studies have linked sleep deprivation with alterations in gene expression that increase the risk for fatty liver disease and insulin resistance. These changes also slow the rate of myelin repair in the brain. Myelin protects the brain, and many experts believe its breakdown is a major force in the process of aging.

More specifically, we know that disrupted sleep can affect DNA methylation. While global DNA methylation is not a precise marker of harm (it depends upon the genes that get methylated), it may hint at systemic disruptions. Children who suffer from obstructive sleep apnea (OSA), a type of sleep disturbance, have increased DNA methylation, which has been linked to inflammation and reduced immune function. People who suffer from insomnia and long-term shift workers also have alterations in DNA methylation.

When it comes to gene expression and sleep, it's a two-way street. The effects of chronic stress on the body's hormonal stress-response systems can induce epigenetic changes in the brain and ultimately impair quality of sleep. Bottom line, the quality and quantity of sleep you achieve matter. In your to-do list for maintaining good health and preventing chronic disease, be sure to include healthy sleep habits along with diet, exercise and optimizing stress management.

9

YOUR

MICROBIOME

Within the gut there is a living jungle; a stable ecosystem that lasts for a life-time. Our unique personal gut flora is one of our lasting inheritances from our mothers. We may have underestimated how important this inheritance is for it seems to have powers that are as yet unknown.

— DAVID BARKER, *NUTRITION IN THE WOMB*

"**N**O MAN IS AN ISLAND," declared the 17th-century poet John Donne, penning what has become one of the most often-quoted statements in literature. The idea is that you're not a self-sufficient individual but rather just one "piece of the Continent, a part of the main." I wonder what Donne would have written if he'd had even an inkling of what that "Continent" really consisted of in biological terms? His vision of humankind comprised physical and certain psychological features. More recently we have learned about the genetic underpinnings of the entity that is you, such as the 23,000 pairs of chromosomes inherited from your parents, as well as DNA. But the truth is, you are much more than even that: a thriving universe of bacteria lives on and inside your body.

The microbes that dwell in your gut contain many trillions of genes, making them much more genetically robust than you are. And — are you ready for this? — scientists say more than half of your body is not human. Those invisible settlers residing in all your covert recesses form the largest part of the individual that is you. In fact, they've been called your "second genome." This reality gives new meaning to the rhetorical question "What is human?"

Your Second Genome

Together your body's bacterial cells and their genes are known as the *microbiome*. This "second genome" is in constant communication with your own genome, so much so that their relationship is described in terms such as *complex ecosystem* and *social network*. And just like your genes, your gut bacteria's genes have the ability to express themselves, meaning they too can turn their volume up or down in response to environmental cues. Therein lies much of bacteria's muscle. While we don't yet understand much about how they actually work, we do know they have the power to modify significant bodily functions, such as your metabolism and even how your brain works.

Your gut microbes are much smarter than you might think. For instance, they can communicate with distant organs (well beyond your gut) to effect changes throughout your body. This impressive skill is known as *microbial signaling*. In simple terms, the bacteria rally their troops to respond to challenges that threaten their well-being — often at the expense of yours. Microbial signaling has been linked with a number of diseases, from nonalcoholic fatty liver disease to obesity and type 2 diabetes, among others.

What does your second genome have to do with your early development? Well, it's quite possible that the bacteria in your gut (and elsewhere) are seeded during your fetal life. This is currently a topic of heated debate among the scientific community, but since 2011, researchers in various parts of the world have been identifying bacteria in the placentas of new mothers, and the evidence seems to be strengthening as time passes. What is clear is that the composition of your microbiome is basically set by the time you celebrate your third birthday, and that makes your microbial ecology a subject of intense developmental

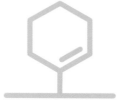

Microbiome:

The collection of bacteria that live in and on your body.

Microbial signaling:

The ability of the microbes that live in your gut to manufacture chemical signals that communicate with distant organs, such as the brain.

THE MICROBIOME IS NOTHING NEW

These days it's difficult to avoid the topic of microbes and how they affect your health. So it seems surprising to learn that most people (even experts) believe that the term *microbiome* didn't enter our vocabulary until 2001. Nobel Prize–winning microbiologist Joshua Lederberg is generally given credit for coining the term and its relative, *microbiota*, in that year. However, in a 2017 paper published in the *Human Microbiome Journal*, immunologist Susan Prescott cites several academic papers in which the term appeared well before the turn of the new millennium. Even cursory research on my part turned up at least two books that support this position. *Microbiota* is, in fact, a term that has been used in the field of microbiology for at least 50 years; it was obscured from view by various other advances in medicine, including the science of genetics.

So why the sudden interest in all these friendly and not-so-friendly bacteria? Scientists have long understood that the bacteria that dwell in and on our bodies affect our health and well-being, but for much of recent history their focus has been on identifying and eliminating pathogens — the bad bacteria that cause infectious diseases. A few adventurers such as Élie Metchnikoff, an embryologist and Nobel laureate who worked out of the Pasteur Institute in Paris around the turn of the 20th century, staked out the other side of the field. Although he is primarily recognized for his work in the field of immunology, toward the end of his career Metchnikoff became keenly interested in gut flora. His interest was sparked by a group of Bulgarian people known for their longevity, which he attributed to their consumption of *Lactobacillus*-rich yogurt.

Dr. Metchnikoff's research led him to conclude that having certain bacteria in the colon could improve health and slow down the aging process. His ideas gained traction in the early part of the 20th century but gradually fell out of favor. As Scott H. Peabody wrote in a 2012 article in *The Lancet*, "The heyday of *Lactobacillus* therapy came to an abrupt end with the advent of sulfa drugs and then antibiotics." With the wisdom of hindsight, it's clear that, after decades of overusing those drugs and the rise of antibiotic resistance, Metchnikoff's interest in bacterial flora was due for a comeback. Now even serious scientists are wondering if we won the battle against infectious disease while losing the war on other fronts.

interest. You and your microbes are engaged in a lifelong process of coevolution that, we are learning, likely has significant impacts on your health.

Health Begins in Your Gut

Experts now tell us that many diseases can be traced back to the health of your gut bacteria. There are good guys and bad guys among them. Most of the players in this network are your allies; *commensal* is the word scientists use to describe these supportive bacteria. However, there are a few bad eggs, such as viruses, some yeasts and other sorts of fungi that need to be restrained. To keep your system humming, you need to take good care of the good guys so they can remain in control.

Studies have compared various types of "good" and "bad" bacteria and haven't found specific combinations that are present in all healthy people. But when it comes to a healthy gut, the key differentiator appears to be bacterial diversity. The more species of bacteria you harbor, the healthier you are likely to be.

Your Very Own Ecosystem

Your mouth, nose, lungs, reproductive organs and skin harbor countless microbes. In addition, you are constantly collecting more, from surfaces, people, pets — basically anything you come in contact with while living your life. Your body hosts trillions of different microbes, but when it comes to your health, the bacteria in your gut probably exert the greatest influence. In medical terms, your gut includes your esophagus, stomach and intestines (small and large). About 1,000 species of bacteria might take up residence there, but only around 150 actually settle in. Each of the species has different strains, and the strains can be quite different genetically. No two people — even identical twins — have the same microbiome. A 2015 study from the Harvard T.H. Chan School of Public Health showed that an individual's microbiome is unique; it identifies them just as DNA and fingerprints do.

As an infant, you arrived in the world quite — but not totally — naked in microbial terms. Until recently it was thought that the womb is a sterile environment and that infants first experience germs in the process of being born. However, we now suspect that isn't correct, and that your mother may have passed on some bacteria to you while you were still in her belly.

If you are very lucky, your mother was raised in what experts call a "high microbial environment" — perhaps an organic farm, complete with animals — that endowed her with an abundance of "good guy" bacteria. You are even luckier if she lived in that lavish landscape while pregnant with you, because those friendly bacteria would have provided a rich starter culture for your own microbiome. Hopefully she didn't need to take any antibiotics while you were gestating, because that would have robbed you of a chunk of your microbial inheritance. And if she consumed a diet of fermented foods, such as yogurt, as well as fiber-rich fruits, vegetables and whole grains, those all enriched your bacterial legacy.

One reward of such biological plenitude is that it reduced your chances of developing allergies while growing up. Research now shows that a pregnant mother's diet (both the specific nutrients it provides and the general pattern, such as many or few fruits and vegetables) and her environment (for instance, breathing clean or polluted air) influence the microbiome of her fetus and, therefore, how its immune system develops.

Microbial Colonization

Your first major experience of what scientists call *microbial colonization* came when you were delivered. How you arrived in the world — via natural childbirth or by caesarean section — played a big role in building the foundation upon which your microbiome developed. For various reasons, when it comes to gut bacteria, diversity is better (see "Dysbiosis," page 279). Babies delivered vaginally acquire communities of bacteria similar to those in their mother's vagina, whereas those delivered via caesarean section pick up a narrower range typically found on the skin. Another factor is chronic maternal stress, which alters vaginal bacteria, negatively affecting the baby's disease risk.

How you were fed is also important. The microbiota of breastfed and bottle-fed babies differ significantly. Among other benefits, breast milk provides an abundance of beneficial bacteria (as many as 600 species, according to one study). A 2017 study published in the journal *JAMA Pediatrics* showed that in the first month of life, babies get almost 30 percent of their gut bacteria from breast milk and about 10 percent from skin contact with the breast. Babies who are breastfed have a higher proportion of beneficial bacteria to protect them from pathogens.

As you grew and explored the world, you were introduced to a wider range of bacteria that, over time, put down roots and proliferated, creating your unique microbial fingerprint that developed in response to your lifestyle and environment. Your microbiome continued to grow rapidly until you were about three years old, when it stabilized. Thereafter, it developed at a slower, steadier pace.

Your Gut and Your Health

Having discovered that more than half of your body isn't human (according to Germany's Max Planck Institutes, only 43 percent of the body is composed of human cells; the remainder is our microbial settlers), you must be wondering whether bacteria, not you, are controlling your life. They might be. For starters, your microbiota is tightly connected with various body systems, including your metabolic and immune systems, as well as your brain, so it shouldn't be surprising to learn that it has been linked with a wide variety of diseases, from allergies and obesity to depression and autism. Your microbiota may also help to explain your distinct experience of daily life. For instance, microbes can modify the effectiveness of a drug and influence whether your liver will be able to detoxify it. And if, like me, you are one of those people mosquitos love, feel free to blame your bacteria. According to Rob Knight, a biologist who specializes in the microbiome, the microbes on our skin produce different chemicals that mosquitos can detect. The insects find some more appealing than others and are attracted to the people who carry the ones they prefer.

Certain disease states can be linked with an unhealthy gut, but we're not sure whether a sickly microbiome is a cause or a consequence of disease. It's probably some of each. Many factors, including your genome, your diet, stress and your lifestyle, impact your microbiome. Over the course of a lifetime, thanks to endless interactions with the environment, the composition of your microorganisms gradually changes. It's not a stretch to imagine that a disease state can shift your bacterial balance into the danger zone. However, we don't understand exactly how gut bacteria impact health. Evidence suggests that bacterial imbalance can initiate a disease process, and laboratory studies (and some human interventions) show that introducing beneficial bacteria can work as a cure. For instance, a 2008 mouse study published in *Nature* proved that a pathogenic bacterium (*Helicobacter hepaticus*) could cause inflammatory bowel disease. When beneficial bacteria (*Bacteroides fragilis*) were introduced, the condition was remedied.

One compelling story about the power of the microbiome to influence health comes from China. In 2006 microbiologist Liping Zhao experimented on himself, monitoring his microbiota and consuming a diet of fermented prebiotic foods (mainly Chinese yam and bitter melon, combined with whole grains) to "cure" his obesity. Over the course of two years he lost 45 pounds (20 kg). His blood pressure, heart rate and cholesterol declined to healthy levels, thanks, he believes, to the proliferation of beneficial gut bacteria generated by his fiber-rich diet. He is currently at Rutgers University in the United States, studying how diet and gut bacteria can be used to alleviate type 2 diabetes.

BACTERIA AND CHRONIC ILLNESS

Since winning the Nobel Prize in Physiology or Medicine in 2005, Barry Marshall and Robin Warren are highly regarded in their fields. However, in 1984 their maverick idea that a spiral-shaped bug could cause a chronic disease was believed to be wacky. First, the stomach was thought to be a sterile environment and therefore uninhabitable by bacteria. In those days, people with ulcers tended to have high levels of stomach acid, which physicians assumed was linked with stress (there was no evidence to support this). So patients were treated with lifelong prescriptions for various types of antacids and possibly even psychotropic medications like antidepressants. The worst cases were treated with surgery, the results of which were far from ideal.

Based on Dr. Warren's work as a pathologist, the two physicians began to suspect that bacteria might play a role in the disease. As he biopsied the stomach linings of patients who had suffered from ulcers, Dr. Warren was noticing an unknown bacteria. It took the two doctors awhile to culture the bacterium, which is now known as *Helicobacter pylori*. For various reasons, Dr. Marshall was forced to drink a dose to test their theory that it was linked with ulcer development. Almost immediately after ingesting the microbe he ended up with gastritis, which he successfully treated with antibiotics. The rest, as they say, is history.

But it's certainly not the end of the story. *H. pylori*, as it's commonly called, is a fairly pervasive type of bacteria. It is particularly prevalent in people who reside in developing countries, where rates approaching 80 percent are common. Perhaps surprisingly, we now know that while many people harbor significant amounts of *H. pylori*, not all of those people have ulcers. That means *H. pylori* does not act alone to cause ulcers. So the question is, what other factors are at work? Does the body have other lines of defense that break down, allowing *H. pylori* to run amok and create ulcers? Basically, the answer is likely yes. As a 2017 review paper published in the *British Journal of Surgery* concluded, the "unrecognized defence factor in the pathogenesis of ulcer disease" is a rich and diverse microbiota.

Your Immune System

Did you know that 70 percent of your immune system is in your gut? Your microbiota has been calibrating your immune system since the day you were born, and likely even before. Moreover, throughout your life your immune system has been shaping the communities of bacteria that reside in and on your body. In fact, your immune system and your microbiota are constantly dancing an intricate *pas de deux*, inspiring, modulating or even undermining each other's performance, based on how life unfolds.

Your body relies on certain bacteria to regulate your immune system. If their numbers are disrupted, it upsets how smoothly the system runs. For instance, bacteria temper how certain immune-system cells, such as toll-like receptors (TLRs), respond to real or imagined threats. Depending on the circumstances, these cells may release inflammatory or anti-inflammatory substances. How they behave is influenced to some extent by your microbiota. Your gut bacteria also help to determine the composition of cell communities. An effective immune system needs an appropriate balance between effector T-cells, which are primed to attack invaders, and regulatory T-cells, which help to tone down the Terminator response. Once again, your microbes help to shape this balance.

Allergies

The diseases most commonly associated with the immune system are allergies. While it's easy to dismiss allergic disease as a mainly localized response — a rash on the skin, runny nose, weepy eyes — immunologist Susan Prescott points out that allergies are "truly a systemic condition." In that regard, a 2005 study published in *Archives of Internal Medicine* provides food for thought. The researchers found that men who suffered from allergic rhinitis or asthma were four times more likely to develop atherosclerosis, the plaque buildup on arteries that may pave the way for a heart attack. A subsequent meta-analysis published in 2017 linked asthma with an increased risk of coronary heart disease, especially in women.

So what's the connection between asthma or allergies, heart disease and your gut? Well, for starters, numerous studies have shown that when people have asthma or allergies, the communities of bacteria in their gut are significantly different from those of nonallergic people. Perhaps not coincidentally, the bacteria in your gut and the products they create have been shown to regulate inflammation. Some bacteria work to prevent inflammation and others support its development. Experts now believe that changes to the microbiota are driving the dramatic rise in inflammatory diseases, such as type 1 diabetes and other autoimmune disorders, in developed countries. Inflammation has also been linked with heart disease.

Autoimmune Diseases

These days the word *epidemic* is being used to describe the increased incidence of autoimmune disorders: conditions in which a person's immune system attacks their own body. Although autoimmune disorders are extremely complex, in recent years researchers have begun to connect the dots between their rising rates and the overgrowth of certain pathogenic gut bacteria. They have also been able to identify links between specific microbes and certain autoimmune diseases, including rheumatoid arthritis and irritable bowel disease.

Celiac disease provides a case in point. Compared to healthy individuals, people with celiac disease have an overabundance of gut bacteria generally associated with inflammation. And, it may be worth noting, people with celiac disease have about 10 times the rate of autoimmune thyroid disorders than the norm.

THE PROCESSED FOOD CONNECTION

For various reasons, researchers have recently begun to wonder if there is a connection between the rising rates of autoimmune disorders and the Western world's love affair with junk food. And it seems there may be. That link is the involvement of a molecule known as *endotoxin*. Endotoxin, which inhabits certain types of bacterial cells, can sometimes "leak" into the bloodstream during the life of the cell or when it dies. So long as endotoxin remains in the wall of the bacterial cell, where it normally resides, it's harmless. However, when it's unleashed into the bloodstream, it provokes inflammation.

What does it take to untether endotoxin? Well, we now know that a typical fast-food meal is likely to do the trick. When researcher Paresh Dandona studied the effects of a high-fat, high-carb McDonald's breakfast, he was shocked to find how quickly blood sugar and levels of C-reactive protein, a measure of inflammation, escalated. He also noticed that his subjects had increased levels of endotoxin, which he concluded had sprung from the bacteria in their gut. The good news is that in subsequent studies, Dr. Dandona found that endotoxins could easily be tamed. All it took was orange juice. When he added a glass of this anti-inflammatory beverage to the meal, his subjects' blood sugar levels and inflammation remained stable.

GASTRIC BYPASS SURGERY AND THE MICROBIOME

Scientists have been researching endotoxin's potential role in chronic disease for decades. It's hard to pin down, but endotoxin has been linked with autoimmune diseases including Crohn's disease, ulcerative colitis and rheumatoid arthritis. (It has also been shown to

THE HYGIENE HYPOTHESIS

My grandmother had a wonderful garden where, as a young child, I spent many happy moments, picking vegetables such as green peas and beans and plucking raspberries from the vines. I enjoyed her garden so much that my mother allowed me to cultivate a little plot near our back porch, where I grew my own radishes. In recent years I've often remembered those experiences because, although I didn't know it then, all that mucking about in the dirt was exposing me to healthy organisms in the soil that were enriching my microbiome.

Prior to the Industrial Revolution, virtually everyone was in constant contact with "good dirt" — the kind I experienced as a child. But once people migrated to urban environments, the balance shifted. Thanks to crowded, unsanitary living conditions, pathogenic bacteria were likely to take control over those that are helpful. Without refrigeration, pathogens had a heyday spoiling food, and poor public sanitation, which exposed people to raw sewage and contaminated drinking water, ensured high rates of infectious disease and, consequently, increased mortality.

In those days scientists were obviously interested in identifying and eradicating the causes of these large-scale problems. Pasteur's discovery that bacteria could spread disease was a paradigm shift; it was supported by the work of other scientists, such as Joseph Lister, who introduced the practice of sanitation to medicine. Along with public health measures like safe drinking water and large waste-management systems, the 20th century became in many ways a successful war against germs.

The problem is, in the course of protecting ourselves from pathogens, we helped to create a macroenvironment that may be shortchanged on beneficial bacteria. Some people think we threw the baby out with the bathwater. The basic premise of the hygiene hypothesis is that the world many of us inhabit is far too clean. (Interestingly, while finishing up this book, I learned that David Barker was an early adopter, if not an initiator, of this term.) A key principle is that when infants and young children are overly protected from exposure to infectious agents, parasites and potentially beneficial microorganisms, proper development of their immune systems is inhibited.

Consider, for instance, that in the developed world babies spend most of their time indoors. Not only do they crawl around on relatively clean floors and drink from sterilized bottles, but it's very likely that at some point in their early life they will be treated with antibiotics. Studies show that these and other typical childhood exposures delay development of the microbiome and suppress development of certain species of bacteria, limiting microbial diversity. One result is higher rates of allergic disease.

The value of a microbe-rich environment in early life was clearly established in a 2016 study published in the *New England Journal of Medicine*. The researchers looked at two groups of children, one from Amish families, who were raised on small, agriculturally diverse farms, and the other from a Hutterite community whose extensive farms were industrialized. The gut bacteria of the Amish children were far richer and more diverse than in the Hutterite group, and they had significantly lower rates of asthma.

play a significant role in the development of atherosclerosis, which helps to explain the connection between immune responses and heart disease.) While this in itself doesn't tell us much about the role of the microbiome in autoimmunity, research into gastric bypass surgery moves us farther along the bread-crumb trail. People who undergo the procedure are usually extremely obese, and researchers have found that, subsequent to the surgery, the levels of endotoxin in their bloodstream plummet.

Research done at Boston's Massachusetts General Hospital helps to explain why the surgery has such a dramatic effect. Rodent studies showed that gastric bypass surgery completely restructured the animals' microbiome, boosting beneficial microbes that not only reduced inflammation but also supported weight loss. This is an important point. After the surgery the rodents could properly metabolize glucose, a finding that suggests the microbiome plays a significant role in influencing metabolic processes.

These days researchers are actively exploring obesity as a trigger for autoimmune disorders. We know that obesity modifies the microbiome (or vice versa), as do certain diets (high-fat, for instance). While we don't understand all the mechanisms, as a 2014 study published in *Current Allergy and Asthma Reports* stated, "It is becoming increasingly clear that the dietary habits in Western societies ('too much,' 'too fatty,' 'too salty') and a high body mass index (BMI) ... constitute risk factors for autoimmune diseases."

Gut Bacteria and Metabolic Illnesses

The connections between gut bacteria and metabolic diseases such as type 2 diabetes and nonalcoholic fatty liver disease (NAFLD) are well established. Microbial imbalance has also been associated with risk factors for heart disease, including high levels of LDL cholesterol and triglycerides. So it's not surprising that researchers are wondering whether interventions directed at "reshaping the gut bacterial landscape" could benefit metabolic disorders.

Although the science is complex, here's a simple example of how this might work: Research tells us that people with type 2 diabetes have reduced levels of bacteria that produce chemicals useful for controlling blood sugar (glucose). When blood sugar levels consistently veer outside an acceptable range, insulin resistance is a likely result. If more of those beneficial bacteria were present, they would produce substances that stimulate the production of insulin, improving glucose utilization. A 2012 rodent study published in *Gastroenterology* showed that when researchers transferred bacteria from lean donors to the intestines of animals with metabolic syndrome, some of the new bacteria in the recipients' microbiota produced a substance that improved their insulin sensitivity.

Dietary interventions may have similar effects. For instance, they can help to keep endotoxin in check. When Dr. Patrice Cani of the Belgian Fund for Scientific Research gave mice a small dose of endotoxin, they became insulin-resistant, the first step in a cascade that moved through obesity and culminated in the development of type 2 diabetes. But if those same mice were fed soluble plant fibers rich in oligosaccharides — found in onions, garlic, legumes and cereal grains — the endotoxin did not invade their bloodstream. The disease process was stopped in its tracks: no inflammation, no insulin resistance, no diabetes. Such foods are known as prebiotics, substances that feed the friendly bacteria in your gut (see page 282).

Bacteria and Weight Loss

The communities of bacteria that reside in the guts of obese people are different from those of people who are lean. The question is, what difference does this make? A 2012 review article in the journal *Nature* showed that how your body digests and transforms food into energy may depend on the composition of your microbiota and the metabolic interactions among its bacterial species. And a small study done in 2018 indicated that these factors play a role in determining whether people will be successful at losing weight. When researchers looked at some participants in the Mayo Clinic Obesity Treatment

Research Program, they found that those who managed to shed pounds had different bacteria from those who were unsuccessful. They also learned that the gene expression of the bacteria differed. In line with the *Nature* review, they concluded that some bacteria influence how the body uses the energy from food, and that this affects an individual's ability to lose weight.

And here's another important point: when obese people lose weight, the balance of their microbiota shifts and their levels of beneficial bacteria increase. Perhaps not coincidentally, the same thing happens when people undergo gastric bypass surgery, as discussed above. This procedure has become quite popular because, in addition to promoting sustained weight loss, it reduces the risk of developing diabetes and cardiovascular disease.

Gut Bacteria, Gene Expression and More

Certain substances in complex carbohydrates feed the bacteria in your gut. Bacteria ferment these substances, producing desirable end products (see "Prebiotics," page 282), which have been shown to influence gene expression. Bacteria also play a role in regulating bile-acid metabolism. Bile acids help your body absorb nutrients and process cholesterol, dietary fats and fat-soluble vitamins, among other functions. In addition, bacteria influence how your body processes choline, a compound that helps to determine how your body handles fats. Your microbes interact with choline in conjunction with certain enzymes. If your microbial ecology is not up to snuff, this process is likely to produce toxic substances, an occurrence that has been linked with the development of NAFLD in mice, as well as with cardiovascular diseases.

Your Second Brain

The health of your microbiome influences every system in your body, including your central nervous system, which consists of the brain and spinal cord. The bacteria in your gut have been in constant communication with your brain likely from the time you were a fetus, and evidence suggests that gut health plays a significant role in mental well-being.

The gut has been called your "second brain." The *gut–brain axis* is a term experts use to define the network connecting the two entities. Much of their direct communication takes place via the vagus nerve, which runs from the brain through the abdomen, but they are also connected through chemical messengers such as hormones and neurotransmitters. Your microbiota helps to direct so much of this gut–brain traffic that recent research suggests the network should be renamed the *brain–gut–microbiota axis*.

The Brain, the Gut and Stress

In a 2012 paper published in *Psychoneuroendocrinology*, researchers found that areas of the brain that regulate stress are particularly susceptible to the influence of gut bacteria and vice versa. One of the body's key stress regulators, the *hypothalamic–pituitary–adrenal* (HPA) axis, can affect microbial composition. For instance, when infants or young children are separated from their mothers, the stress induces long-term changes to their HPA axis, and by day three of the separation at least one type of beneficial gut bacteria has declined significantly.

Attachment bonds play an important role in early childhood development. Both human and animal studies have connected separation anxiety in young offspring with long-term effects on the microbiome. They have also shown that early-life trauma or stress can precede the development of irritable bowel syndrome, a common gastrointestinal condition that has recently been linked with intestinal microbiota.

Mental Health

Exciting research regarding the microbiome involves its role in promoting mental health. Microbial imbalances have been linked with several disorders, including common conditions like anxiety and depression. Gut bacteria can produce neurotransmitters such as serotonin, dopamine, norepinephrine, GABA (gamma-aminobutyric acid) and acetylcholine, which help to regulate mood. The neurotransmitters serotonin and dopamine are known as the "happy hormones" because (not surprisingly) they help to make you happy. Norepinephrine triggers your fight-or-flight response, helping your brain think clearly or making your heart beat faster in order to cope with stress. GABA has been called "nature's Valium" for its ability to soothe anxiety, and acetylcholine supports memory and certain cognitive skills, among other benefits. Consequently, researchers are looking at ways to improve gut bacteria with a view to preventing and treating psychiatric disorders.

When certain gut bacteria digest certain foods, they produce substances known as short-chain fatty acids (SCFAs). Among their many benefits, SCFAs help your brain function better. One study provided a pill delivering *Bifidobacterium longum*, a bacterium associated with SCFA production, to 22 healthy men for a month. The subjects who consumed the bacterium reported feeling less stressed than the control group, who took a placebo. Blood tests showed that the group who took the *Bifidobacterium* had reduced levels of the hormone cortisol, which is related to stress. When measured by an electroencephalogram (EEG), their visual memory was also found to have improved slightly. See page 283 for more information on SCFAs.

The Autism Connection

Autism spectrum disorder encompasses a range of complex conditions, some of which may be connected to the immune system and possibly the microbiome. Skeptics suggest that autism is a neurodevelopmental disorder, and therefore it is unlikely that its roots lie in the microbiome. However, we now have a rapidly expanding body of evidence linking gut bacteria with the brain, and there is a growing awareness that, in some cases, altered intestinal bacteria may contribute to autism. Over 70 percent of children with autism also have digestive symptoms. Stool samples of children with autism showed lower levels of SCFA production, and the more severe the autism, the more likely it was that the child would also have digestive problems. Some researchers believe that autistic children have different types of gut bacteria than neurotypical children, and that restoring a healthy balance in their microbiome could be helpful in treating the condition.

IS MY DOG A PROBIOTIC?

Don't get annoyed with your dog when she tracks dirt into the house. Say thank you, because she has increased the microbial diversity of your environment. If you have children, she has helped to improve their health. Studies show that children who grow up with a dog in the house are less likely to develop immune-system illnesses such as allergies and asthma. Being exposed to a dog during the first three months of life, when a baby's immune system is in active development mode, is particularly helpful. A dog brings valuable bacteria (according to one study, 56 different types) into the environment, stimulating the infant's immune system and making it more resistant to potential allergens later in life. Although some of these species may not be beneficial, many are ones the infant wouldn't otherwise encounter, and most experts agree that the benefits of canine companionship outweigh the risks.

Here's another win: the emotional bond you feel with your dog may have biological benefits. Some scientists have speculated that your gut bacteria may be involved in the feelings of well-being derived from hanging out with your dog. Your bacteria enjoy getting together with their new friends, and they express themselves by producing mood-altering neurotransmitters that make you happy too.

Who Lives Here?

What determines which bacteria take up residence in your gut? It's a combination of your genes and environmental factors. Where you live is very important; scientists say they can identify where you reside (or have lived for an extended period of time) by the bacteria that inhabit your gut. Studies have also linked dietary patterns with the types of bacteria that cluster together to dominate your microbial community.

Numerous other factors contribute to your evolving microbiome, including:

- **Hygiene.** Cleaner is not necessarily better (see page 272).
- **Antibiotic use.** It kills off friendly bacteria along with pathogens and reduces bacterial diversity.
- **Chronic stress.** Stress is damaging because it creates disruptions that throw off the microbial balance, reducing diversity.
- **Exposure to toxins.** Environmental toxins, such as air pollution, heavy metals or polychlorinated biphenyls (PCBs), can affect bacterial composition and reduce diversity. Studies have also linked glyphosate, a pesticide used with genetically modified seeds, to a disruption of gut bacteria that may have long-reaching associations with numerous modern diseases.
- **Pets.** Contact with animals usually expands bacterial diversity.
- **The air you breathe.** Dust is particularly potent, delivering huge amounts of bacteria. It is estimated that we inhale about 800,000 bacteria daily. Dust is diverse in its bacterial composition, and scientists are now actively interested in the relationship between a household's microbes and its human inhabitants' health.
- **Physical activity.** Sedentary behavior has been shown to affect the bacterial composition of the gut.

Diet and Your Microbiome

While we haven't worked out a formula for the ideal microbiome, we do know diet plays a major role in determining the types of bacteria that inhabit your gut, as well as their relative representation. For instance, if your diet is heavily weighted toward meat and dairy, shifting the focus toward fiber-rich plant foods will immediately boost the quality of your microbiome. A 2014 study published in the journal *Nature* reported that after only one day of a plant-focused diet, the quantity of beneficial bacteria in participants' guts improved, as did the gene expression of their resident species.

DYSBIOSIS

In a 2014 paper published in *Cell Metabolism*, microbiologists Justin and Erica Sonnenburg suggested that the microbiota of a typical human living in the Western world (even one deemed to be healthy) is dysbiotic, which means it's lacking in beneficial bacteria. When the balance in gut bacteria is disrupted, the effects are systemic. Dysbiosis has been linked with a wide variety of conditions, ranging from obesity and type 2 diabetes to atherosclerosis and even cancer.

The Sonnenburgs blame this pervasive problem on a low intake of *microbiota-accessible carbohydrates*. Although fiber is by far the most prevalent of these substances, the category also includes oligosaccharides, which are found in fibrous plant foods, such as leeks and Jerusalem artichokes, as well as in breast milk. Researchers are in the process of expanding the list of dietary components that qualify as prebiotics (see page 282) to include various healthy fats (polyunsaturated fatty acids and conjugated linoleic acid) as well as certain phytochemicals in plant foods. Studies show that a diet rich in these nutritious substances can reshape your microbiota, although their potential benefits depend on two things: the amount consumed and the bacteria that already live in your gut.

Other research indicates that your microbiome can go south almost as quickly. A mouse study published in the journal *Microbiome* in 2019 linked short-term consumption — for as little as two weeks — of a "Westernized" diet (high in animal fats and low in fiber) with a shift in gut bacteria toward a ratio commonly associated with low-grade inflammation and glucose intolerance. In addition, researchers noted changes in the expression of certain genes associated with inflammation. The effects of the diet were systemic and consistent with physiological changes connected with the onset of obesity. Equally significant, the researchers found that the diet undermined the immune system of the mice, reducing their ability to fight infectious disease.

Good Bacteria Dislike Junk Food

In the interest of scientific research, British geneticist Tim Spector allowed his son to consume nothing but processed food for 10 days. Although he had strongly suspected the diet would negatively affect the microbial diversity in his son's gut, he wasn't prepared

Fiber, Your Gut and Your Health

By the turn of the new millennium, most people were aware of the connections between chronic conditions such as obesity, cardiovascular disease and type 2 diabetes and the so-called Western lifestyle, which is characterized by a high intake of nutrient-poor processed foods. Among their deficiencies, these foods are very low in dietary fiber, a type of indigestible carbohydrate found in plant foods. Fiber can be broken down into two main groups: soluble and insoluble. Today scientists are looking at the possibility that fiber-deficient diets may play a significant role in many of the diseases of our time.

Soluble Fiber

Soluble fiber combines with water to make a gel-like substance that has specific health benefits. It helps to regulate the speed at which you digest food, supporting nutrient absorption. Because your body doesn't absorb soluble fiber easily, it binds to excess cholesterol and helps to eliminate it from your body. Depending on your intake, soluble fiber has been shown to reduce both total and LDL ("bad") cholesterol by as much as 10 percent.

Soluble fiber also slows down the rate at which your body absorbs dietary sugar. If you are at risk for prediabetes or diabetes, it can help keep your blood glucose levels under control. A small study published in *Science* in 2018 showed that people with type 2 diabetes who consumed a high-fiber diet increased the growth of specific strains of gut bacteria that produce short-chain fatty acids (SCFAs). These SCFAs signaled other hormones that promote insulin production and help to control appetite. The subjects improved their HgA1c levels — a measure of how well blood sugar is controlled — and lost weight.

Soluble fiber is found in whole grains — especially oats, barley and amaranth — peas, beans, lentils, nuts, seeds (including flax seeds and chia seeds) and some fruits and vegetables.

Insoluble Fiber

Unlike soluble fiber, insoluble fiber does not dissolve in water, which means it works to keep your digestion humming, in part by increasing the bulk of your stool, which helps to keep you regular and prevents constipation. Sources of insoluble fiber include whole grains, beans, seeds, most vegetables (especially dark leafy greens, cruciferous vegetables, asparagus and celery) and fruits (especially raspberries, pears and apples).

Eat Both Types

It makes sense to include an abundance of both types of fiber in your daily diet. In addition to helping you to feel fuller at meals, they have positive effects on blood sugar, cholesterol and overall digestion. However, it is impossible to get enough fiber if you consume a diet high in processed foods. Refined grains and processed meats and fats contain little or no dietary fiber, and animal foods have none. Foods that do not provide fiber need to be balanced with an abundance of plant-based foods to ensure adequate intake of this nutrient.

Fiber and Your Gut

In the 1960s scientists became curious about the links between dietary fiber and health. Researchers found, for instance, that African people had much lower rates of colorectal cancer, diabetes and heart disease than people in the West, and also consumed high-fiber diets. In hunter-gatherer societies, people typically ingest more than 150 grams of fiber every day. Back then, scientists had few insights into how eating fiber-rich foods led to reduced rates of certain diseases. Now they believe that the microbes that live in our guts and relish gobbling up fiber may play a key role.

Most people living in the industrialized world don't consume enough fiber to properly nurture their helpful little microorganisms. And according to Justin and Erica Sonnenburg, two microbiologists (who happen to be married) at Stanford University's School of Medicine, over the years the variety of microbes living in our guts has shrunk dramatically thanks to our fiber-deficient diet.

As an aside, it's interesting to speculate how much of a role our society's fondness for white bread played in killing off resident species. A small study published in 2013 in the *ISME Journal* found that eating more whole grains for a mere four weeks increased the populations of "good bacteria" in their subjects' guts. Did having more bacterial diversity improve the health of these people? When the researchers looked at various metabolic and immunological markers, they concluded that the answer was yes. They could see definite improvements to glucose and lipid metabolism, as well as benefits to the immune system. Compared to some other high-fiber foods, whole grains seemed to have a unique capacity for increasing microbial diversity. The researchers speculated that this could be because of their "compositional complexity," which may interest a wider variety of bacteria than those attracted by fiber alone.

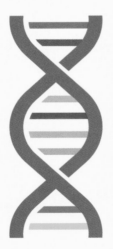

for how rapidly those effects would materialize and how impactful the shift would be. By day four of his fast-food diet, his son felt terrible. As he commented in a program aired on CBC's *The Nature of Things* in 2017, he felt like he was hungover after every meal. Meanwhile, his scientist father was diligently sending daily stool samples to a lab for analysis. The results were equally surprising. After 10 days, nearly half of the bacterial species in his son's gut had been completely wiped out.

We don't fully understand why processed food has such an immediate negative effect on the gut microbiome. A common assumption is that its high-calorie, high-fat, nutrient-poor nature is to blame, but research suggests that other components may also play a role. Mouse studies indicate that the detrimental effects may stem from common food additives like emulsifiers. These substances, which are ubiquitous in processed foods, have been shown to affect bacterial composition in the gut, altering metabolism. Artificial sweeteners have similar effects.

Prebiotics

Prebiotics are foods for the friendly bacteria in your gut, helping them to proliferate and promote health. Prebiotics include certain carbohydrates, such as inulin, pectin, resistant starch and some that have unpronounceable names like fructo-oligosaccharides and galacto-oligosaccharides. Good food sources of fiber-rich prebiotics include onions, garlic, leeks, bananas, Jerusalem artichokes, chicory root, jicama, dandelion greens, whole grains and legumes.

Prebiotic substances remain undigested until they reach your colon, where they are fermented and gobbled up by the bacteria that reside there. The bacteria break down the indigestible compounds, in the process creating health benefits for you, their host. For instance, they generate certain vitamins (B_{12} and K) and may increase calcium absorption in your gut, thereby improving bone density and helping to prevent osteoporosis. They also produce short-chain fatty acids. SCFAs are of great interest to scientists these days, not only for their role in gut health but also for their apparent contribution to health and well-being overall.

PHYTONUTRIENTS

While fiber is a key contributor to a healthy microbiome (see "Fiber, Your Gut and Your Health," page 280), recent research suggests that other substances, including phytonutrients, may also play significant roles in maintaining your bacterial ecology. Phytonutrients are chemicals produced by plants; like traditional nutrients, they help to keep you healthy.

They also act like prebiotics by interacting with certain microbes.

In their book *The Secret Life of Your Microbiome*, Susan Prescott and Alan C. Logan noted that certain phytonutrients have an "exceptional" ability to promote the growth of beneficial bacteria. Within this category, polyphenols are particularly effective. These substances are found in a wide variety of foods, mostly fruits and vegetables (especially red and yellow vegetables), but also nuts, seeds, herbs, spices and chocolate, among others.

Although polyphenols have been linked with many health benefits, they tend not to be readily available to the body. Prescott and Logan cited a 2016 animal study that suggested the typical Western diet may affect the body's ability to metabolize polyphenols, which are broken down by intestinal and liver enzymes as well as by bacterial degradation. Diets high in processed foods foster dysbiosis (see page 279), and a high ratio of unfriendly gut bacteria undermines the body's ability to extract the beneficial compounds from polyphenols. On the other hand, friendly microbes, including those belonging to the *Lactobacillus* and *Bifidobacterium* species, help to make polyphenols more bioavailable. Happily, this is a two-way street: foods that are particularly rich in polyphenols promote the growth of beneficial bacteria.

Another benefit of polyphenols is that they can help to increase levels of anti-inflammatory omega-3 fatty acids in the body while reducing inflammatory omega-6s. Obtaining omega-3 fatty acids from plant foods can be challenging. The process of converting ALA to EPA and DHA is notoriously inefficient (it can be as low as 8 percent). But we are now learning that when beneficial bacteria digest polyphenols, they produce new biologically active chemicals that facilitate the conversion process.

SHORT-CHAIN FATTY ACIDS

When the bacteria in your gut break down the indigestible compounds in foods, SCFAs are among the substances they create. Scientific interest in these molecular messengers has been heating up because more and more evidence suggests they influence health and well-being far beyond the gastrointestinal tract. They may, for instance, help your body to synthesize and absorb some essential nutrients. We are just beginning to understand how this complex ecosystem works, but it seems likely that we may have uncovered just the tip of the iceberg when it comes to the benefits of SCFAs.

The three most significant SCFAs are acetate, propionate and butyrate. Together they make up roughly 95 percent of your body's SCFA content. Research into allergic airways disease has linked protection against asthma specifically to the SCFAs acetate and propionate. Mouse studies suggest that maternal diet during pregnancy influences gut microbiota and fetal gene expression in ways that may encourage or suppress allergic airways disease. In a 2015 article published in *Nature Communications*, the researchers suggested that asthma may have developmental origins, resulting from low levels of SCFAs produced by the mother.

About 20 years ago, scientists began to recognize that SCFAs — butyrate in particular — have anti-inflammatory benefits. Butyrate supports the function of your regulatory T-cells, which, among other benefits, help to keep your immune system in check. Butyrate also helps to prevent metabolic syndrome and may improve insulin sensitivity. Moreover, it appears to protect against colorectal cancer, possibly by inhibiting the activity of histone deacetylase, an enzyme that can promote cancer growth. Butyrate is particularly helpful for people with gastrointestinal problems such as irritable bowel syndrome (IBS) and Crohn's disease, perhaps because it strengthens the integrity of the intestinal lining. While we don't fully understand exactly how this all works, we do know that butyrate increases the activity of certain genes, which likely plays a role in its beneficial effects.

Probiotics

As many as 1,000 species of bacteria live in a healthy gut. As noted, you can actively encourage the growth of beneficial bacteria by feeding them a diet high in fruits, vegetables, whole grains, legumes, nuts and seeds. But there is another powerful way to give your microbiome a boost, and that is by consuming microorganisms called probiotics.

Probiotics are friendly microbes known to benefit health. In addition to bacteria, a common species of yeast, *Saccharomyces boulardii*, is among the microbes considered a probiotic. *S. boulardii* can be used to treat and to help prevent a number of gastrointestinal problems, including traveler's diarrhea and IBS. It has also been shown in clinical trials to help prevent and treat highly problematic *Clostridium difficile* infections, which are usually acquired in hospital settings. In general, probiotics are helpful in treating intestinal conditions, skin allergies and respiratory tract infections.

FERMENTED FOODS

Long before we discovered refrigeration, fermentation was used to preserve food. But bacteria weren't identified in this process until 1857, when the chemist Louis Pasteur discovered that living organisms — yeast and bacteria — were responsible for fermentation. The yeast and bacteria convert the carbohydrates and sugar in food and drinks into by-products that act as preservatives. As it turns out, these by-products may have benefits far beyond their ability to preserve food.

284

Although some studies do not show a clear benefit from eating fermented foods, we do know that they help to make some nutrients more bioavailable. Essentially, fermentation jump-starts the process of digestion, predigesting the carbs, proteins and fats. This makes it easier for your body to absorb the nutrients the foods provide.

In addition, fermentation reduces the levels of so-called antinutrients in food. These compounds bind to minerals, making them less available to your body. Phytic acid is a case in point. While this substance, which is found in seeds, grains and legumes, is known to have certain health benefits, it also binds to minerals such as iron, zinc and calcium in the digestive tract, making them less available to your body. Fermenting foods lowers the levels of this antinutrient, increasing the bioavailability of the minerals.

Emerging evidence, although weak at this point, suggests that consuming fermented foods may also benefit your central nervous system. Scientists are only speculating on why, but it's possible that the new chemicals created by the fermentation process may have neuroprotective effects.

Another benefit is that some of the by-products created by fermentation may encourage the growth of friendly bacteria. Regularly consuming probiotics in the form of fermented foods appears to be a quick way to boost the number of "good" bacteria that reside in your gut and improve bacterial diversity. Fermented foods include some dairy products (yogurt, kefir, cheese), vegetables (sauerkraut, kimchi, pickles), soy products (miso, tempeh, soy sauce), whole grains (sourdough bread) and tea (kombucha).

We have traditionally assumed that commercially prepared foods are deficient in beneficial bacteria and yeast because they are processed at high heat, which destroys any living organisms. However, recent research indicates that although living microbes are preferable, friendly bacteria need not be alive to have beneficial effects. For instance, a study of 118 people showed that consuming a pasteurized milk product increased numbers of *Bifidobacterium* species in their guts. Other studies have produced similar results with *Lactobacillus* bacteria.

Since encouraging bacterial diversity is a key strategy for promoting gut health, it likely makes sense to consume different types of fermented foods. However, a word of caution is necessary: improperly fermented foods can be deadly. If you are fermenting at home, carefully follow the food safety instructions.

PROBIOTIC SUPPLEMENTS

While fermented foods typically provide more bacterial species than supplements, a probiotic supplement might be useful, particularly if you need to avoid certain species of

WHERE THE BAD GERMS CONGREGATE

Understanding the role of the microbiome in disease prevention is a relatively new and important area of research. Not only does it have a bearing on how we manage many chronic diseases, but it is also relevant to the treatment of critical illness. Acute situations such as heart attack or stroke, as well as trauma (think burns and serious accidents), are known to have an immediate and intense effect on the microbiome. This disruption is likely to be worsened by a hospital stay.

Several years ago I had a relatively minor procedure that involved an overnight stay in the hospital. I have vivid memories of my doctor warning me that my time in the hospital was in itself a risk factor associated with my treatment, increasing my chances of developing a health-care-associated infection (HAI). About 10 percent of people who spend any time in an intensive care unit contract an HAI, and 90 percent of these infections are caused by pathogenic bacteria. Hospitals are where the bad bugs love to hang out.

Pathogenic bacteria are primed to strike when you are at your most vulnerable to succumbing to infection. By the time you are admitted to a hospital, your immune system is likely already weakened, either by the wear and tear of living with a chronic condition or by the stress associated with an acute event, such as surgery. Sepsis, a potentially deadly infection associated with surgery, is caused by bacteria that commonly live in the bloodstream. Doctors suspect that the stress of surgery, coupled with physiological changes associated with critical illness, alters the microbiota, affecting other body systems, and that sepsis can be an end result.

On admission to hospital you are perched precariously at the top of a slippery slope. You are already sick, or certainly not functioning at your best. Many standard "evidence-based" hospital practices further weaken your microbiome. These include routine courses of antibiotics, which are known to rapidly annihilate microbial diversity. While we don't have an abundance of information on the effects of other drugs, a 2018 study published in *Scientific Reports* found that just one day of morphine treatment resulted in dysbiosis, including an alarming increase in pathogenic bacteria and a loss of bacteria associated with stress tolerance. In addition, numerous tests and procedures require a period of fasting, which deprives you of nutrients that nourish your beneficial bacteria.

And don't forget, your bacteria are busy watching out for themselves. Some types of pathogenic bacteria are primed to spot weakness and will exploit your debility. As Robert Martindale, a professor of surgery at Oregon Health & Science University, told me in an interview, "Bacteria sense when your body is stressed — say, from surgery or another acute experience — and they will take advantage of your vulnerability. Take *E. coli*, for instance. This bacterium is usually harmless, but when you are stressed, it can transform itself into a pathogenic strain. Beneficial *E. coli* lives happily in the lining of the intestines. When it becomes pathogenic, it will destroy the intestinal lining and invade your bloodstream."

Perhaps not coincidentally, Dr. Martindale also has an undergraduate degree in nutrition. He has been focused on preventing surgery-related infections for many years, and that interest led him into the realm of probiotics. He has been a pioneer in prescribing probiotics when patients are undergoing surgery.

Clostridium difficile is the most common cause of hospital-based infection and can lead to death in high-risk individuals. It is a major problem worldwide and a growing concern, because hypervirulent strains are now emerging. Dr. Martindale was one of the authors of a 2018 study published in the *American Journal of Surgery* that looked at various approaches to reducing the incidence of *C. difficile*. Based on a sample of 6,000 trauma patients, the researchers found that the most significant reduction resulted from a combination of antibiotics and probiotics. They also discovered that the timing of delivery was critical. "It's important to start the probiotics along with the antibiotics," Dr. Martindale told me. "The patients who started both simultaneously had virtually no chance [0.7 percent] of developing *C. difficile*. The longer they delayed the probiotics, the greater the risk. After five days, there was no benefit at all."

Large overview studies of the benefits of probiotics with regard to surgery have produced mixed results. Dr. Martindale believes that's because they haven't asked the right questions. "Probiotics are not a one-size-fits-all solution," he noted. "You need to pick your bacteria and tailor them to your specific problem. For instance, if you're having colon surgery, the *Lactobacillus* strain has been shown to be beneficial. *Lactobacillus* and *Bifidobacterium* species in combination work best for stomach surgery. If you give the probiotic presurgery, it's been shown to decrease infection risk and reduce the time spent in hospital."

bacteria (some strains are problematic for people who have difficulty tolerating histamine, for instance). And a supplement that provides specific types of bacteria might be helpful if you are trying to treat certain conditions, such as diarrhea and inflammatory bowel disease.

Current research suggests that probiotic supplements are useful only as long as you continue to provide the supplement; the bacteria's ability to colonize appears limited. However, they may have an indirect influence, perhaps by initiating processes that favor the proliferation of friendly species and thus helping to create a more balanced microbiome. They may also be useful in helping to stabilize microbial disruptions, such as those provoked by the use of antibiotics.

Physical Activity

Although diet plays a major role in the flora of your microbiome, it isn't the only factor that nurtures good bacteria and keeps the bad varieties in check. It has long been known that exercise can alter the microbial composition of your gut. Current research is revealing that there is a difference between lean and obese people in terms of how these shifts take shape. A 2018 study published in *Medicine & Science in Sports & Exercise* followed up on mouse studies that showed improving rodents' microbiota through exercise increased their ability to resist pathogens. Thirty-two humans who did not exercise (about half of whom were obese) were recruited for the study; the subjects were instructed to remain on their usual diets. After six weeks of an exercise program that gradually increased in intensity, the lean participants showed statistically significant higher concentrations of beneficial bacteria species that produce SCFAs, along with higher concentrations of SCFAs in their intestines. The researchers could also identify differences in the gene expression of the bacteria in those subjects. However, higher concentrations of SCFAs and similar changes in gene expression were not observed in the obese participants, who showed only modest (not statistically significant) increases in their SCFA-producing bacteria.

All of the participants were told to stop exercising once the program was completed, and after six weeks their gut bacteria were assessed again. At that point most of the benefits of the exercise program had dissipated. The researchers concluded that exercise benefits not only the composition of gut bacteria but also how they function, and that those benefits depend on body weight status.

An Intricate Web

When I began working on this book I did not intend to write about the microbiome, even though I've been fascinated by the subject since it began to appear on my radar about 10 years ago. David Barker did not write much about it, perhaps because the research was still in its nascent stages when he passed away in 2013. And since the traditional wisdom was that the womb is a sterile environment, bacteria didn't seem relevant to the developmental origins of health and disease. Now, however, it seems increasingly likely that mothers do transmit some of their microbiota to a developing fetus, and that a child's microbiome is pretty well developed by the age of three.

The science is still evolving, but I don't have the slightest doubt that microbes play a significant role in human health. They certainly influence how the immune system and metabolism function, and they communicate constantly with the brain, affecting mood and possibly even more unlikely conditions, such as the experience of chronic pain. While it's challenging to establish direct causality, imbalances in gut bacteria have been implicated in numerous disease states.

We now know that the composition of our gut bacteria can be influenced by diet. We also have an abundance of evidence that processed foods are bad for the microbiome. It's probably not surprising that the approach for nourishing your gut bacteria aligns with a basic message about preventing disease that runs throughout this book. To paraphrase Michael Pollan, author of *Food Rules: An Eater's Manual*, eat whole foods, mostly plants, and not too much. And don't ingest "foodish" products with names your great-grandmother wouldn't recognize as food, like those containing chemical additives or food derivatives. Without a doubt, that's the best strategy for promoting health and resisting disease — not only now, but for generations to come.

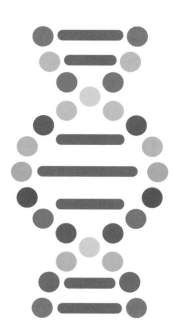

EPILOGUE

I am a part of all that I have met.

— ALFRED, LORD TENNYSON, *ULYSSES*

I often wonder if David Barker was ever in awe of the amazing journey his research took after the Barker hypothesis was published in 1986. His gut instinct — that heart disease and infant mortality were somehow linked — sent scientists traveling down many long and winding roads, from identifying low birth weight as a harbinger of adult illness to the cutting-edge epigenetic research being conducted today. And yet, despite the dramatic differences between early statistical observations and current genome-wide studies, they have all led to the same conclusion: early life makes a major contribution to the development of chronic disease.

First and foremost is the involvement of poor nutrition, which zigzags through the fabric of chronic illness like a wayward thread, its effects taking hold at both an individual and a collective level. Development in the womb is largely dependent on the nourishment a fetus receives during this critical period. Moreover, we now know that when malnutrition is prolonged over several generations, diseases begin to show up as historical phenomena. Examples include the Stroke Belt in the American South and the runaway rates of diabetes in previously nonindustrialized nations with long histories of poorly nourished people, such as India and China.

While it's clear that poor nutrition plays a key role in the legacy of chronic disease, the long-term effects of a hardscrabble life also take an undeniable toll. A wide body of research links various disturbances in early life with poor health later on. Childhood exposure to experiences such as abuse, neglect and domestic violence have major impacts on an adult's physical and mental health. A field of study known as "the social origins of illness" has arisen around this reality.

Today income disparity — the dramatic and growing gap between those at the top of the economic scale and those who struggle on a daily basis just to make ends meet — is a major concern. Numerous studies have examined the impact of a minimum-wage existence on a person's health; although the results are mixed, some general conclusions have emerged. First, surviving on scarce resources is relentlessly draining. If you must work constantly just to provide the bare necessities, it can be impossible to meet other needs, such as finding time to relax, eating healthy food or obtaining essential medical care. And the resulting stress can lead people to make poor decisions. For instance, even small increases in the minimum wage — as little as $1 an hour — decrease the likelihood that people on a low income will smoke.

Low income has been specifically linked with obesity, a connection that began to show up in earnest about 30 years ago, according to a 2018 study published in the open-access journal *Palgrave Communications*. Using data from both Europe and the United States, the researchers found that obesity "disproportionately affects the poor" thanks to the "overabundance of inexpensive food calories combined with decrease in daily physical activity." In addition, people who are poor, especially in proximity to others who are much better off, experience chronic stress, which negatively impacts their health on many different fronts.

A study published in *Lancet Public Health* in 2018 concluded that income disparity is affecting life expectancy. In 2016 the poorest people in England could expect to live to the age of 78.8 if they were women and 74 if they were men. But life expectancy for the most affluent people was significantly greater: women were likely to reach 86.7 years of age, and men 83.8. Perhaps even more chilling, the researchers found that children younger than five from the poorest families were 2.5 times more likely to die than children from well-off families.

Commenting on the report, its senior author, Majid Ezzati, an expert on the risk factors for disease at the population level, called the current climate "a perfect storm of factors that can impact on health and that are leading to poor people dying younger." He specifically noted food insecurity as a contributing factor. For various reasons, including affordability, nutrient-deficient processed foods are more accessible to the poorest people in countries with wide income disparity. This is especially true in the United States, which appears to have the highest level of economic inequality among developed countries.

We now have more than enough evidence to conclude that socioeconomic equity plays a key role in the development of chronic disease. Consider a study published in the *American Journal of Public Health* in 2016. It determined that, in the United States, raising the minimum wage to a dollar above the federally mandated level would decrease the number of low-birth-weight babies by 1 to 2 percent and would reduce the infant mortality rate by 4 percent. It's fascinating that economists who actively debate the merits of increasing the minimum wage don't take public health outcomes into consideration. They seem to be unaware of the long-term economic payoffs associated with preventing disease before it develops.

Simply stated, people need a healthy start in life. The food a mother eats while she is pregnant and the environment surrounding her offspring for the first thousand days of life play a key role in their health as an adult. So the question is, why aren't we doing everything possible to ensure that pregnant women and children are well nourished? An extensive body of research supports the importance of early intervention — the earlier, the better. Finland, for instance, was able to reduce an extremely high infant mortality rate to one of the lowest in the world (today about 2.3 babies out of every 1,000 births) thanks to its excellent prenatal care programs, which include the much-lauded "baby box."

The United States has the highest infant mortality of any Western country (6.5 per 1,000 in 2016), but rather than introducing a national prenatal care program, legislators are more likely to cut taxes and take an axe to programs that benefit women and children. Many also appear blind to studies that show a high rate of return, including significant improvements to academic performance, on interventions such as school meal programs. Not only is this approach breathtakingly inhumane, it's very shortsighted. Over the long term, it's extremely expensive because it spawns high rates of chronic illnesses, which are costly to treat.

The numbers are alarming and should serve as a wake-up call. What happens in pregnancy is dependent on what happened before. We need to take better care of women and children to make sure that future generations live healthier lives. We can begin that process by identifying and implementing public health policies that will improve nutrition for all mothers, infants and children. Ultimately, this will benefit us all, by helping to create a more equitable and healthy society.

GLOSSARY

ADIPOSITY: The state of being morbidly overweight (obese). Abdominal adiposity (also known as visceral fat) is associated with even greater health risks than obesity because it affects major organs, such as the liver and pancreas.

ALLELE: One of two versions of the same gene, depending on the DNA base sequence of paired nucleotides.

ALLOSTATIC LOAD: The long-term wear and tear on the systems that help the body adapt to environmental impacts, such as stress. When these impacts are persistent, the allostatic systems become overloaded, predisposing an individual to illness.

ALLOSTATIC SYSTEMS: Systems that help to keep the body on an even keel in response to environmental impacts.

BEHAVIORAL EPIGENETICS: The application of epigenetic principles to effects related to behavior (broadly speaking), such as parenting, stress and socioeconomic status. This relatively new science can help us determine how nurture shapes nature.

BIOACTIVE COMPOUNDS: Chemicals in foods that work with your body to promote health.

BODY MASS INDEX (BMI): A measure of body fat determined by your weight and height, used as a tool to determine if you are overweight.

CHROMOSOME: The part of a cell that resides in its nucleus and contains the genes. Humans have 46 chromosomes, 23 from each parent.

COMMENSAL: A term used to describe the "friendly" bacteria that inhabit your microbiota.

DEVELOPMENTAL ORIGINS OF HEALTH AND DISEASE (DOHAD): A body of research focused on identifying the links between in utero conditions and lifelong health.

DNA (DEOXYRIBONUCLEIC ACID): The main constituent of chromosomes, DNA carries genetic information, ensuring that a cell precisely replicates itself when it divides.

DNA METHYLATION: A chemical reaction that takes place in cells when a methyl group attaches to DNA, changing the expression of the gene to which is it attached. *Hypomethylation* refers to the state of being undermethylated; *hypermethylation* means being overmethylated.

DNA SEQUENCING: The order in which the four nucleotides are strung together on the DNA molecule.

DYSBIOSIS: An unhealthy imbalance in the species of bacteria living in the gut, favoring those that are harmful.

ENDOCRINE DISRUPTORS: A group of toxins, including chemicals that turn up in many familiar products, that have been shown to have a negative impact on gene expression, potentially setting the stage for disease development.

ENDOCRINE SYSTEM: The body system comprising all the glands that produce hormones.

ENDOCRINOLOGY: The study of hormones.

ENDOTOXIN: A molecule that resides in bacterial cells. It may "leak" into the bloodstream in response to negative stimulants and is released when the cell dies.

ENERGY-DENSE: Also known as *calorie-dense*. A term used to define food that is high in calories but low in nutrients in proportion to its weight.

ENZYMES: Molecules present throughout the body that speed up certain chemical reactions in cells. Enzymes help to ensure that the various body systems — such as digestion, metabolism, muscles and the central nervous system — function properly.

EPIDEMIOLOGY: The study of disease patterns in populations of people, with a view toward identifying the underlying causes of illness.

EPIGENETIC: With its prefix from the Greek word *epi*, which means "in addition to," this word relates to factors in addition to DNA base sequence that influence the function of genes.

EPIGENETIC INHERITANCE: The biological transmission to offspring of changes to gene expression resulting from epigenetic modifications.

EPIGENETIC MODIFICATION: A dynamic process influencing gene expression that acts like a kind of biological memory, stamping life experience on cells and genomes.

EPIGENETIC TAGS: Chemical tags added to DNA that record the effects of experience, changing gene expression.

EPIGENETICS: A biological process resulting in heritable changes (those passed on to cells of the same type as they divide) that are transmitted to future generations.

EPIGENOME: The network of compounds surrounding our genes, which interacts with our environment, altering gene expression in response to external influences.

FERTILITY: In males, the sperms' ability to fertilize an egg; in females, the ability to become pregnant.

GENE EXPRESSION: A complex process by which genetic information is converted into instructions for making molecules the body can use, such as proteins. It is influenced by epigenetic changes.

GENE REGULATION: The process of turning genes on or off, up or down, in the course of gene expression.

GENOME: The genetic material that comprises a human being, consisting primarily of genes and DNA.

GENOME-WIDE ASSOCIATION STUDIES (GWAS): Observational studies that scan the genomes of individuals with a view toward identifying genetic variations linked with particular diseases.

GUT FLORA: The bacteria that live in your esophagus, stomach and intestines.

HISTONE ACETYLATION: A specific type of histone modification involving the addition of a chemical group known as an acetyl.

HISTONE MODIFICATION: An epigenetic process whereby histones (a type of protein) are modified by certain chemical groups, influencing gene expression.

HORMONE: A chemical messenger that operates at the cellular level. Hormones are secreted by the endocrine glands (for example, the adrenals and thyroid).

HPA (HYPOTHALAMIC-PITUITARY-ADRENAL) AXIS: A body system that links parts of the brain with the adrenal glands, which are located in the kidneys. This system plays a key role in the body's response to stress.

100-YEAR EFFECT: The idea that an individual's complete package of DNA is shaped long before conception, in part because the egg from which someone develops was created in their mother's ovaries when she was still a fetus in their grandmother's womb.

HUNGER/OBESITY PARADOX: The apparently contradictory circumstance whereby hunger and obesity exist simultaneously in the same person and/or household. It has been linked with food insecurity.

HYPOTHALAMUS: The part of the brain that regulates appetite satiety and metabolism.

INSULIN RESISTANCE: A state in which the body gradually loses its ability to process insulin.

INTERGENERATIONAL INHERITANCE: *See* epigenetic inheritance.

INTRAUTERINE GROWTH RESTRICTION (IGR): A condition whereby a fetus is smaller than the norm due to factors such as poor maternal nutrition.

IN UTERO: In the uterus (womb), before birth.

KETONE BODIES: Compounds produced when fat is metabolized.

KETOSIS: The state in which a body burns fat because it does not have an adequate supply of glucose for energy.

LIPOTOXICITY: The buildup of fat in tissues, where it has a negative impact on organs such as the heart and liver.

LOW BIRTH WEIGHT (LBW): A condition that describes newborn babies who weigh less than 5 pounds 8 ounces (2,500 g). David Barker's early research identified LBW as a marker for increased risk of diseases such as obesity, type 2 diabetes and heart disease.

MENDELIAN INHERITANCE: A concept based on Gregor Mendel's experiments with pea plants, which showed that traits are passed on through generations in a regular manner, thanks to what we now know to be genes.

METABOLISM: The chemical processes that break down the nutrients in food and transform them into the energy required to keep the body functioning.

METABOLIZE: The process of breaking down nutrients so they can be used by the body.

METHYL DONOR: Nutrients, like folate and vitamin B$_{12}$, that when metabolized support the process of DNA methylation.

METHYL GROUP: A type of molecular structure that occurs in many compounds. *See also* DNA methylation.

MICROBIAL COLONIZATION: The process of acquiring the communities of bacteria that constitute your microbiome.

MICROBIAL DIVERSITY: Variety in the species of bacteria living on and in an organism, an abundance of which is thought to contribute to good health.

MICROBIAL SIGNALING: The ability of the microbes that live in your gut to communicate with distant organs, such as the brain.

MICROBIOME: The collection of bacteria that live in and on your body.

MICROBIOTA-ACCESSIBLE CARBOHYDRATES: Substances, including fiber and oligosaccharides, that nourish beneficial bacteria.

MULTIFACTORIAL DISEASES: Diseases involving hundreds of genes, each making a small contribution to disease development, which may also involve epigenetic influences.

NEUROTRANSMITTER: A chemical that helps to regulate mood, such as serotonin or dopamine.

NUCLEOTIDE: A chemical compound that is the basic structural unit of DNA. The DNA double helix consists of four nucleotides: adenine (A), thymine (T), cytosine (C) and guanine (G).

NUCLEOTIDE SEQUENCING: When cells divide, the complementary base pairing rule states that the four nucleotides bond with a specific partner — A with T, and C with G — to form base pairs. Variations in this sequencing produce single-nucleotide polymorphisms (SNPs).

NUTRIENT-DENSE: Describing food that provides a high ratio of nutrients in relation to its weight.

NUTRI-EPIGENOMICS: The study of how nutrients affect gene expression.

NUTRIGENOMICS: The study of gene–nutrient interactions, directed toward understanding how genetic variations affect how the body absorbs, stores and uses nutrients.

OBESOGENIC: Contributing to obesity.

OBESOGENIC ENVIRONMENT: An environment in which factors that encourage obesity are plentiful.

OBESOGENS: Chemical compounds found in common products, such as processed foods, pesticides and prescription medications, that affect gene expression, encouraging the metabolism to store fat.

ONCOGENES: Genes that have been altered from the norm, either by mutation or by increased expression, with the potential to initiate the growth of cancer cells.

PATHOGEN: A disease-causing microorganism, including viruses and some types of bacteria and fungi.

PENETRANCE: The likelihood that a person will develop a disease based on carrying a particular genetic mutation. The higher the penetrance, the more probable that the carrier will develop the disease. Some single gene disorders have 100 percent penetrance.

PHARMACOGENOMIC TESTS: Tests that use an individual's genes to help predict their response to drug therapy.

PHARMACOGENOMICS: The study of how genes influence the body's response to pharmaceutical drugs.

PHENOTYPE: The manifestation of an organism's characteristics or traits, resulting from its genotype and accumulated environmental impacts.

PHYTOESTROGEN: A form of estrogen that occurs naturally in plants, commonly found in soy products.

PLACENTAL INSUFFICIENCY: A complication in pregnancy whereby the placenta cannot deliver adequate nutrition and/or oxygen to the fetus.

PREBIOTICS: Foods that feed the friendly bacteria in your gut.

PREFRONTAL CORTEX: A part of the brain associated with what experts call "executive function." It is strongly linked with personality and social behavior, and matures in adolescence.

PROBIOTICS: Good bacteria, often found in foods, that directly benefit health.

PROGENITOR CELLS: Related to stem cells but more focused in their potential to differentiate into specific cell types. This is an emerging concept, and a precise definition is still evolving.

REACTIVE OXYGEN SPECIES (ROS): A type of unstable molecule containing oxygen, often called a "free radical." Traditional wisdom is that when ROS build up, they cause cellular damage, a process often compared to rust collecting on a car. However, recent research suggests that in some contexts these substances may be beneficial.

RNA: A molecule that, like DNA, is a nucleic acid that plays important roles in biological processes, such as regulating genes and how they are expressed.

RNA EXPRESSION: *See* RNA signaling.

RNA MODULATION: *See* RNA signaling.

RNA SIGNALING: An epigenetic process involving a specific molecule that has numerous subsets, with many different functions. These include microRNAs, which regulate gene expression.

SENESCENCE: The state that cells reach when they stop dividing but do not die.

SHORT-CHAIN FATTY ACIDS (SCFAS): Beneficial substances produced by gut bacteria in the process of digestion.

SINGLE GENE DISORDERS: Diseases that result from a mutation in a specific gene.

SINGLE-NUCLEOTIDE POLYMORPHISMS (SNPS): The most common type of genetic variation, SNPs are normal modifications that occur throughout an individual's DNA. They occur when the base sequence of paired nucleotides does not conform to the base pairing rule — for instance, when A pairs with C in a certain section of DNA. SNPs are particularly useful for studying gene-related phenomena, such as reactions to pharmaceuticals and disease risk, as well as for tracking ancestry.

SOCIOECONOMIC STATUS (SES): A family or individual's standing in the community based on the complete measure of factors such as occupation, income and education.

STEM CELL: A cell with the potential to develop into many different kinds of cells.

TELOMERASE: An enzyme, often referred to as "anti-aging," that maintains telomeres, helping to keep them long.

TELOMERES: Bits of DNA at the end of a chromosome that protect it during the process of replication.

TRANSCRIPTION: The first step of gene expression, whereby a gene's DNA sequence is copied to make RNA.

TRANSGENERATIONAL INHERITANCE: *See* epigenetics.

TUMOR-SUPPRESSOR GENES: Genes that work in a variety of ways to prevent the development and growth of cancer cells.

VISCERAL FAT: *See* adiposity.

ACKNOWLEDGMENTS

MANY PEOPLE HAVE BEEN helpful in transforming this material from a multitude of scattershot ideas into a book. First and foremost is Bob Moore. You may know him as the friendly face on the Bob's Red Mill packages of whole grains. I know him as someone whose passion for the power of good nutrition is, quite simply, inspirational. I owe a big debt of thanks to Bob for introducing me to the work of David Barker, as well as for his encouragement and support throughout the process of researching and writing this book.

Dr. Kent Thornburg, a highly esteemed scientist at Oregon Health & Science University, graciously wrote the foreword. He also read the manuscript in its entirety to ensure scientific accuracy. Like the best editors, he wielded his red pencil lightly but with laser-like precision. Epidemiologists Dr. Johan Eriksson of the University of Helsinki in Finland and Dr. Caroline Fall at the University of Southampton in England also reviewed large chunks of material. Thank you all for your kindness and support, and for sharing your expertise and your delightful stories about David Barker. Any errors that may have crept in are entirely my own.

Dr. Julie Briley and Dr. Courtney Jackson are naturopathic doctors, cofounders of the Food as Medicine Institute at the National University of Natural Medicine in Portland, Oregon, and joint authors of the excellent book *Food as Medicine Everyday*. They worked closely with me in developing the nutrition information in this book. In the process, they taught me a lot about some of the complex interactions between nutrients and the human body, for which I am very grateful. Dr. Robert Martindale was extremely helpful in providing invaluable background information on the microbiome and its impact on health.

As always, the editorial and design team at Robert Rose was exceptional. Kudos to Gillian Watts, indexer and copy editor extraordinaire, and, of course, my editor, Sue Sumeraj, who is delightful to work with. The design for this book is particularly noteworthy. Special thanks to Laura Palese and Kevin Cockburn for their superlative work.

I'd also like to thank the marketing team at Robert Rose, especially Kelly Glover and Megan Brush, as well as Scott Manning and Abby Wellhouse of Scott Manning & Associates.

And, of course, my family. My daughter, Meredith, a talented editor who read early drafts and offered valuable suggestions that helped steer me in the right direction. And last but certainly not least, my husband, Bob, for his constant support and ongoing commitment to good dinners and fresh flowers.

REFERENCES

Key Sources in the Developmental Origins of Health and Disease

Bagby SP. Developmental origins of renal disease: Should nephron protection begin at birth? *Clin J Am Soc Nephro* 4, no. 1 (2009): 10–13.

Bagby SP. Maternal nutrition, low nephron number and hypertension in later life: Pathways of nutritional programming. *J Nutr* 137, no. 4 (2007): 1066–72.

Barker D. The midwife, the coincidence, and the hypothesis. *BMJ* 327, no. 7429 (2003): 1428–30.

Barker DJ. Fetal origins of coronary heart disease. *BMJ* 311, no. 6998 (1995): 171–74.

Barker DJ, Eriksson JG, Forsén T, Osmond C. Fetal origins of adult disease: Strength of effects and biological basis. *Int J Epidemiol* 31, no. 6 (2002): 1235–59.

Barker DJ, Forsén T, Eriksson JG, Osmond C. Growth and living conditions in childhood and hypertension in adult life: A longitudinal study. *J Hypertens* 20, no. 10 (2002): 1951–56.

Barker DJ, Martyn CN, Osmond C, et al. Growth in utero and serum cholesterol concentrations in adult life. *BMJ* 307, no. 6918 (1993): 1524–27.

Barker DJ, Osmond C. Infant mortality, childhood nutrition and ischaemic heart disease in England and Wales. *Lancet* 1, no. 8489 (1986): 1077–81.

Barker DJ, Osmond C, Forsén TJ, et al. Trajectories of growth among children who have coronary events as adults. *N Engl J Med* 353, no. 17 (2005): 1802–9.

Barker DJ, Thornburg KL. The obstetric origins of health for a lifetime. *Clin Obstet Gynecol* 56, no. 3 (2013): 511–19.

Barker DJ, Thornburg KL. Placental programming of chronic diseases, cancer and lifespan: A review. *Placenta* 34, no. 10 (2013): 841–85.

Barker DJ, Winter PD, Osmond C, et al. Weight in infancy and death from ischaemic heart disease. *Lancet* 2, no. 8663 (1989): 577–80.

Barker DJP. *Nutrition in the Womb: How Better Nutrition During Development Will Prevent Heart Disease, Diabetes and Stroke*. Southampton, UK: D.J. Barker, 2008.

Cooper C, Eriksson JG, Forsén T, et al. Maternal height, childhood growth and risk of hip fracture in later life: A longitudinal study. *Osteoporos Int* 12, no. 8 (2001): 623–29.

Eriksson J, Forsén T, Tuomilehto J, et al. Catch-up growth in childhood and death from coronary heart disease: Longitudinal study. *BMJ* 318, no. 7181 (1999): 427–31.

Eriksson J, Forsén T, Tuomilehto J, et al. Early growth and coronary heart disease in later life: Longitudinal study. *BMJ* 322, no. 7292 (2001): 949–53.

Eriksson J, Forsén T, Tuomilehto J, et al. Fetal and childhood growth and hypertension in adult life. *Hypertension* 36, no. 5 (2000): 790–94.

Eriksson JG, Kajantie E, Osmond C, et al. Boys live dangerously in the womb. *Am J Hum Biol* 22, no. 3 (2010): 330–35.

Eriksson JG, Kajantie E, Thornburg KL, et al. Mother's body size and placental size predict coronary heart disease in men. *Eur Heart J* 32, no. 18 (2011): 2297–2303.

Eriksson JG, Lindi V, Uusitupa M, et al. The effects of the Pro12Ala polymorphism of the peroxisome proliferator-activated receptor-gamma2 gene on insulin sensitivity and insulin metabolism interact with size at birth. *Diabetes* 51, no. 7 (2002): 2321–24.

Forsén T, Eriksson JG, Tuomilehto J, et al. Mother's weight in pregnancy and coronary heart disease in a cohort of Finnish men: Follow up study. *BMJ* 315, no. 7112 (1997): 837–40.

Heijmans BT, Tobi EW, Stein AD, et al. Persistent epigenetic differences associated with prenatal exposure to famine in humans. *Proc Natl Acad Sci U S A* 105, no. 44 (2008): 17046–49.

Johnson LSB, Salonen M, Kajantie E, et al. Early life risk factors for incident atrial fibrillation in the Helsinki Birth Cohort Study. *J Am Heart Assoc* 6, no. 6 (2017).

Lucas A. Long-term programming effects of early nutrition — implications for the preterm infant. *J Perinatol* 25, suppl. 2 (2005): S2–6.

Lucas A. Programming by early nutrition: An experimental approach. *J Nutr* 128, suppl. 2 (1998): 401–6S.

Northstone K, Golding J, Davey Smith G, et al. Prepubertal start of father's smoking and increased body fat in his sons: Further characterisation of paternal transgenerational responses. *Eur J Hum Genet* 22, no. 12 (2014): 1382–86.

Pembrey M, Saffery R, Bygren LO, and Network in Epigenetic Epidemiology. Human transgenerational responses to early-life experience: Potential impact on development, health and biomedical research. *J Med Genet* 51, no. 9 (2014): 563–72.

Pembrey ME, Bygren LO, Kaati G, et al. Sex-specific, male-line transgenerational responses in humans. *Eur J Hum Genet* 14, no. 2 (2006): 159–66.

Phillips DI, Barker DJ, Hales CN, et al. Thinness at birth and insulin resistance in adult life. *Diabetologia* 37, no. 2 (1994): 150–54.

Polderman TJ, Benyamin B, de Leeuw CA, et al. Meta-analysis of the heritability of human traits based on fifty years of twin studies. *Nat Genet* 47, no. 7 (2015): 702–9.

Ravelli AC, van der Meulen JH, Michels RP, et al. Glucose tolerance in adults after prenatal exposure to famine. *Lancet* 351, no. 9097 (1998): 173–77.

Perälä M-M, Moltchanova E, Kaartinen NE, et al. The association between salt intake and adult systolic blood pressure is modified by birth weight. *Am J Clin Nutr* 93, no. 2 (2011): 422–26.

Roseboom T, de Rooij S, Painter R. The Dutch famine and its long-term consequences for human health. *Early Hum Dev* 82, no. 8 (2006): 485–91.

Roseboom TJ, van der Meulen JH, Osmond C, et al. Plasma lipid profiles of adults after prenatal exposure to the Dutch famine. *Am J Clin Nutr* 72, no. 5 (2000): 1101–6.

Roseboom TJ, van der Meulen JH, Ravelli AC, et al. Effects of prenatal exposure to the Dutch famine on adult disease in later life: An overview. *Mol Cell Endocrinol* 185, no. 1–2 (2001): 93–98.

Thornburg KL, Marshall N. The placenta is the center of the chronic disease universe. *Am J Obstet Gynecol* 213, no. 4, suppl. (2015): S14–20.

Thornburg KL, Shannon J, Thuillier P, Turker MS. In utero life and epigenetic predisposition for disease. *Adv Genet* 71 (2010): 57–78.

Tobi EW, Goeman JJ, Monajemi R, et al. DNA methylation signatures link prenatal famine exposure to growth and metabolism. *Nat Commun* 5 (2014): 5592.

Waterland RA, Jirtle RL. Transposable elements: Targets for early nutritional effects on epigenetic gene regulation. *Mol Cell Biol* 23, no. 15 (2003): 5293–300.

Winder NR, Krishnaveni GV, Veenaj SR, et al. Mother's lifetime nutrition and the size, shape and efficiency of the placenta. *Placenta* 32, no. 11 (2011): 806–10.

Selected References by Chapter

CHAPTER 1

Epstein D. How an 1836 famine altered the genes of children born decades later. Gizmodo, 26 August 2013. https://io9.gizmodo.com/how-an-1836-famine-altered-the-genes-of-children-born-d-1200001177.

Gardner MJ, Winter PD, Barker DJP. *Atlas of Mortality from Selected Diseases in England and Wales, 1968–1978.* Chichester, UK: Wiley, 1984.

Gillman MW, Rich-Edwards JW. The fetal origin of adult disease: From sceptic to convert. *Paediatr Perinat Epidemiol* 14, no. 3 (2000): 192–93.

Hall SS. Small and thin: The controversy over the fetal origins of adult health. *New Yorker*, 19 November 2007: 52–57.

Li J, Liu S, Li S, et al. Prenatal exposure to famine and the development of hyperglycemia and type 2 diabetes in adulthood across consecutive generations: A population-based cohort study of families in Suihua, China. *Am J Clin Nutr* 105, no. 1 (2017): 221–27.

CHAPTER 2

Alam MT, Zelezniak A, Mülleder M, et al. The metabolic background is a global player in *Saccharomyces* gene expression epistasis. *Nat Microbiol* 1 (2016): 15030.

Besingi W, Johansson A. Smoke-related DNA methylation changes in the etiology of human disease. *Hum Mol Genet* 23, no. 9 (2014): 2290–97.

Carey N. *The Epigenetics Revolution: How Modern Biology is Rewriting Our Understanding of Genetics, Disease and Inheritance.* New York: Columbia University Press, 2013.

Choi SW, Friso S. Epigenetics: A new bridge between nutrition and health. *Adv Nutr* 1, no. 1 (2010): 8–16.

Crider KS, Bailey LB, Berry RJ. Folic acid food fortification: Its history, effect, concerns, and future directions. *Nutrients* 3, no. 3 (2011): 370–84.

Denham J. Exercise and epigenetic inheritance of disease risk. *Acta Physiol (Oxf.)* 222, no. 1 (2018).

YOU ARE WHAT YOUR GRANDPARENTS ATE

Fenech M, El-Sohemy A, Cahill L, et al. Nutrigenetics and nutrigenomics: Viewpoints on the current status and applications in nutrition research and practice. *J Nutrigenet Nutrigenomics* 4, no. 2 (2011): 69–89.

Francis, RC. *Epigenetics. How Environment Shapes Our Genes*. New York: W.W. Norton & Company, 2011.

Jorgensen RA. Epigenetics: Biology's quantum mechanics. *Front Plant Sci* 2 (2011): 10.

Lee HJ, Hore TA, Reik W. Reprogramming the methylome: Erasing memory and creating diversity. *Cell Stem Cell* 14, no. 6 (2014): 710–19.

McDade TW, Ryan C, Jones MJ, et al. Social and physical environments early in development predict DNA methylation of inflammatory genes in young adulthood. *Proc Natl Acad Sci U S A* 114, no. 29 (2017): 7611–16.

Mukherjee S. *The Gene: An Intimate History*. New York: Scribner, 2016.

Pavlidis C, Patrinos GP, Katsila T. Nutrigenomics: A controversy. *Appl Transl Genom* 4 (2015): 50–53.

Pembrey M, Saffery R, Bygren LO, et al. Human transgenerational responses to early-life experience: Potential impact on development, health and biomedical research. *J Med Genet* 51, no. 9 (2014) 563–72.

Rodgers AB, Morgan CP, Bronson SL, et al. Paternal stress exposure alters sperm microRNA content and reprograms offspring HPA stress axis regulation. *J Neurosci* 33, no. 21 (2013): 9003–12.

Sharma P, Dwivedi S. Nutrigenomics and nutrigenetics: New insight in disease prevention and cure. *Indian J Clin Biochem* 32, no. 4 (2017): 371–73.

Spannhoff A, Kim YK, Raynal NJ, et al. Histone deacetylase inhibitor activity in royal jelly might facilitate caste switching in bees. *EMBO Rep* 12, no. 3 (2011): 238–43.

Vinci T, Robert JS. Aristotle and modern genetics. *J Hist Ideas* 66, no. 2 (2005): 201–21.

CHAPTER 3

Coglin A. Childhood poverty leaves its mark on adult genetics. *New Scientist*, 26 October 2011. www.newscientist.com/article/dn20255-childhood-poverty-leaves-its-mark-on-adult-genetics.

Kanherkar RR, Bhatia-Dey N, Csoka AB. Epigenetics across the human lifespan. *Front Cell Dev Biol* 2 (2014): 49.

Rajakumar K. Pellagra in the United States: A historical perspective. *South Med J* 93, no. 3 (2000): 272–77.

Reynolds CM, Gray C, Li M, et al. Early life nutrition and energy balance disorders in offspring in later life. *Nutrients* 7, no. 9 (2015): 8090–111.

Skogen JC, Overland S. The fetal origins of adult disease: A narrative review of the epidemiological literature. *JRSM Short Rep* 3, no. 8 (2012): 59.

CHAPTER 4

Adler NE, Boyce T, Chesney MA, et al. Socioeconomic status and health: The challenge of the gradient. *Am Psychol* 49, no. 1 (1994): 15–24.

Danese A, Pariante CM, Caspi A, et al. Childhood maltreatment predicts adult inflammation in a life-course study. *Proc Natl Acad Sci U S A* 104, no. 4 (2007): 1319–24.

Di Q, Dai L, Wang Y, et al. Association of short-term exposure to air pollution with mortality in older adults. *JAMA* 318, no. 24 (2017): 2446–56.

Favé M-J, Lamaze FC, Soave D, et al. Gene-by-environment interactions in urban populations modulate risk phenotypes. *Nat Commun* 9, no. 1 (2018): 827.

Goodman S. Tests find more than 200 chemicals in newborn umbilical cord blood. *Scientific American*, 2 December 2009. www.scientificamerican.com/article/newborn-babies-chemicals-exposure-bpa.

Ho SM, Johnson A, Tarapore P, et al. Environmental epigenetics and its implication on disease risk and health outcomes. *ILAR J* 53, no. 3–4 (2012): 289–305.

Hodges RE, Minich DM. Modulation of metabolic detoxification pathways using foods and food-derived components: A scientific review with clinical application. *J Nutr Metab* 2015 (2015): 760689.

James D, Devaraj S, Bellur P, et al. Novel concepts of broccoli sulforaphanes and disease: Induction of phase II antioxidant and detoxification enzymes by enhanced-glucoraphanin broccoli. *Nutr Rev* 70, no. 11 (2012): 654–65.

Jurewicz J, Radwan M, Wielgomas B, et al. Human semen quality, sperm DNA damage, and the level of reproductive hormones in relation to urinary concentrations of parabens. *J Occup Environ Med* 59, no. 11 (2017): 1034–40.

Kiani J, Imam SZ. Medicinal importance of grapefruit juice and its interaction with various drugs. *Nutr J* 6 (2007): 33.

Kirchhoff R, Beckers C, Kirchhoff GM, et al. Increase in choleresis by means of artichoke extract. *Phytomedicine* 1, no. 2 (1994): 107–15.

Ku LC, Smith PB. Dosing in neonates: Special considerations in physiology and trial design. *Pediatr Res* 77, no. 1-1 (2015): 2–9.

Lee CH, Wettasinghe M, Bolling BW, et al. Betalains, phase II enzyme-inducing components from red beetroot (*Beta vulgaris* L.) extracts. *Nutr Cancer* 53, no. 1 (2005): 91–103.

Lu C, Toepel K, Irish R, et al. Organic diets significantly lower children's dietary exposure to organophosphorus pesticides. *Environ Health Perspect* 114, no. 2 (2006): 260–63.

Lucassen PJ, Naninck EF, van Goudoever JB, et al. Perinatal programming of adult hippocampal structure and function: Emerging roles of stress, nutrition and epigenetics. *Trends Neurosci* 36, no. 11 (2013): 621–31.

Obschonka M, Stuetzer M, Rentfrow PJ, et al. In the shadow of coal: How large-scale industries contributed to present-day regional differences in personality and well-being. *J Pers Soc Psychol* 155, no. 5 (2018): 903–27.

Ouellet-Morin I, Wong CC, Danese A, et al. Increased serotonin transporter gene (SERT) DNA methylation is associated with bullying victimization and blunted cortisol response to stress in childhood: A longitudinal study of discordant monozygotic twins. *Psychol Med* 43, no. 9 (2013): 1813–23.

Parker N, Wong AP, Leonard G, et al. Income inequality, gene expression, and brain maturation during adolescence. *Sci Rep* 7, no. 1 (2017): 7397.

Powell ND, Sloan EK, Bailey MT, et al. Social stress up-regulates inflammatory gene expression in the leukocyte transcriptome via ß-adrenergic induction of myelopoiesis. *Proc Natl Acad Sci U S A* 110, no. 41 (2013): 16574–79.

Sarapas C, Cai G, Bierer LM, et al. Genetic markers for PTSD risk and resilience among survivors of the World Trade Center attacks. *Dis Markers* 30, no. 2–3 (2011): 101–10.

Swartz JR, Hariri AR, Williamson DE. An epigenetic mechanism links socioeconomic status to changes in depression-related brain function in high-risk adolescents. *Mol Psychiatry* 22, no. 2 (2017): 209–14.

Yehuda R, Cai G, Sarapas C, et al. Gene expression patterns associated with posttraumatic stress disorder following exposure to the World Trade Center attacks. *Biol Psychiatry* 66, no. 7 (2009): 708–11.

Yehuda R, Engel SM, Brand SR, et al. Transgenerational effects of posttraumatic stress disorder in babies of mothers exposed to the World Trade Center attacks during pregnancy. *J Clin Endocrinol Metab* 90, no. 7 (2005): 4115–18.

Zanger UM, Schwab M. Cytochrome P450 enzymes in drug metabolism: Regulation of gene expression, enzyme activities, and impact of genetic variation. *Pharmacol Ther* 138, no. 1 (2013): 103–41.

CHAPTER 5

Briley J, Jackson C. *Food as Medicine Everyday: Reclaim Your Health with Whole Foods*. Portland, OR: NUNM Press, 2016.

Chiu YH, Williams PL, Gillman MW, et al. Association between pesticide residue intake from consumption of fruits and vegetables and pregnancy outcomes among women undergoing infertility treatment with assisted reproductive technology. *JAMA Intern Med* 178, no. 1 (2018): 17–26.

Cole ZA, Gale CR, Javaid MK, et al. Maternal dietary patterns during pregnancy and childhood bone mass: A longitudinal study. *J Bone Miner Res* 24, no. 4 (2009): 663–68.

Donkin I, Barrès R. Sperm epigenetics and influence of environmental factors. *Mol Metab* 14 (2018): 1–11.

Goodman S. Tests find more than 200 chemicals in newborn umbilical cord blood. *Scientific American*, 2 December 2009. www.scientificamerican.com/article/newborn-babies-chemicals-exposure-bpa.

Greenberg JA, Bell SJ, Ausdal WV. Omega-3 fatty acid supplementation during pregnancy. *Rev Obstet Gynecol* 1, no. 4 (2008): 162–69.

Houfflyn S, Matthys C, Soubry A. Male obesity: Epigenetic origin and effects in sperm and offspring. *Curr Mol Biol Rep* 3, no. 4 (2017): 288–96.

McGuire S. WHO guideline: Vitamin A supplementation in pregnant women. Geneva: WHO, 2011. *Adv Nutr* 3, no. 2 (2012): 215–16.

McMahon LP. Iron deficiency in pregnancy. *Obstet Med* 3, no. 1 (2010): 17–24.

Moore TG, Arefadib N, Deery A, West S. *The First Thousand Days: An Evidence Paper*. Parkville, Victoria: Centre for Community Child Health, Murdoch Children's Research Institute, 2017.

Mulligan ML, Felton SK, Riek AE, Bernal-Mizrachi C. Implications of vitamin D deficiency in pregnancy and lactation. *Am J Obstet Gynecol* 202, no. 5 (2010): 429.e1–9.

Niinistö S, Takkinen HM, Erlund I, et al. Fatty acid status in infancy is associated with the risk of type 1 diabetes-associated autoimmunity. *Diabetologia* 60, no. 7 (2017): 1223–33.

Nugent BM, O'Donnell CM, Epperson CN, Bale TL. Placental H3K27me3 establishes female resilience to prenatal insults. *Nat Commun* 9, no. 1 (2018): 2555.

Prescott S. *Origins: Early-Life Solutions to the Modern Health Crisis*. Crawley: University of Western Australia, 2015.

Watkins AJ, Dias I, Tsuro H, et al. Paternal diet programs offspring health through sperm- and seminal plasma-specific pathways in mice. *Proc Natl Acad Sci U S A* 115, no. 40 (2018): 10064–69.

CHAPTER 6

Adolescent Brain Cognitive Development Study. https://abcdstudy.org.

Belsky DW, Moffitt TE, Baker TB, et al. Polygenic risk and the developmental progression to heavy, persistent smoking and nicotine dependence: Evidence from a 4-decade longitudinal study. *JAMA Psychiatry* 70, no. 5 (2013): 534–42.

Casey BJ, Jones RM, Hare TA. The adolescent brain. *Ann N Y Acad Sci* 1124 (2008): 111–26.

Dahm CC, Chomistek AK, Jakobsen MU, et al. Adolescent diet quality and cardiovascular disease risk factors and incident cardiovascular disease in middle-aged women. *J Am Heart Assoc* 5, no. 12 (2016).

Dong Y, Pollock N, Stallmann-Jorgensen IS, et al. Low 25-hydroxyvitamin D levels in adolescents: Race, season, adiposity, physical activity, and fitness. *Pediatrics* 125, no. 6 (2010): 1104–11.

El Baza F, AlShahawi HA, Zahra S, AbdelHakim RA. Magnesium supplementation in children with attention deficit hyperactivity disorder. *Egypt J Med Hum Genet* 17, no. 1 (2016): 63–70.

Estes ML, McAllister AK. Maternal immune activation: Implications for neuropsychiatric disorders. *Science* 353, no. 6301 (2016): 772–77.

Finegersh A, Rompala GR, Martin DI, Homanics GE. Drinking beyond a lifetime: New and emerging insights into paternal alcohol exposure on subsequent generations. *Alcohol* 49, no. 5 (2015): 461–70.

Fisher MM, Eugster EA. What is in our environment that effects puberty? *Reprod Toxicol* 44 (2014): 7–14.

Friedman RA. What cookies and meth have in common. *New York Times*, 30 June 2017. www.nytimes.com/2017/06/30/opinion/sunday/what-cookies-and-meth-have-in-common.html.

Georgieff MK. Nutrition and the developing brain: Nutrient priorities and measurement. *Am J Clin Nutr* 85, no. 2 (2007): 614S–20S.

Hakim D. Are Honey Nut Cheerios healthy? We look inside the box. *New York Times*, 10 November 2017. www.nytimes.com/2017/11/10/business/honey-nut-cheerios-sugar.html.

Harrington R. Does artificial food coloring contribute to ADHD in children? *Scientific American*, 27 April 2015. www.scientificamerican.com/article/does-artificial-food-coloring-contribute-to-adhd-in-children.

Henriksen TB, Hjollund NH, Jensen TK, et al. Alcohol consumption at the time of conception and spontaneous abortion. *Am J Epidemiol* 160, no. 7 (2004): 661–67.

Johnson AD, Markowitz AJ. Associations between household food insecurity in early childhood and children's kindergarten skills. *Child Dev* 89, no. 2 (2018): e1–e17.

Konofal E, Lecendreux M, Arnulf I, Mouren MC. Iron deficiency in children with attention-deficit/hyperactivity disorder. *Arch Pediatr Adolesc Med* 158, no. 12 (2004): 1113–15.

Likes R, Madl RL, Zeisel SH, Craig SA. The betaine and choline content of a whole wheat flour compared to other mill streams. *J Cereal Sci* 46, no. 1 (2007): 93–95.

Lomniczi A, Ojeda SR. The emerging role of epigenetics in the regulation of female puberty. *Endocr Dev* 29 (2016): 1–16.

Lowette K, Roosen L, Tack J, Vanden Berghe P. Effects of high-fructose diets on central appetite signaling and cognitive function. *Front Nutr* 2 (2015): 5.

Milne E, Greenop KR, Scott RJ, et al. Parental alcohol consumption and risk of childhood acute lymphoblastic leukemia and brain tumors. *Cancer Causes Control* 24, no. 2 (2013): 391–402.

Moss M. *Salt Sugar Fat: How the Food Giants Hooked Us.* Toronto: McClelland & Stewart, 2013.

Page KA, Chan O, Arora J, et al. Effects of fructose vs glucose on regional cerebral blood flow in brain regions involved with appetite and reward pathways. *JAMA* 309, no. 1 (2013): 63–70.

Rendeiro C, Masnik AM, Mun JG, et al. Fructose decreases physical activity and increases body fat without affecting hippocampal neurogenesis and learning relative to an isocaloric glucose diet. *Sci Rep* 5 (2015): 9589.

Taubes G. *The Case Against Sugar.* New York: Alfred A. Knopf, 2016.

World Health Organization. Adolescent development. www.who.int/maternal_child_adolescent/topics/adolescence/development/en.

World Health Organization. *Nutrition in Adolescence: Issues and Challenges for the Health Sector.* Geneva: WHO, 2005.

CHAPTER 7

Arnason TG, Bowen MW, Mansell KD. Effects of intermittent fasting on health markers in those with type 2 diabetes: A pilot study. *World J Diabetes* 8, no. 4 (2017): 154–64.

Basaranoglu M, Basaranoglu G, Bugianesi E. Carbohydrate intake and nonalcoholic fatty liver disease: Fructose as a weapon of mass destruction. *Hepatobiliary Surg Nutr* 4, no. 2 (2015): 109–16.

Berger S, Raman G, Vishwanathan R, et al. Dietary cholesterol and cardiovascular disease: A systematic review and meta-analysis. *Am J Clin Nutr* 102, no. 2 (2015): 276–94.

Buric I, Farias M, Jong J, et al. What is the molecular signature of mind-body interventions? A systematic review of gene expression changes induced by meditation and related practices. *Front Immunol* 8 (2017): 670.

CARDIoGRAMplusC4D Consortium. Large-scale association analysis identifies new risk loci for coronary artery disease. *Nat Genet* 45, no. 1 (2013): 25–33.

Chrysohou C, Panagiotakos DB, Pitsavos C, et al. Adherence to the Mediterranean diet attenuates inflammation and coagulation process in healthy adults: The ATTICA Study. *J Am Coll Cardiol* 44, no. 1 (2004): 152–58.

Cohen HW, Hailpern SM, Fang J, Alderman MH. Sodium intake and mortality in the NHANES II follow-up study. *Am J Med* 119, no. 3 (2006): 275.e7–14.

Cohen S, Janicki-Deverts D, Doyle WJ, et al. Chronic stress, glucocorticoid receptor resistance, inflammation, and disease risk. *Proc Natl Acad Sci U S A* 109, no. 16 (2012): 5995–99.

Conti P, Shaik-Dasthagirisaeb Y. Atherosclerosis: A chronic inflammatory disease mediated by mast cells. *Cent Eur J Immunol* 40, no. 3 (2015): 380–86.

Corbin KD, Zeisel SH. Choline metabolism provides novel insights into non-alcoholic fatty liver disease and its progression. *Curr Opin Gastroenterol* 28, no. 2 (2012): 159–65.

Dalgaard K, Landgraf K, Heyne S, et al. Trim28 haploinsufficiency triggers bi-stable epigenetic obesity. *Cell* 164, no. 3 (2016): 353–64.

Danese A, Pariante CM, Caspi A, et al. Childhood maltreatment predicts adult inflammation in a life-course study. *Proc Natl Acad Sci U S A* 104, no. 4 (2007): 1319–24.

De Long NE, Holloway AC. Early-life chemical exposures and risk of metabolic syndrome. *Diabetes Metab Syndr Obes* 10 (2017): 101–9.

de Munter JS, Hu FB, Spiegelman D, et al. Whole grain, bran, and germ intake and risk of type 2 diabetes: A prospective cohort study and systematic review. *PLoS Med* 4, no. 8 (2007): e261.

Denham J. Exercise and epigenetic inheritance of disease risk. *Acta Physiol (Oxf)* 222, no. 1 (2018).

de Vocht F, Suderman M, Tilling K, et al. DNA methylation from birth to late adolescence and development of multiple-risk behaviours. *J Affect Disord* 227 (2018): 588–94.

Dhurandhar NV, Thomas D. The link between dietary sugar intake and cardiovascular disease mortality: An unresolved question. *JAMA* 313, no. 9 (2015): 959–60.

Di Ciaula A, Portincasa P. Fat, epigenome and pancreatic diseases: Interplay and common pathways from a toxic and obesogenic environment. *Eur J Intern Med* 25, no. 10 (2014): 865–73.

Dimitrov S, Hulteng E, Hong S. Inflammation and exercise: Inhibition of monocytic intracellular TNF production by acute exercise via ß2-adrenergic activation. *Brain Behav Immun* 61 (2017): 60–8.

DiNicolantonio JJ, O'Keefe JH, Lucan SC. Added fructose: A principal driver of type 2 diabetes mellitus and its consequences. *Mayo Clin Proc* 90, no. 3 (2015): 372–81.

Dje N'Guessan P, Riediger F, Vardarova K, et al. Statins control oxidized LDL-mediated histone modifications and gene expression in cultured human endothelial cells. *Arterioscler Thromb Vasc Biol* 29, no. 3 (2009): 380–86.

Dongiovanni P, Anstee QM, Valenti L. Genetic predisposition in NAFLD and NASH: Impact on severity of liver disease and response to treatment. *Curr Pharm Des* 19, no. 29 (2013): 5219–38.

Gilbert ER, Liu D. Anti-diabetic functions of soy isoflavone genistein: Mechanisms underlying effects on pancreatic ß-cell function. *Food Funct* 4, no. 2 (2013): 200–212.

Godfrey KM, Sheppard A, Gluckman PD, et al. Epigenetic gene promoter methylation at birth is associated with child's later adiposity. *Diabetes* 60, no. 5 (2011): 1528–34.

Harburg E, Gleibermann L, Roeper P, et al. Skin color, ethnicity, and blood pressure I: Detroit blacks. *Am J Public Health* 68, no. 12 (1978): 1177–83.

Herrera BM, Lindgren CM. The genetics of obesity. *Curr Diab Rep* 10, no. 6 (2010): 498–505.

Huang T, Xu M, Lee A, et al. Consumption of whole grains and cereal fiber and total and cause-specific mortality: Prospective analysis of 367,442 individuals. *BMC Med* 13 (2015): 59.

Hyppönen E, Virtanen SM, Kenward MG, et al. Obesity, increased linear growth, and risk of type 1 diabetes in children. *Diabetes Care* 23, no. 12 (2000): 1755–60.

Jamal O, Aneni EC, Shaharyar S, et al. Cigarette smoking worsens systemic inflammation in persons with metabolic syndrome. *Diabetol Metabol Syndr* 6 (2014): 79.

Jerram ST, Dang MN, Leslie RD. The role of epigenetics in type 1 diabetes. *Curr Diab Rep* 17, no. 10 (2017): 89.

Johnson LSB, Salonen M, Kajantie E, et al. Early life risk factors for incident atrial fibrillation in the Helsinki Birth Cohort Study. *J Am Heart Assoc* 6, no. 6 (2017).

Karachanak-Yankova S, Dimova R, Nikolova D, et al. Epigenetic alterations in patients with type 2 diabetes mellitus. *Balkan J Med Genet* 18, no. 2 (2016): 15–24.

Knip M, Simell O. Environmental triggers of type 1 diabetes. *Cold Spring Harb Perspect Med* 2, no. 7 (2012): a007690.

Kuneš J, Vaněčková I, Mikulášková B, et al. Epigenetics and a new look on metabolic syndrome. *Physiol Res* 64, no. 5 (2015): 611–20.

Lebenthal E, Bier DM. Novel concepts in the developmental origins of adult health and disease. *J Nutr* 137, no. 4 (2007): 1073–75.

Loucks EB, Lynch JW, Pilote L, et al. Life-course socioeconomic position and incidence of coronary heart disease: The Framingham Offspring Study. *Am J Epidemiol* 169, no. 7 (2009): 829–36.

Lu W, Li S, Li J, et al. Effects of omega-3 fatty acid in nonalcoholic fatty liver disease: A meta-analysis. *Gastroenterol Res Pract* 2016: 1459790.

Maintz L, Novak N. Histamine and histamine intolerance. *Am J Clin Nutr* 85, no. 5 (2007): 1185–96.

Martinelli N, Girelli D, Malerba G, et al. FADS genotypes and desaturase activity estimated by the ratio of arachidonic acid to linoleic acid are associated with inflammation and coronary artery disease. *Am J Clin Nutr* 88, no. 4 (2008): 941–49.

McDade TW, Ryan C, Jones MJ, et al. Social and physical environments early in development predict DNA methylation of inflammatory genes in young adulthood. *Proc Natl Acad Sci U S A* 114, no. 29 (2017): 7611–16.

Moore LL, Singer MR, Bradlee ML. Low sodium intakes are not associated with lower blood pressure levels among Framingham Offspring Study adults. *FASEB J* 31, no. 1 (suppl.) (2017).

Mujahid MS, Diez Roux AV, Morenoff JD, et al. Neighborhood characteristics and hypertension. *Epidemiology* 19, no. 4 (2008): 590–98.

Neuschwander-Tetri BA. Carbohydrate intake and nonalcoholic fatty liver disease. *Curr Opin Clin Nutr Metab Care* 16, no. 4 (2013): 446–52.

Newby PK, Maras J, Bakun P, et al. Intake of whole grains, refined grains, and cereal fiber measured with 7-d diet records and associations with risk factors for chronic disease. *Am J Clin Nutr* 86, no. 6 (2007): 1745–53.

Osmond C, Kajantie E, Forsén TJ, et al. Infant growth and stroke in adult life: The Helsinki Birth Cohort Study. *Stroke* 38, no. 2 (2007): 264–70.

Pacana T, Sanyal AJ. Vitamin E and non-alcoholic fatty liver disease. *Curr Opin Clin Nutr Metab Care* 15, no. 6 (2012): 641–48.

Reynolds CM, Gray C, Li M, et al. Early life nutrition and energy balance disorders in offspring in later life. *Nutrients* 7, no. 9 (2015): 8090–111.

Romero-Gómez M, Zelber-Sagi S, Trenell M. Treatment of NAFLD with diet, physical activity and exercise. *J Hepatol* 67, no. 4 (2017): 829–46.

Saben JL, Boudoures AL, Asghar Z, et al. Maternal metabolic syndrome programs mitochondrial dysfunction via germline changes across three generations. *Cell Rep* 16, no. 1 (2016): 1–8.

Sahyoun NR, Jacques PF, Zhang XL, et al. Whole-grain intake is inversely association with the metabolic syndrome and mortality in older adults. *Am J Clin Nutr* 83, no. 1 (2006): 124–31.

Singh GM, Micha R, Khatibzadeh S, et al. Estimated global, regional, and national disease burdens related to sugar-sweetened beverage consumption in 2010. *Circulation* 132, no. 8 (2015): 639–66.

Stephenson K. Cholesterol-lowering "portfolio diet" also reduces blood pressure, study finds. St Michael's Hospital, 7 November 2015. www.stmichaelshospital.com/media/detail.php?source=hospital_news/2015/20151107_hn.

Straub JM, New J, Hamilton CD, et al. Radiation-induced fibrosis: Mechanisms and implications for therapy. *J Cancer Res Clin Oncol* 141, no. 11 (2015): 1985–94.

Tedders SH, Fokong KD, McKenzie LE, et al. Low cholesterol is association with depression among US household population. *J Affect Disord* 135, nos. 1–3 (2011): 115–21.

Thériault S, Lali R, Chong M, et al. Polygenic contribution in individuals with early-onset coronary artery disease. *Circ Genom Precis Med* 11, no. 1 (2018): e001849.

Thompson R, Allam AH, Lombardi GP, et al. Atherosclerosis across 4000 years of human history: The Horus study of four ancient populations. *Lancet* 381, no. 9873 (2013): 1211–22.

van der Ploeg HP, Chey T, Korda RJ, et al. Sitting time and all-cause mortality risk in 222,497 Australian adults. *Arch Intern Med* 172, no. 6 (2012): 494–500.

van Dijk SJ, Tellam RL, Morrison JL, et al. Recent developments on the role of epigenetics in obesity and metabolic disease. *Clin Epigenetics* 7 (2015): 66.

Vickers MH. Developmental programming and transgenerational transmission of obesity. *Ann Nutr Metab* 64, suppl. 1 (2014): 26–34.

Weigel C, Veldwijk MR, Oakes CC, et al. Epigenetic regulation of diacylglycerol kinase alpha promotes radiation-induced fibrosis. *Nat Commun* 7 (2016): 10893.

Wijarnpreecha K, Thongprayoon C, Ungprasert P. Coffee consumption and risk of nonalcoholic fatty liver disease: A systematic review and meta-analysis. *Eur J Gastroenterol Hepatol* 29, no. 2 (2017): e8–e12.

Yajnik CS. The thin-fat man: Pilgrim's progress. Diabetes Unit, King Edward Memorial Hospital & Research Centre, Pune. www.kemdiabetes.org/About_Landing.html.

Yajnik CS, Fall CH, Coyaji KJ, et al. Neonatal anthropometry: The thin-fat Indian baby. The Pune Maternal Nutrition Study. *Int J Obes Relat Metab Disord* 27, no. 2 (2003): 173–80.

CHAPTER 8

Archer T. Epigenetic changes induced by exercise: Commentary. *J Reward Defic Syndr* 1, no. 2 (2015): 71–74.

Biswas A, Oh PI, Faulkner GE, et al. Sedentary time and its association with risk for disease incidence, mortality and hospitalization in adults: A systematic review and meta-analysis. *Ann Intern Med* 162, no. 2 (2015): 123–32.

Braicu C, Mehterov N, Vladimirov B, et al. Nutrigenomics in cancer: Revisiting the effects of natural compounds. *Semin Cancer Biol* 46 (2017): 84–106.

Brown BM, Peiffer JJ, Martins RN. Multiple effects of physical activity on molecular and cognitive signs of brain aging: Can exercise slow neurodegeneration and delay Alzheimer's disease? *Mol Psychiatry* 18, no. 8 (2013): 864–74.

Busch C, Burkard M, Leischner C, et al. Epigenetic activities of flavonoids in the prevention and treatment of cancer. *Clin Epigenetics* 7 (2015): 64.

Buxton JL, Walters RG, Visvikis-Siest S, et al. Childhood obesity is associated with shorter leukocyte telomere length. *J Clin Endocrinol Metab* 96, no. 5 (2011): 1500–5.

Chilton WL, Marques FZ, West J, et al. Acute exercise leads to regulation of telomere-associated genes and microRNA expression in immune cells. *PLoS One* 9, no. 4 (2014): e92088.

de Jager CA, Oulhaj A, Jacoby R, et al. Cognitive and clinical outcomes of homocysteine-lowering B-vitamin treatment in mild cognitive impairment: A randomized controlled trial. *Int J Geriatr Psychiatry* 27, no. 6 (2012): 592–600.

de la Monte SM, Wands JR. Alzheimer's disease is type 3 diabetes: Evidence reviewed. *J Diabetes Sci Technol* 2, no. 6 (2008): 1101–13.

Entringer S, Epel ES, Kumsta R, et al. Stress exposure in intrauterine life is associated with shorter telomere length in young adulthood. *Proc Natl Acad Sci U S A* 108, no. 33 (2011): e513–18.

Heidinger BJ, Blount JD, Boner W, et al. Telomere length in early life predicts lifespan. *Proc Natl Acad Sci U S A* 109, no. 5 (2012): 1743–48.

Heneka MT, Carson MJ, El Khoury J, et al. Neuroinflammation in Alzheimer's disease. *Lancet Neurol* 14, no. 4 (2015): 388–405.

Lahiri DK, Zawia NH, Greig NH, et al. Early-life events may trigger biochemical pathways for Alzheimer's disease: The "LEARn" model. *Biogerontology* 9, no. 6 (2008): 375–79.

McNeely E, Mordukhovich I, Staffa S, et al. Cancer prevalence among flight attendants compared to the general population. *Environ Health* 17, no. 1 (2018): 49.

O'Toole PW, Jefferey IB. Gut microbiota and aging. *Science* 350, no. 6265 (2015): 1214–15.

Rajagopalan P, Jahanshad N, Stein JL, et al. Common folate gene variant, MTHFR C677T, is associated with brain structure in two independent cohorts of people with mild cognitive impairment. *Neuroimage Clin* 1, no. 1 (2012): 179–87.

Raqib R, Alam DS, Sarker P, et al. Low birth weight is associated with altered immune function in rural Bangledeshi children: A birth cohort study. *Am J Clin Nutr* 85, no. 3 (2007): 845–52.

Robinson MM, Dasari S, Konopka AR, et al. Enhanced protein translation underlies improved metabolic and physical adaptations to different exercise training modes in young and old humans. *Cell Metab* 25, no. 3 (2017): 581–92.

Shalev L, Entringer S, Wadhwa PD, et al. Stress and telomere biology: A lifespan perspective. *Psychoneuroendocrinology* 38, no. 9 (2013): 1835–42.

Sharma S, Kelly TK, Jones PA. Epigenetics in cancer. *Carcinogenesis* 31, no. 1 (2010): 27–36.

Shin S, Sung J, Joung H. A fruit, milk and whole grain dietary pattern is positively associated with bone mineral density in Korean healthy adults. *Eur J Clin Nutr* 69, no. 4 (2015): 442–48.

Wang F, Meng J, Zhang L, et al. Morphine induces changes in the gut microbiome and metabolome in a morphine dependence model. *Sci Rep* 8, no. 1 (2018): 3596.

Wang LS, Kuo CT, Cho SJ, et al. Black raspberry-derived anthocyanins demethylate tumor suppressor genes through the inhibition of DNMT1 and DNMT3B in colon cancer. *Nutr Cancer* 65, no. 1 (2013): 118–25.

Yuan JM, Koh WP, Sun CL, et al. Green tea intake, ACE gene polymorphism and breast cancer risk among Chinese women in Singapore. *Carcinogenesis* 26, no. 8 (2005): 1389–94.

CHAPTER 9

Ackerman J. The ultimate social network. *Sci Am* 306, no. 6 (2012): 36–43.

Alam MT, Zelezniak A, Mülleder M, et al. The metabolic background is a global player in *Saccharomyces* gene expression epistasis. *Nat Microbiol* 1 (2016): 15030.

Alverdy JC, Hyoju SK, Weigerinck M, Gilbert JA. The gut microbiome and the mechanisms of surgical infection. *Br J Surg* 104, no. 2 (2017): e14–e23.

Bommiasamy AK, Connelly C, Moren A, et al. Institutional review of the implementation and use of a *Clostridium difficile* infection bundle and probiotics in adult trauma patients. *Am J Surg* 215, no. 5 (2018): 825–30.

Chassaing B, Koren O, Goodrich JK, et al. Dietary emulsifiers impact the mouse gut microbiota promoting colitis and metabolic syndrome. *Nature* 519, no. 7541 (2015): 92–96.

Courage KH. Fiber-famished gut microbes linked to poor health. *Scientific American*, 23 March 2015. www.scientificamerican.com/article/fiber-famished-gut-microbes-linked-to-poor-health1.

David LA, Maurice CF, Carmody RN, et al. Diet rapidly and reproducibly alters the human gut microbiome. *Nature* 505, no. 7484 (2014): 559–63.

Desai MS, Seekatz AM, Koropatkin NM, et al. A dietary fiber-deprived gut microbiota degrades the colonic mucus barrier and enhances pathogen susceptibility. *Cell* 167, no. 5 (2016): 1339–53.

Duda-Chodak A, Tarko T, Satora P, Sroka P. Interaction of dietary compounds, especially polyphenols, with the intestinal microbiota: A review. *Eur J Nutr* 54, no. 3 (2015): 325–41.

Exteberria U, Fernández-Quintela A, Milagro FI, et al. Impact of polyphenols and polyphenol-rich dietary sources on gut microbiota composition. *J Agric Food Chem* 61, no. 40 (2013): 9517–33.

Ghanim H, Sia CL, Upadhyay M, et al. Orange juice neutralizes the proinflammatory effect of a high-fat, high-carbohydrate meal and prevents endotoxin increase and Toll-like receptor expression. *Am J Clin Nutr* 91, no. 4 (2010): 940–49.

Goldsmith JR, Sartor RB. The role of diet on intestinal microbiota metabolism: Downstream impacts on host immune function and health, and therapeutic implications. *J Gastroenterol* 49, no. 5 (2014): 785–98.

Holscher HD. Dietary fiber and prebiotics and the gastrointestinal microbiota. *Gut Microbes* 8, no. 2 (2017): 172–84.

Hooper LV, Littman DR, Macpherson AJ. Interactions between the microbiota and the immune system. *Science* 336, no. 6086 (2012): 1268–73.

Indrio F, Martini S, Francavilla R, et al. Epigenetic matters: The link between early nutrition, microbiome, and long-term health development. *Front Pediatr* 5 (2017): 178.

Jones ML, Ganopolsky JG, Martoni CJ, et al. Emerging science of the human microbiome. *Gut Microbes* 5, no. 4 (2014): 446–57.

Jorgensen RA. Epigenetics: Biology's quantum mechanics. *Front Plant Sci* 2 (2011): 10.

Las Heras V, Clooney AG, Ryan FJ, et al. Short-term consumption of a high-fat diet increases host susceptibility to *Listeria monocytogenes* infection. *Microbiome* 7, no. 1 (2019): 7.

Liu H, Fu Y, Wang K. Asthma and risk of coronary heart disease: A meta-analysis of cohort studies. *Ann Allergy Asthma Immunol* 118, no. 6 (2017): 689–95.

Manzel A, Muller DN, Hafler DA, et al. Role of "Western diet" in inflammatory autoimmune diseases. *Curr Allergy Asthma Rep* 14, no. 1 (2014): 404.

Martínez I, Lattimer JM, Hubach KL, et al. Gut microbiome composition is linked to whole grain-induced immunological improvements. *ISME J* 7, no. 2 (2013): 269–80.

Nicholson JK, Holmes E, Kinross J, et al. Host-gut microbiota metabolic interactions. *Science* 336, no. 6086 (2012): 1262–67.

Parker W. The "hygiene hypothesis" for allergic disease is a misnomer. *BMJ* 348 (2014): g5267.

Prescott SL, Logan AC. *The Secret Life of Your Microbiome: Why Nature and Biodiversity Are Essential to Health and Happiness*. Gabriola Island, BC: New Society, 2017.

Schroeder BO, Bäckhed F. Signals from the gut microbiota to distant organs in physiology and disease. *Nat Med* 22, no. 10 (2016): 1079–89.

Shapiro H, Thaiss CA, Levy M, Elinav E. The cross talk between microbiota and the immune system: Metabolites take center stage. *Curr Opin Immunol* 30 (2014): 54–62.

Spector T. "It Takes Guts." Episode of *The Nature of Things*. Directed by L. Eisen. Toronto: 90th Parallel Productions/CBC. Broadcast 26 August 2017.

Suez J, Korem T, Zeevi D, et al. Artificial sweeteners induce glucose intolerance by altering the gut microbiota. *Nature* 514, no. 7521 (2014): 181–86.

Thorburn AN, McKenzie CI, Shen S, et al. Evidence that asthma is a developmental origin disease influenced by maternal diet and bacterial metabolites. *Nat Commun* 6 (2015): 7320.

Thursby E, Juge N. Introduction to the human gut microbiota. *Biochem J* 474, no. 11 (2017): 1823–36.

INDEX

parabens, 90
Pardee, Arthur, 52
Pasteur, Louis, 272, 284
pasteurization, 285
paternal origins of health and
    disease (POHaD), 100
pathogens, 269, 272, 286–87,
    297
Paus, Tomas, 84–85, 89
PCBs (polychlorinated
    biphenyls), 90, 145
Peabody, Scott H., 265
pellagra, 61
Pembrey, Marcus, 30, 36–38,
    101, 206
penetrance, 64, 298
personality, 72–95
pesticides, 90–91, 94, 122–23,
    144–45, 242. See also food,
    organic
Peters, Sanne, 210
pets, 277, 278
pharmacogenomics, 50, 91,
    298
phenotype, 36, 298
phosphorus, 247
phthalates, 95, 144–45
phytic acid, 285
phytoestrogen, 242, 298
phytonutrients, 240, 279,
    282–83. See also specific
    nutrients
Pima Indians, 188
placenta, 27, 59, 60, 63, 106,
    108–13
    insufficiency of, 121, 127,
        298
    male fetuses and, 112–13
    physical characteristics,
        109–10
    role in pregnancy, 62, 109
    sperm and, 100–101
plasticity, 60, 69, 106, 109,
    137, 229
Pollan, Michael, 289
polycyclic aromatic
    hydrocarbons (PAHs), 240
polycystic ovary syndrome
    (PCOS), 103
polyphenols, 77, 231, 239, 283
portfolio diet, 203, 208
potassium, 66, 202, 220

poverty, 17, 74, 151–53
    and brain development,
        134–35, 144
    and diet, 148, 292
    and disease incidence, 17, 61,
        205, 216
    health effects, 84, 85,
        198–99, 292, 293
    and heart disease, 19, 84,
        206, 219, 292
PPAR-gamma (protein), 195
Prader-Willi syndrome, 37
prebiotics, 173, 274, 282–84, 298
    and SCFAs, 131, 282
    sources, 247, 279, 282
preconception, 98–105
preeclampsia, 110, 209
pregnancy
    alcohol and, 69–70, 101, 104,
        116–17, 121, 218
    diet during, 58–61, 99–100,
        113–20, 141, 283–84
    father and, 66, 100–101, 105,
        106, 122, 167
    folate and, 44, 114
    nausea in, 113, 116
    obesity and, 124–25, 166–67,
        218
    preparing for, 99, 102–4
    smoking and, 89, 120–21
    stress during, 60, 75–76,
        82–83, 112–13, 267
    trauma and, 63, 76, 80
    first trimester, 113, 116–17
    second trimester, 117–18
    third trimester, 118–19
    weight gain during, 124–26
prenatal care, 25, 26, 293
Prescott, Susan, 140, 174, 182,
    183, 199, 245, 265. See also
    specific works
    on allergies, 131, 132, 270
    on inflammation, 214, 216
Pritikin diet, 214
probiotics, 173, 284–85, 298
    health benefits, 213, 247, 287
    in pregnancy, 141, 142
    as supplements, 173, 285, 288
propionate, 283
prostate cancer, 231, 237, 241
protein, 51, 77–78, 93, 250. See
    also specific proteins

proton pump inhibitors, 257
pseudoagouti, 46
PTSD (post-traumatic stress
    disorder), 76, 80–83. See
    also trauma
puberty. See adolescence
public health, 25–26, 58, 272,
    292
    programs for, 25, 26, 84, 153,
        293
PUFAs (polyunsaturated fatty
    acids), 105, 214
Purnell, Jonathan, 156–57

Q

quercetin, 92

R

radiation therapy, 221
reactive oxygen species (ROS),
    221, 232, 258, 298
resilience, 77, 83, 225
resveratrol, 195, 239
Reynolds, Clare, 176
rheumatoid arthritis, 41, 246
rice, 66–67
Rich-Edwards, Janet W., 21–22
RNA, 43, 298
RNA modulation, 87, 298
RNA signaling, 43, 298
Roseboom, Tessa, 22, 23, 63,
    70
Roundup (chlorpyrifos), 90–91,
    94
royal jelly, 47, 48
Russell, Edmund, 49

S

Saccharomyces boulardii, 284
salt, 200–201, 241
Salt Sugar Fat: How the Food
    Giants Hooked Us (Moss),
    78, 148
sarcopenia, 248–52
    obesity and, 249, 252
    preventing, 250–51
SCFAs. See short-chain fatty
    acids
schizophrenia, 41, 76, 101

Library and Archives Canada Cataloguing in Publication

Title: You are what your grandparents ate : what you need to know about nutrition, experience, epigenetics & the origins of chronic disease / Judith Finlayson ; foreword by Dr. Kent Thornburg.

Names: Finlayson, Judith, author. | Thornburg, Kent L., writer of foreword.

Description: Includes bibliographical references and index.

Identifiers: Canadiana 20190115467 | ISBN 9780778806332 (hardcover)

Subjects: LCSH: Medical genetics—Popular works. | LCSH: Epigenetics—Popular works. | LCSH: Chronic diseases—Genetic aspects—Popular works. | LCSH: Chronic diseases—Etiology—Popular works. | LCSH: Health—Popular works. | LCSH: Nutrition—Popular works.

Classification: LCC RB155 .F56 2019 | DDC 616/.042—dc23